ADHD AND FETAL ALCOHOL SPECTRUM DISORDERS (FASD)

ADHD AND FETAL ALCOHOL SPECTRUM DISORDERS (FASD)

KIERAN D. O'MALLEY
EDITOR

Nova Science Publishers, Inc.
New York

For permission to use material from this book please contact us:
Telephone 631-231-7269; Fax 631-231-8175
Web Site: http://www.novapublishers.com

NOTICE TO THE READER

The Publisher has taken reasonable care in the preparation of this book, but makes no expressed or implied warranty of any kind and assumes no responsibility for any errors or omissions. No liability is assumed for incidental or consequential damages in connection with or arising out of information contained in this book. The Publisher shall not be liable for any special, consequential, or exemplary damages resulting, in whole or in part, from the readers' use of, or reliance upon, this material.

Independent verification should be sought for any data, advice or recommendations contained in this book. In addition, no responsibility is assumed by the publisher for any injury and/or damage to persons or property arising from any methods, products, instructions, ideas or otherwise contained in this publication.

This publication is designed to provide accurate and authoritative information with regard to the subject matter covered herein. It is sold with the clear understanding that the Publisher is not engaged in rendering legal or any other professional services. If legal or any other expert assistance is required, the services of a competent person should be sought. FROM A DECLARATION OF PARTICIPANTS JOINTLY ADOPTED BY A COMMITTEE OF THE AMERICAN BAR ASSOCIATION AND A COMMITTEE OF PUBLISHERS.

Library of Congress Cataloging-in-Publication Data
ADHD and fetal alcohol spectrum disorders (FASD) Kieran D. O'Malley (editor).
    p. ; cm.
Includes bibliographical references and index.
ISBN 13 978-1-59454-573-3
ISBN10 1-59454-573-1
1. Fetal alcohol syndrome. 2. Attention-deficit hyperactivity disorder. 3. Alcohol--Physiological effect.   I. O'Malley, Kieran D.
[DNLM: 1. Fetal Alcohol Syndrome. 2. Attention Deficit and Disruptive Behavior Disorders. 3. Developmental Disabilities. 4. Human Development.   WQ 211 A234 2006]
RG628.3.F45A34   2006
618.3'26861--dc22   2006011607

Published by Nova Science Publishers, Inc. ✦ New York

CONTENTS

Preface   **vii**

Chapter 1   Fetal Alcohol Spectrum Disorders: An Overview   **1**
                     Kieran D.O'Malley

Chapter 2   Infant, Toddler and Young Child Systems of Care for Patients with
                     Fetal Alcohol Spectrum Disorders (FASD) and Their Families   **25**
                     Kieran D. O'Malley

Chapter 3   Sensory Integration and Sensory Processing Disorders   **39**
                     Tracy Jirikowic

Chapter 4   Pathophysiology of ADHD in Patients with ADHD and Fetal
                     Alcohol Spectrum Disorders. The Role of Medication   **51**
                     Kieran D.O'Malley

Chapter 5   The Role of Therapeutic Intervention with Substance Abusing
                     Mothers: Preventing FASD in the Next Generation   **69**
                     Therese Grant, Julie Youngblood Pedersen,
                     Nancy Whitney and Cara Ernst

Chapter 6   Neuropsychological Profiles of Children and Adolescents with Fetal
                     Alcohol Spectrum Disorders and ADHD   **95**
                     Donald S. Massey and Valerie J. Massey

Chapter 7   Adult Neuropsychology of Fetal Alcohol Spectrum Disorders   **103**
                     Kathy Page

Chapter 8   Sexually Inappropriate Behavior in Patients with Fetal Alcohol
                     Spectrum Disorders   **125**
                     Natalie Novick-Brown

Chapter 9   Identifying and Treating Social Communication Deficits in School-
                     Age Children with Fetal Alcohol Spectrum Disorders   **161**
                     Truman E. Coggins, Geralyn R. Timler and Lesley B. Olswang

Chapter 10   FASD and ADHD: The Nuts and Bolts of Diagnosis and Treatment
in the Real World   **179**
Phil Mattheis

Chapter 11   Muti-Modal Management Strategies Through the Lifespan   **199**
Kieran D. O'Malley

Chapter 12   Fetal Alcohol Spectrum Disorders (FASD) in the Adult:
Vulnerability, Disability, or Diagnosis - A Psychodynamic
Perspective   **217**
Arthur K. Sullivan

Index   **249**

PREFACE

This multi-author book will discuss the history and clinical presentation of Fetal Alcohol Spectrum Disorders (FASD) i.e. Fetal Alcohol Syndrome (FAS) and Alcohol Related Neurodevelopmental Disorder (ARND). These developmental neuropsychiatric disorders result from prenatal exposure to alcohol during any gestational period of pregnancy. The book will particularly address the co-occurring presence of ADHD in patients with FASD. ADHD is the most frequent neuropsychiatric presentation of FASD throughout the lifespan and it is particularly difficult to manage because the underlying pathophysiology is related to prenatal neurotoxic brain injury. Although prenatal alcohol exposure, and the resulting FASD, is recognized as the commonest preventable cause of intellectual disability, many clinicians and educators are not aware that 75 to 80% of the patients with FASD have I.Q.s over 70. Thus, the neuropsychiatric presentation of FASD can often be unrecognized or misunderstood. FASD are the true clinical masqueraders' and ADHD is their most likely disguise!

The authors are all experienced professionals from a wide range of disciplines working throughout the USA and Canada. They have been involved in the diagnosis, research and management of FASD for many years and this book will bring their collective knowledge regarding management from infancy to adulthood to an inter-professional audience.

This book has had a fairly long gestation. It began over 2 years ago when I was entrenched in the world of academic medicine at the University of Washington, in Seattle. It is seeing the light of day as I am rapidly becoming immersed in the life and work of another world, namely Belfast, Northern Ireland. Ironically the relevance of the book has taken on new significance as Ireland and the U.K are places where some studies have shown that 80 to 85% of women drink during pregnancy and the rates of binge drinking among young women (and young men) are the highest in Europe.

The clinical thrust of linking ADHD and Fetal Alcohol Spectrum Disorders, either Fetal Alcohol Syndrome (FAS) or Alcohol Related Neurodevelopmental Disorder (ARND) was informed by collective clinical knowledge of 15 to 20 years dealing with these patients. It had become clearly apparent that prenatal exposure to alcohol had an immediate, but also sustained effect, on the infant through childhood to adulthood. The commonest clinical presentation of patients of whatever age was a picture most aptly described by ADHD.There were problems, however. How could clinicians capture the clinical essence of infants who were exposed to alcohol during pregnancy but theoretically too young to be described as ADHD. It was here that the Zero to Three classification of infant and early childhood mental health disorders came to the rescue. In this classification system there is a diagnostic category most suited to the FASD population.. Hence the recognition that Regulatory Disorders of Infancy are really the harbingers of later and commonly life long struggles with ADHD in patients with FASD.

Commonly infants, children and adults with FASD are dismissed as just reflecting 'nurture' not 'nature' . Popular belief still would have us think that these children are just the common and garden variety of children of alcoholics (CAO), and their behaviors are easily explained by the chaotic rearing environments in which they grew up. But it is not so simple.

Over 30 years of painstaking animal research and equally well grounded epidemiological research has quietly teased out the role of nature. The FASD population may also come from chaotic, violent backgrounds, but they may also not come from these backrounds. Their ADHD-like behaviors may, in fact, directly reflect the effect of neurotoxic brain damage on the developing central nervous system.

The book has a beginning, a middle and an end. It starts with a general overview of FASD, and then moves into infancy and early childhood. Along the way, professionals from varied disciplines attest to the multi-faceted complexity of FASD. Parent/child support, sensory integration, language therapy, neuropsychology all have their critical roles to play. FASD are not ' doc in a box' conditions. They subscribe to the well recognized wisdom of generations of the management of developmental disability, and it is only through a marriage of different professionals can adequate care be provided.The meat of the book involves dealing with uncomfortable behaviors such as aggression and ADHD when underlying brain damage makes medication unpredictable, or sexually inappropriate impulsive behaviors, or again the inability to express emotions in acceptable verbal language (alexithymia). The book ends with a review of multi-modal management strategies, offering a panoply of ideas and techniques which are often needed to approach such a patient population.

This book has no pretensions to academia. The authors are all well qualified and recognized in their fields. They command years of collective, varied clinical experience, and it was my hope that they would offer a template for management in the context of a reluctance of government agencies in the USA (NIH) or the UK (MRC) to become involved in outcome studies of the practical management of FASD.Sometimes it seemed that FASD patients were not just orphans in their own right but also orphans from modern medicine. Their challenges seen as too vague, too complex.

So here is a book that analyses the ins and outs of ADHD as it appears in FASD, and offers a range of insights into understanding and management.

Science, as life, overtakes us. We are now on a new threshold of understanding in FASD as the effect of prenatal alcohol on genetic transcription and imprinting is being explored. We enter an uncertain generation where we will see genetic shifts maybe caused by prenatal binge drinking passing from generation to generation , and often coupled with the added neurotoxic damage of active prenatal alcohol exposure in the current generation. As I sit in Belfast amidst a plethora of these children I cannot help but wonder where are the public health doctors of our modern era?

Every book is personal and this is no more so than others. I would like to acknowledge my touchstone, my late father Patrick Pearse O'Malley (RIP) a neuropsychiatrist who founded the Mater Infirmorium Hospital Psychiatric Department, Belfast in 1946, and Professor Ann Streissguth in Seattle for inspiring me. Finally, I would like to thank Nancy

Mills my critical eye, confidante and partner over the book's pre-conception, embryo and lifetime.

In: ADHD and Fetal Alcohol Spectrum Disorders (FASD)   ISBN: 1-59454-573-1
Editor: Kieran D. O'Malley, pp. 1-23   © 2008 Nova Science Publishers, Inc.

Chapter 1

FETAL ALCOHOL SPECTRUM DISORDERS: AN OVERVIEW

Kieran D.O'Malley [*]

INTRODUCTION

The association between prenatal alcohol exposure and its teratogenic effect on the developing fetus was first observed in Nantes, France by paediatrician Paul Lemoine in 1968. He described similar dysmorphic facial features and growth delays in 127 infants of mothers who had drank alcohol during their pregnancies. The clear central nervous system sequelae and associated physical manifestations from prenatal alcohol were elaborated upon and named the Fetal Alcohol Syndrome in two classic papers from Seattle by David Smith, Ken Jones, Christy Ulleland and Ann Streissguth in 1973.The Seattle group described eight unrelated infants from three different ethnic groups all born to mothers who were chronic alcoholics. Thus, it was established that prenatal alcohol exposure caused facial dysmorphology, growth delays and central nervous system abnormalities The current diagnostic criteria for Fetal Alcohol Syndrome still incorporates this triad of clinical effects, namely, dysmorphic facial features, growth retardation and central nervous system abnormalities The essential principles of the teratogenic effects of prenatal alcohol involve;

i)   The dosage of alcohol (the agent) even a low dosage may be teratogenic,
ii) The timing(trimester) of the exposure during pregnancy. Each trimester of pregnancy has specific teratogenic effects, the 1st trimester , facial dysmorphology and growth deficiencies and the 2nd and 3rd trimester exposure has the most insidious effect on CNS development, especially the neurotransmitter development.

---

[*] Kieran D.O'Malley M.B., D.A.B.P.N.(P); Lecturer / Adjunct Faculty, Dept. of Psychiatry and Behavioral Sciences and Henry M. Jackson School of International Studies. 22727 84th Ave W. Edmonds. WA 98026; Contact: omalley.kieran@gmail.com

iii) Medical factors particular to the mother (or host). These include the chronicity of alcoholism in the mother and her general nutritional status, as well as the protective factor of her specific genetic endowment. The group of infants and children who did not show the full Fetal Alcohol Syndrome were initially described as displaying Fetal Alcohol Effects (FAE).

Over twenty years later in 1996 the U.S. Institute of Medicine described 3 different conditions related to prenatal alcohol exposure, Full FAS, Partial FAS and Alcohol Related Neurodevelopmental Disorder (ARND). The ARND condition replacing the older FAE descriptive term. More recently the full clinical range of clinical effects associated with a range of alcohol exposure have been described under the umbrella title of FAS Spectrum Disorder initially described and documented by O'Malley and Hagerman in 1998, and subsequently refined to Fetal Alcohol Spectrum Disorder(s) (FASD) by O'Malley and Streissguth.in 2000. A recent consensus statement from NOFAS (National Organization of Fetal Alcohol Syndrome) and the FASD Centre of Excellence in FASD in Washington DC, April 15th 2004 states: " Fetal Alcohol Spectrum Disorders (FASD) is an umbrella term describing the range of effects that can occur in an individual whose mother drank alcohol during pregnancy. These effects may include physical, mental, behavioral, and /or learning disabilities with possible lifelong implications. The term FASD is not intended for use as a clinical diagnosis."

Thus the essence of understanding patients with FASD is to appreciate that they are not just the children of alcoholics (COA) or adult children of alcoholics (ACOA), where many of the behaviors and psychiatric disorders are learned and reflective of the chaotic and/or abusive home-rearing environment. The FASD population of patients are presenting clinical features related to the teratogenic effect of alcohol on the developing brain, irrespective of the home-rearing environment. FASD are now recognized as chronic developmental and neuropsychiatric disorders with two conditions, Fetal Alcohol Syndrome (FAS) and Alcohol Related Neurodevelopmental Disorder (ARND). Although FASD are true developmental disorders, as Streissguth and colleagues have shown in 1996, at least 70-75% of the patients have a normal IQ and it is the deficit in functional ability that is the kernel of the disability. Clinical experience is showing that the functional disability is more commonly related to the co-morbid neurospychiatric disorder (O'Malley 2005).

Recent interest has evolved in exploring the epigenetic component to Fetal Alcohol Spectrum Disorders. Epigenetics deals with regulatory mechanisms of gene activity and inheritance that are independent of changes in the nucleotide sequence of DNA(Pembrey 2002). The epigenetic mechanisms are in turn controlled by genes whose products encode the enzymes needed for DNA methylation, RNA regulatory apparatus and histone modifications to name a few. Already epigenetic factors have been shown to have a role in medical diseases, as well as in psychiatric diseases such as Schizophrenia and Alcohol Dependence (Song et al 2003, Waterland et al 2003, Tchurikov 2005). Current research has shown an association between alcohol dependence and GABA (A) receptors which is modulated by genetic imprinting (Song et al 2003). Genetic imprinting is the phenomenon whereby one or two alleles are preferentially expressed, dependent on its parent of origin. The association between psychiatric disorders, including alcohol dependence, and FASD has been documented by Baer et al in1998 and Barr et al 2006.

Genetic imprinting is one of the key areas of epigenetics that is currently being studied in FASD. The essence of genetic imprinting involves the encoding of gene methylation patterns which have been shown to differ between paternally and maternally derived alleles(Tchurikov 2005). Subsequently, the transmission of gene expression from parental to daughter cells commonly occurs through DNA methylation. The level of DNA methylation sharply decreases during early embryogenesis of mammals. However, it recovers later due to what is called de-novo methylation. A number of regulatory proteins , including DNA methyl transferases (DNMT), histone modifying enzymes (acetylases and deacetylases) and methyl CpG binding proteins, have been identified as involved in this epigenetic process(Tchurikov 2005).

The DNA methylation has been shown to be decreased in response to folate, zinc methionine/choline insufficiencies often associated with excessive alcohol intake. The relevance of the DNA hyomethylation in FASD relates to the possibility that this could result in the activation of genes that are normally inactivated. This key balance between gene silencing and gene activation has been postulated as the mechanism underpinning inappropriate gene transcription. Thus the major liver pathway of oxidative metabolism of ethanol which involves production of acetaldehyde by cytosolic alcohol dehydrogenase is accompanied by the reduction of NAD to NADH. This reduction alters the cellular redox state by decreasing the NAD/NADH ratio, and may result in gene activation with subsequent changes in gene expression. Many of these ideas are still speculative and further research will uncover their veracity. Nevertheless, at the present time there is a scientific belief that medical disorders, cancer or diabetes and psychiatric disorders, schizophrenia or alcohol dependence, may have their roots in epigenetic factors in the pregnant adult woman as well potentially her offspring. This would make FASD a mutagenic disorder, and necessitate a re-visitation of the effect of alcohol on the male spermatozoa involved in fertilization especially it's possible effect on male DNA or RNA(Anway et al 2005).

EPIDEMIOLOGY

There have been differing analysis of the incidence and prevalence of FASD. Varying prevalence figures have been estimated for FAS from Cleveland, 4.6 per 1000 live births, 1.3 to 4.8 per 1000 live births in Roubaix, France and 2.8 per 1000 live births in Seattle. However, a recent estimate of the prevalence of FAS and ARND was 9.1 per 1000 live births in Seattle (Sampson et al 1997). In contrast a recent extensive survey, of 922 first-grade students, aged 5 to 7 years, in 12 elementary schools in a South African community produced an incidence of more than 40 cases of FAS per 1,000 births among this population.

The varying rates have been attributed to higher maternal alcoholism, and binge drinking in particular, in some geographical areas. Also some researchers have postulated that there may be genetic differences in susceptibility to alcohol based on the individual's liver metabolism, specifically the alcohol dehydrogenase and acetaldehyde dehydrogenase pathways which metabolize alcohol. The challenges for more consistent mapping of incidence and prevalence of FASD will depend on the increasing awareness of the more common subtype ARND which is traditionally underestimated or even ignored because of the absence of facial dysmorphic features.

The University of Washington's Secondary Disability Study in 1996 showed no gender difference in parent or caregiver report of ADHD in 6 to 11.9 year old children with either FAS or FAE (ARND). This is significant as boys commonly show ADHD symptoms 4 to 5 times more commonly than girls. This suggests that the ADHD resulting from prenatal alcohol exposure is distributed equally between the genders.(O'Malley et al 2006)

There have been no scientific studies showing an increase in mortality due to FASD. However, it is beginning to be recognized clinically that depression with suicidal attempts and impulsivity can lead to premature deaths in young adult FASD patients (Huggins and O'Malley 2004).

ETIOLOGY AND PATHOGENESIS

The etiology of FASD is clearly the teratogenic effect of prenatal alcohol exposure on the developing fetus. It remains to be seen if prenatal alcohol exerts its long term clinical effect as a mutagen. Nevertheless, the developmental and neuropsychiatric clinical presentation of this teratogenic effect has been shown to be effected by *genetic factors* which modulate a woman's susceptibility to having a baby with FASD. Studies have demonstrated that certain genetic traits have a protective effect on alcohol abusing pregnant women decreasing her likelihood of having a baby with full FAS. Also *environmental factors,* influence the clinical presentation of FASD. So a child raised in a stable and nuturant home, or in a stable environment when 8 to 12 years of age displays less adverse risk outcomes (Streissguth , et al, 2004). Whereas a child exposed to early abandonment, multiple foster home placements, or physical or sexual abuse shows much more complicated overlapping psychiatric disorders. Some of which include Post Traumatic Stress Disorder or Reactive Attachment Disorder.

The diffuse CNS effects of prenatal alcohol begin with the nerve cell. There may be direct toxic effect on nerve cells, producing cell death with massive apoptotic neurodegeneration in the developing brain (Olney, et al 2000). It can also and disrupt astrocyte, glial cell and neuronal migration and maturation (Phillips , 1994, Guerri and Renau-Piqueras, 1997, Streissguth , 1997). Other work has studied the effect of alcohol on inhibiting L1, an immunoglobulin cell adhesion molecule that promotes cell–cell adhesion, cell migration and synaptic plasticity (Sutherland , et al, 1997, Ikonomidou , et al 2000).Finally, recent research has pointed out the selective loss of complexin proteins in the frontal cortex of rats prenatally exposed to alcohol which may have parallels in future human studies (Barr, et al 2005).The possible role of complexin protein in psychiatric disorders has been explored by Sawada and colleagues in 2002 and 2005.

Structural brain damage in severe FASD has been reviewed using autopsy reports of early infant deaths. Diffuse structural brain changes reported included severe brain malformations with hydrocephalus, microcephaly, enlarged ventricles, cerebellar hypoplasia, corpus callosal agenesis, and hetertopias (pockets of arrested migration of groups of cells (Streissguth 1997, Hagerman 1999).

Brain imaging (MRI, CAT SCAN) techniques have enabled mapping of brain abnormalities in patients with less severe forms of FASD. Microcephaly is consistently seen. The corpus callosum appears to be the area of the brain most commonly affected by prenatal alcohol. Researchers have demonstrated morphological changes in the shape of the corpus callosum. The caudate, which is important for working memory and executive function cognition is the area most affected in the basal ganglion. The cerebellum can be smaller, especially the anterior cerebellar vermis (vermal bodies I through V) compared to controls. Lastly, the hippocampus has been shown to be decreased in shape and volume (Mattson, et al 1994, Riley, et al 1995, Sowell, et al, 1996, Swayze, et al 1997, Hagerman 1999, Bookstein, et al 2001).

Neurotransmitter development is disrupted by prenatal alcohol exposure. Deficits have been found in the dopaminergic, noradrenergic, serotonergic, GABAergic, cholinergic, glutaminergic and histaminergic. The dopaminergic and noradrenergic system deficits most likely are connected with the ADHD presentation of patients with FASD. Previous rat research has demonstrated that the D1 receptors of the mesolimbic dopamine system are more affected by prenatal alcohol than the nigrostriatal or tegmental dopamine D1 receptor system. Ongoing research is analyzing the clinical effect of the prenatal alcohol disruption of the balance between the inhibitory, GABA, and the excitatory Glutaminergic neurotransmitters (Hannigan 1996).

Neurophysiological abnormalities have been demonstrated to be sequelae of prenatal alcohol exposure. They were initially described by Lemoine and colleagues in 1968. Recent work in the 1990's has reported the increased prevalence of temporal lobe dysrhythmia and complex partial seizure disorder in FASD children and adolescents. All these patients responded to carbamazepine(O'Malley and Barr 1998). Animal research has shown the kindling of seizures due to the effect of prenatal alcohol on the GABA ergic cells in the hippocampus. which lowers the seizure threshold.(Bonthius et al 2001) This is borne out in humans where it appears GABA agents have good efficacy for FASD patients with seizure disorder .

DIAGNOSTIC CLINICAL FEATURES OF FASD

Developmental Impairments

The developmental disability of FASD is a Complex Learning Disorder affecting multiple domains of functioning including working memory, attention, impulsivity, learning, interpersonal relatedness, social skills and language development. The patient's complex Learning Disorder is coded under AXIS II in DSM- IV T-R. It often includes a Mathematics Disorder (315.1), and/ or Disorder of Written Expression (315.2) and/or Reading Disorder(315.0), and. evidence of a Mixed Receptive/Expressive Language Disorder(315.32) with specific deficits in social cognition and social communication. Sometimes a more generic coding of Cognitive Disorder NOS (249.9) or Learning Disorder NOS (315.9) may suffice as initial clinical descriptions.

A standardized intellectual functioning assessment is the first step in assessing the cognitive function i.e. WPPSSI or WISC –IV. The deficits in functional development are best quantified by standardized instruments such as the Vineland Adaptive Behavioral Scale (VABS). This shows varying deficits in daily living skills, socialization and communication. It is important to remember that 70 to 75% of patients with FASD are not mentally retarded, so the developmental disability is commonly seen in the context of a normal I.Q.

Developmental disability in FASD is also seen in gross and fine motor delays which can be coded Developmental Coordination Disorder(315.4).

Neuropsychiatric Impairment

Neither of the current diagnostic nomenclature DSM-IV T-R or ICD- 10 acknowledge the neurodevelopmental or neuropsychiatric disorders resulting from prenatal alcohol exposure. However, there is a general category called Mental Disorders due to a General Medical Condition which can be used to describe FASD and their co-morbid psychiatric presentation. Each descriptor has a code which can then be used for re-imbursement through the different medical insurance companies, for example:

- Mood Disorder due to general medical condition of prenatal alcohol exposure with evidence of FAS (293.83)
- Anxiety Disorder due to general medical condition of prenatal alcohol exposure with evidence of PFAS(293.84)
- Psychotic Disorder due to general medical condition of prenatal alcohol exposure with evidence of ARND (293.8x)
- Personality Change due to general medical condition of prenatal alcohol exposure with evidence of ARND (310.1). The personality changes include , Labile, Disinhibited, or Paranoid.

ICD-10. has similar categories which can be used as descriptors for patients with FASD, and also facilitate re-imbursement. In this instance the terms are:

- Catatonic Disorder due to a general medical condition of prenatal alcohol exposure with evidence of FAS
- Personality Change due to a general medical condition of prenatal alcohol exposure with evidence of ARND

Patients with FASD can present clinical symptoms from infancy/young childhood. The clinical presentation is described using the Zero to Three Diagnostic Classification (Zero to three 1994). This classification has been developed to describe psychiatric disorders in the under three year old population , which is not included in the more commonly used DSM IV T-R classification. AXIS I disorders cover the major psychiatric disorders in the infant or young child. The AXIS II component analyses the relationship between the mother or care provider and the infant or young child. The psychiatric diagnoses reflect the CNS sensory integration problems that are pathognomonic of FASD in infancy. The Zero to Three classification is less widely known in primary care environments, but has been developed since 1994 and is well validated and used commonly in the early childhood mental health world (DC:O-3R 2005).

Infants and young children with FASD commonly demonstrate Regulation Disorders of Sensory Processing which are characterized by difficulties in tolerating environmental stimuli, co-ordinating basic motor movements or in approaching and interacting with others in their immediate environment. Three types of Regulation Disorder are seen:

i)   Hypersensitive : Type A Fearful / Cautious or Type B Negative Defiant may present in the FASD infant or young child by becoming upset very easily, crying, irritable with no clear cause .i.e. sometimes the force of the water jet from a shower may precipitate an episode of marked distress.

ii) Hypopsensitive /Underresposive (either Withdrawn and Difficult to engage or Self-Absorbed) may be evidenced by the appearance of marked avoidance and withdrawal in social situations. Also the young child may show little reactive to visual or auditory cues

iii) Sensory Stimulation –Seeking /Impulsive may be seen in the infant or young child's pervasive high motor activity and almost ceaseless motion. Often the infant or young child shows dangerous impulsivity and is quite accident prone.

Other psychiatric disorders which can be seen are: Disorders of Affect of Infancy and Early Childhood are diagnosed when the infant or young child shows emotional incontinence with overwhelming crying or giddiness.

Anxiety Disorders of Infancy and Early Childhood are diagnosed if the infant or young child has a panic attack with hyperventilation in a common social situation i.e. a mother takes a toy away from the young child.

Finally the psychiatric disorders may be of a Secondary nature due to environmental stressors such as Reactive Attachment Disorder of Infancy or Early Childhood related to separation from birth mother or multiple foster home placements.

The AXIS II diagnostic frame of the Zero to Three Classification is equally important in obtaining a holistic clinical picture of the infant or young child with FASD, as it addresses the immediate safety, security and organization in the nurturing environment.

All the relationships listed are relevant, but the commonest ones are:

1. Overinvolved; where the mother/careprovider often interferes with the infant or young child's goals or desires i.e. inhibits the young child's developmental progress by doing everything for him/her.

2. Underinvolved, where the mother/careprovider is insensitive to the infant or young child's needs.

3. Anxious/Tense, where the mother/careprovider is very anxious in parenting and appears to create anxiety in the child because of inconsistent parenting cues about basic issues such as feeding.

4. Angry/ Hostile, where the actual handling of the infant or young child is quite rough or abrupt with very little patience. Also where there appears to be resentment of the infant or young child's developmental needs.

5. Disorganized, where the birth mother may have FASD herself and is cognately disorganized, impulsive and is unpredictable in parenting. Thus this type of relationship highlights the risk of parental neglect due to cognitive, neurodevelopmental reasons.

While all of these types be observed in the infant/ young child dyadic relationship, none specifically characterizes this relationship. Nevertheless, the Disorganized paradigm is frequently observed due to the birth mother having one of the FASD herself, or due to severe

Regulatory Disorder in the infant or young child with FASD which also creates major parenting challenges.

LATER CHILDHOOD, ADOLESCENCE AND YOUNG ADULTHOOD

The psychiatric course of FASD in childhood and adulthood has been documented by a number of studies in the USA and Canada using standardized psychiatric assessments such as the SCID or psychiatric specialist clinical evaluation. This is truly where it is seen that FASD is the great 'masquerader' as it presents itself in the form of many common psychiatric disorders.

The most common AXIS I (Primary Psychiatric) disorders were, ADHD, Mood Disorder, Anxiety Disorder, Alcohol or Drug Dependence, PDD and Psychotic Disorder The largest series of 57 patients showed that 64% had two AXIS I diagnoses and 19% patients had three AXIS I diagnose (Famy et al 1998,O'Malley 2001).

So diagnostic codes such as: ADHD, Predominantly Inattentive Type, due to prenatal alcohol exposure with evidence of ARND (314.00) or Major Depressive Disorder, Recurrent with mood- incongruent psychotic features due to prenatal alcohol exposure with evidence of FAS (296.3x) may be used to describe the FASD. Recent clinical observation has delineated a subgroup of adult FASD patients who display Schizoaffective Disorder features either Depressed type or Bipolar type.

As well, the psychiatric disorder may be Secondary due to environmental stressors, such as PTSD after physical or sexual abuse.

The most common AXIS II (Personality) Disorders seen were, Avoidant, Dependent, Schizoid, Passive/Aggressive and Borderline. Furthermore, at least 50 % of those with AXIS 11 Personality Disorders had more than one .Thus it appears that patients with FASD demonstrate multiple personality diagnoses not conforming to the classical DSM IV –T-R clusters A, B or C.

Overall there was no significant difference between the AXIS I and AXIS II diagnoses in the FAS or ARND subtypes of FASD populations. Thus the presence or absence of facial dysmorphology or growth features did not seem to be clinically correlated to the psychiatric presentation of this neurodevelopmental disorder.

SUMMARY

The clinical features of FASD may be divided into to two broad categories (Tables 1 and 2):

1. Fetal Alcohol Syndrome (FAS) .
2. Alcohol Related Neurodevelopmental Disorder (ARND) (adapted from Stratton and colleagues, Institute of Medicine, classification).

The neuropsychiatric condition most problematic to diagnose and understand is the Alcohol Related Neurodevelopmental Disorder (ARND). However, with a clear significant history of prenatal alcohol exposure it should be possible to grade the clinical severity of the possible ARND.

Mild ARND (Also known as Alcohol Related Neurobehavioral Disorder in Dysmorphology assessments), evidence of Complex Learning Disorder, commonly including Mathematics Disorder, with or without Mixed Receptive/ Expressive language disorder, evidence of Psychiatric Disorder such as ADHD, inattention type with Impulsivity or Mood or Panic disorder, deficits in adaptive functioning and or executive functioning.

Moderate ARND Evidence of Complex Learning Disorder with or without borderline intellectual functioning or mental retardation. Chronic psychiatric disorder unresponsive to standard medication. or behavioral/psychological management approaches. neuropsychological deficits in working memory, executive functioning, judgment and decision-making, significant deficits in adaptive functioning.

Severe ARND (Also known as Static Encephalopathy in Dysmorphology assessments) Evidence of structural brain dysfunction or seizure disorder.

(Sources: Stratton et al 1996, Streissguth 1997, Astley and Clarren 1997, Coggins et al 1998, Streissguth and O'Malley 2000, Kapp and O'Malley 2001)

Table 1. Anatomic and Functional Characteristic's of FAS vs ARND (O'Malley 2005)

	FAS	ARND
Confirmed maternal alcohol exposure	Yes	Yes
Evidence of a characteristic pattern of facial anomalies	short palpebral fissures flat upper lip flattened philtrum flat midface	No characteristic pattern of facial anomalies
Evidence of Growth retardation	low birth weight (less than 3rd percentile for height and weight), decelerating weight over time not due to nutrition, disproportional low weight to height.	No or little growth retardation
Structural Brain Abnormalities	decreased cranial size at birth, microcephaly, partial or complete agenesis of the corpus callosum, cerebellar hypoplasia,decreased hippocampal size	decreased cranial size at birth, microcephaly, partial or complete agenesis of the corpus callosum, cerebellar hypoplasia, decreased hippocampal size
neurophysiological abnormalities	complex partial seizure disorder, absence seizure, other seizure	complex partial seizure disorder, absence seizure, or other seizure
Gross Motor Function	poor tandem gait, positive romberg test, balance problems	poor tandem gait, positive romberg test, balance problems
Fine Motor Function	Constructional apraxia, ideomotor apraxia, poor hand-eye co-ordination, intentional tremor, motorically disorganized in the under 5 year age group	Constructional apraxia, ideomotor apraxia, poor hand- eye co-ordination, intentional tremor, motorically – disorganized in the under 5 year age group
Sensory Function	abnormal sensation upper or lower limbs, neurosensory hearing loss, abnormal visual, auditory, gustatatory, olfactory or tactile sensations, including hallucinations, includes craving touch and can make the patient a victim of a false accusation of sexually inappropriate behavior	abnormal sensation upper or lower limbs,neurosensory hearing loss, abnormal auditory, visual, gustatatory, olfactory, or tactile sensations, including hallucinations, includes craving touch and can make the patient a victim of a false accusation of sexually inappropriate behavior

As well, this age group of patients with FASD experience a host of social dysfunctions or what have been called Secondary Disabilities through their lifespan. (Streissguth et al 1996). For example, inappropriate sexual behaviors occurred in 45%, 43% had a disrupted school experience and 42% have had trouble with the law (including incarceration). Other authors have commented on the psychiatric and social dysfunction in adolescents and adults with FASD in the absence of clear diagnostic criteria, decreased awareness even among psychiatrists, and standardized therapeutic interventions (Nowicki 1992, Brown 1993, Streissguth and O'Malley 2000) See Table 3.

Table 2. Behavioral, Cognitive and Language Characteristics of FAS vs ARND

	FAS	ARND
Behavioral	attentional problems, visual and auditory poor impulse control working memory problems poor adaptive functioning	attentional problems, visual and auditory poor impulse control working memory problems poor adaptive functioning
Cognitive	complex learning disorders With inability to link cause and effect Specific deficits in mathematical skills Marked split between verbal and performance IQ, over 12-15 points Poor capacity for abstraction and metacognition, deficits in school performance poor insight impaired judgment	complex learning disorders with inability to link cause and effect specific deficits in mathematical skills marked split between verbal and performance IQ, over 12-15 points poor capacity for abstraction and metacognition deficits in school performance poor insight impaired judgment
Language	Deficits in higher level receptive and expressive language i.e. the patient does not fully comprehend the "gist".of a social situation -impairment in social interaction -problems in social perception ,cognition and communication -problems in expressing emotions, Alexithymia,where the patient does not have the words to express feelings and acts them out, or expresses them, physically (O'Malley 2004).	deficits in higher level receptive and expressive language i.e.the patient does not fully comprehend the "gist" of a social situation -impairment in social interaction -problems in social perception, cognition and communication -problems in expressing emotions, Alexithymia, where the patient does not have the words to express feelings and acts them out,or expresses them, physically.

Table 3. Psychiatric and Social Dysfunction with FASD

Problem	Percentage of Patients with FASD
Mental Health/Psychiatric Problems	94%
Problems with Employment	80%
Patient in Dependent Living	80%
Inappropriate Sexual Behavior	45%
Disrupted School Experience	43%
Trouble with the Law	42%
Confinement for a Crime	35%
Mental Hospital Admission	23%
Drug/ Alcohol In-Patient Treatment Admission	15%

Adapted from Streissguth et al 1996, Gideon et al 2003.

CO-MORBIDITY IN FASD: DUAL AND TRIPLE DIAGNOSIS

Co-morbidity is the rule rather than the exception in patients with FASD. It often begins in infancy , continues through the lifespan , and may change over time due to environmental stressors.

The infants, children, adolescents and adults with FASD present the features of a *Dual Diagnosis* condition i.e. Developmental Disorder with co-morbid Neuropsychiatric Disorder. The psychiatric disorder may also have a familial component due to the presence of Depression, Bipolar Disorder or Schizophrenia in the birth mother or birth father. Patients with common developmental disabilities such as Autistic Spectrum Disorder, Down's Syndrome or Aspergers Disorder have a range of psychiatric disorders from 40 to 60%, whereas, the patients with FASD have a prevalence of psychiatric/ mental health disorders through the lifespan of 90-94%. Therefore, the developmental disorder of the FASD inevitably co-morbidly occurs with a neuropsychiatric disorder.

There has been extensive animal research on prenatal alcohol exposure which has formed a basis for the understanding of the aetiology of the co-morbid neuropsychiatric disorders in FASD. The co-morbid ADHD, for example, may originate in the effect that pre natal alcohol has on the developing dopaminergic neurotransmitter system. Previous animal studies have demonstrated that prenatal alcohol interferes with the development of the mesolimbic dopamine D1 receptors which have been shown to regulate attention, impulsivity , and to some extent, affect

The co-morbid Mood Disorders may relate to prenatal alcohol modulating the development of the suprachiasmatic nucleus (SCN), the master circadian pacemaker, as well as disrupting the developing serotonergic neurotrasmitter system.(Sher 2003)

Co-morbid Anxiety Disorders, including Panic Attacks, may have their origins in the prenatal alcohol disruption of the balance between the developing excitatory (glutaminergic) and inhibitory (GABAergic) neurotransmitters (Ikonomidou , et al 2000).

As an added clinical complication the co-morbid conditions are often not unitary. So FASD may present with developmental disorder features of PDD or Asperger's Disorder and it may be hard to unravel where the FASD ends and the other begins. Similarly the neuropsychiatric presentation of FASD may not just be one psychiatric disorder but a combination of AXIS I and AXIS disorders , i.e. ADHD with co-morbid Mood Disorder and personality features of avoidant and dependent.(O'Malley 2003)

A number of authors have pointed out that in the adolescent and adult years FASD can present features of a *Triple Diagnosis* i.e. Developmental Disorder with co-morbid Neuropsychiatric Disorder and co-morbid Alcohol or Substance Use Disorder. (commonly Alcohol Dependence). Prenatal alcohol exposure has been shown to increase the prevalence of co-morbid alcohol abuse in adolescents and young adults with FASD by as much as threefold. This is higher than the influence of family history of alcoholism. This alcohol craving due to chemical sensitization of the developing brain by prenatal alcohol had been demonstrated repeatedly in animal work. This work has also postulated that the co-morbid alcohol abuse and dependence related to the prenatal priming of dopamine transmission in the Nucleus Accumbens among other basal ganglion structures (Baer et al 2003, Kapp and O'Malley 2001).

DSM IV –TR criteria: Alcohol Abuse (305.00) Alcohol Dependence (303.90) Polysubstance Dependence (304.80).

It is important to assess the probability of FASD in adolescents or adults with Alcohol or Substance Use Disorder as the standard group counseling approach is commonly not a good fit for this developmental population. As the Alcohol Dependence in FASD may have an organic etiology, medication such as Naltrexone may be a critical part of the Alcohol/Substance Dependence management. Furthermore, careful diagnostic attention to the co-morbid Alcohol or Substance Dependence issues in this neurodevelopmental population offers an opportunity to connect with more appropriate advocacy and clinical services, such as the Parent Child Assistance Programme developed by Grant, Streissguth and colleagues for substance abusing women and children, who also have FASD.(Grant et al 1999)

Table 4. Alcohol Related Birth Defects (ARBD) With FASD

Body Part	Alcohol Related Birth Defect
EYE	• Visual impairment • Strabismus • Ptosis • Optic nerve hypoplasia • Refractive problems secondary to small eye globes • Tortuosity of the retinal arteries
EAR	• Conductive hearing loss secondary to recurrent otitis media • Sensory- neural hearing loss • Central auditory processing abnormalities related to brain damage in brainstem and cortical areas that process auditory information
TEETH	• Orthodontic Problems
HEART	• Aberrant great vessels • Atrial septal defects • Ventricular septal defects • Tetralogy of Fallot
KIDNEY	• Ureteral duplications • Hydronephrosis • Horseshoe kidneys • Hypoplastic kidneys • Aplastic or Dysplastic kidneys
SKELETAL	• Clindodactyly • Hypoplastic nails • Shortened fifth digits • Radioulnar synostosis • Kippel-Feil syndrome • Pectus excavatum and pectus carinatum • Hemivertebrae • Scoliosis

Table adapted from Stratton et al 1996, Streissguth 1997, Hagerman 1999, Koren et al 2003.

Finally, it is equally critical to remember that prenatal alcohol cause effects on organ and system development in the body so co-morbid medical problems are relatively common. These co-morbid medical problems vary in prevalence from 5% for renal abnormalities to 50% with visual impairment. Collectively they are called *Alcohol Related Birth Defects* (ARBD) and include structural abnormalities in the eye, ear, heart , kidney, liver and skeletal system. These conditions are coded under AXIS III of the DSM IV –T-classification. The co-morbid medical problems are important in general medical differential diagnosis as they are not primary medical disorders. Also they are important to be aware of in the monitoring of psychotropic medication n patients with FASD (Table 4).

DIFFERENTIAL DIAGNOSIS

The commonest clinical conditions which need to be considered and out-ruled are:

1. Genetic Disorders
2. Medical Disorders

1.a. **Genetic syndromes with dysmorphic features.** Some genetic disorders with dysmorphic features may have faces that resemble FAS or PFAS. A genetic assessment of the patient is prudent if there are atypical dysmorphic features.

-   Velo-Cardio Facial Syndrome (VCFS); can show flattening of mid facial features structures that are similar to FAS. However, children with VCFS do not generally have a thin upper lip or flat philtrum , but have a long face, large nose with a large tip, high nasal root, small ears and narrow squinting eyes.
-   Fragile X Syndrome: These patients have a long face with a slightly increased head circumference, a large jaw with large protruding ears.
-   -Downs Syndrome (Trisomy 21); have the pathognomonic mongoloid features, with also upward slanting eyes, epicanthus and wide nasal bridge
-   -Williams Syndrome; show elfin-like faces with full prominent cheeks, a widemouth and a flat nasal bridge, but do not have the classical FAS dysmorphic facial, features.

b. **Genetic Syndromes without dysmorphology**. These syndromes would not be mistaken for FAS, PFAS , but it might be hard to differentiate such syndromes from ARND. These syndromes include:

-   -Autistic Spectrum Disorder, and Pervasive Developmental Disorder
-   -Aspergers Disorder

These children or adolescents may display poor social relatedness, obsessive pre-occupations with topics such as computers, hyper or hypo/hyper-responsiveness to sensory stimuli and soft neurological signs with motor clumsiness and coordination problems. They might well be differentiated by the well documented history of prenatal alcohol exposure in the effected patient. The organically-driven pervasive impulsivity and ADHD symptomatology which exists throughout the lifespan is also a discriminating clinical feature of the ARND patient population.

Nevertheless, it has been recognized for over 10 years that patients with FASD can present with either Autistic or Asperger's Disorder symptoms as their primary clinical presentation (Nanson, et al 1990).

2. Medical disorders, presenting psychiatric disorders that may be confused with, or even potentially mask, the FASD diagnosis. These medical disorders should be considered and out ruled before a diagnosis of a neuropsychiatric disorder associated with the FASD is considered.

The medical disorders can begin in infancy as a result of hypoxia in labour or a difficult delivery. It is always important to review other prenatal toxins such as nicotine, cocaine or even prescription drugs such as the SSRIs. All of these medical conditions can lead to a wide variety of non-specific motor, cognitive and behavioral problems which need to be distinguished from ARND. As well as that, certain seizure disorders, more commonly Complex Partial or Absence, may have their origins in prenatal alcohol exposure and be a primary neurological presentation of the ARND. Acute medical disorders such as hyperthyroiditis, infectious diseases, encephalitis or even meningitis may present acute psychiatric symptomatology, either of a delirium or psychotic nature, which may mask the underlying ARND.

Finally some chronic medical conditions can present complex neuropsychiatric or neurological disorders, including panic disorder, psychosis, dementia and seizures, that need to be considered in the differential assessment of a patient with possible ARND. They include; metabolic or endocrine disorders i.e. uremia, liver or thyroid disease, infectious diseases, including HIV associated early-onset dementia, or even a cerebral tumour (for a complete list see O'Malley 2003).

ASSESSMENT OF FASD

Infants, children, adolescents and adults with FASD present problems of a Dual Diagnosis nature e.g. developmental disability due to prenatal exposure to alcohol and psychiatric disorder (of a primary or secondary nature). However as well, adolescents and adults with FASD may present a Triple Diagnosis clinical picture, namely a combination of developmental disability, psychiatric disorder and an addictive disorder. The Addictive disorder being related to the chemical sensitization of the developing brain by prenatal alcohol exposure (Baer et al 1998, Baer et al 2003)

The first step is to evaluate the Developmental Disability that is a legacy of the prenatal alcohol exposure. When assessing a child or even adolescent with possible FASD it is important to be sensitive to their capacity to make up stories because of their deficits in working memory .So the patient can confabulate to fill in the gaps in a personal history narrative. As well the patient may be very suggestible to leading questions. This is especially problematic if the assessment is in the context of a `sexually compromising behavior or legal situation. No patient should be assessed without collateral information from parent or caregiver. Also, as so many of these children and adolescents are in social service custody, it is essential to obtain clear, unambiguous directions from the state social worker as to the role, context and expectations of the clinical assessment.

The clinical dysmorphology and developmental disability assessment used at the University of Washington FAS-DPN clinic is one appropriate screening method. This assessment involves a review of the mother's pregnancy history, a clinical dysmorphological examination, see FAS and PFAS criteria in clinical features section, cognitive and language assessment, Occupational Therapy assessment using the mini-neurological examination.

Infant assessment is more specialized and needs an infant trained primary care physician. with particular attention to basic growth, height and head circumference parameters. The assessment obviously involves the parent or caregiver in a true dyadic assessment to quantify the all interactional and attachment issues. This assessment can often bring forth the `immediate unpredictability and management problems with the infant and the need for ancillary professional support. or even respite care.

This screening assessment quantifies and subtypes the Developmental Disability resulting from the prenatal alcohol exposure. The distinction between the subtypes of FASD is the initial stage of diagnostic evaluation i.e. FAS or ARND.

Table 5. Medical Consultation for Patients with FASD

1. Diagnostic Assessment of the Dual Diagnosis, i.e. Developmental Disability and Psychiatric Disorder, with referral to psychiatrist if probable psychiatric disorder.
2. Blood assays CBC, LFT, TSH, B. glucose, serum creatinine, blood lead
3. Electrocardiogram especially if taking medication.
4. OT assessment especially under 5 and early childhood. Assess for sensory integration and gross / fine motor function.
5. Arrange Intellectual Testing WPPSSI or WISC IV as age appropriate. WAIS in adult to quantify if developmental disability is associated with mental retardation.
6. Sleep Deprived EEG if clinical evidence of possible seizure disorder, especially if intermittent explosiveness or episodes of 'drifting off' seen as ADHD, inattention type
7. Medical consultations as needed e.g. neurologist, paediatrician for general health care if marked developmental disability
8. Public Health referral for pregnant teenager or young adult with FASD. Connection to advocate for help with the arrival of new baby and prevent alcohol/ drug usage in pregnancy.
9. Screening of FASD teenager or young adult for alcohol usage in pregnancy using BARC, TWEAK, or GGT. Haemaglobin Acetaldehyde Adduct. Blood tests.

Sources: Stratton et al 1997, Streissguth and O'Malley 2000, 2003, O'Malley 2003.

It is also imperative to quantify the co-morbid Psychiatric Disorder. A thorough psychiatric evaluation should be done by a mental health professional or, ideally, a child/adolescent psychiatrist. This assessment should include a complete review of previous medication dosage response and general medical status. This evaluation includes specific attention to issues of Reactive Attachment Disorder or Post Traumatic Stress Disorder, as patients with FASD are at high risk for abandonment, removal from birth parents, multiple foster care placements, or early-onset physical or sexual abuse .As these children and even adolescents often have problems expressing their feelings in words (Alexithymia) non-verbal assessment techniques such as drawing, painting , structured and unstructured play or sandtray are necessary assessment skills (Gardner 1993).

The medical status is important because of the prevalence of Alcohol Related Birth Defects (ARBD), which are a legacy of prenatal alcohol exposure. Prenatal alcohol can affect the skeletal system, cardiac, renal and liver as well as the eye development. The holistic diagnostic assessment which quantifies the Dual Diagnosis i.e. Developmental Disability and Psychiatric Disorder helps greatly in relieving some of the caregiver burden as. adoptive or foster parents are often are blamed as the cause of the child's behavioral problems due to their poor parenting. It also gives direction to ongoing advocacy with both birth and adoptive or foster parents as the assessment clarifies the role of organic brain dysfunction in the child or adolescent's clinical presentation (see Tables 5 and 6).

Table 6. Psychiatric and Psychological Assessment of FASD

1. Clarification of Dual Diagnosis i.e. developmental disability, FAS or ARND subtype and psychiatric presentation i.e. ADHD or Mood Disorder
2. Consideration of Triple Diagnosis in Adolescent or Adult .i.e. Addictive Disorder
3. Medication review with attention to previous drug response and presumptive co-morbid psychiatric diagnoses.
4. Intellectual Testing if not already performed or over 3 years old. WPPSI –R, WISC IV as age appropriate, or WAIS in adult.
5. Speech and Language testing with emphasis on Discourse Analysis (especially social cognition and social communiation).
6. Family Functioning Assessment essential to establish impact of child/ adolescent with FASD on the family system .
7. MRI of brain to assess corpus callosum, hippocampus or cerebellum, especially if low IQ, marked split, over 15 in Verbal/ performance IQ, unresponsiveness to medication. Or case where patient is in forensic/ jail system.
8. Vineland Adaptive Behavior Scales (VABS) to quantify functional disability in activities of daily living, socialization and communication., especially useful if IQ over 70.
9. Neuropsychological testing especially useful for patient with ARND and normal or above average IQ. This establishes the neurocognitive deficits in executive functioning, working memory, impulsivity and personal and social judgment.
10. Case management planning with involvement of social worker to establish support for family/ caregiver, including regular planned respite care and, in-home support or 1on 1 mentorship for teenager (includes job coach).
11. School management meeting to advocate for adequate special education services, especially vocational and work experience in junior high and high school years
12. If Adult case management meeting with DDD or PDD services to establish guardianship, payee (or trusteeship) Pts. with FASD are more likely to qualify for mental health disability funding as their IQ is often over 70.

Sources: King et al 1998, O'Malley and Streissguth 2000and 2003, Lemay et al 2003 , Goren et al 2003.

VIGNETTES

The age, gender and ethnicity of these patients have been altered to protect their identity.

1. DM is a 12-year-old Caucasian boy of Irish/ Scottish heritage, is in custody of his birth father and stepmother. His birth mother drank heavily throughout his pregnancy and also had a pattern of binge drinking, at least 5 –6 beers at the weekend. The birth mother is still drinking and only sees DM in supervised visits. Both his parents had finished high school and his father was a house painter (see table 7).

Although he was born by Breech presentation at 38 weeks gestation he had no birth anoxia and no history of neonatal problems. His birth weight was 7 lbs. His developmental milestones were normal for sitting, standing and walking, but he had a history of speech delay and had seen a speech therapist for 2 years from 7 to 9 years of age. A WISC III done at 9 years showed a 24-point difference between verbal and Performance IQ. His verbal IQ was 70 and his Performance IQ was 94 Reading was at 7th percentile, Spelling at the 4th percentile and Mathematics at the 1st percentile.

He was diagnosed as ADHD by a pediatrician at 7 years of age and was treated with methylphenidate for 5 years with mixed success; The dosage of the medication kept increasing and at psychiatric assessment when 12 years of age he was taking 45 mgs of methylphenidate a day, or almost 2 mgs per kilogram. His height and weight were at the 3 rd percentile and head circumference at the 50th percentile. He had FAS dysmorphic features and fulfilled the criteria for full FAS. Patients with FASD are particularly at risk for the negative growth and sleep effects of psychostimulants, especially methylphenidate. X ray for bone age showed that his bone age was 3 years behind his chronological age. Growth hormone was low, less than 0.1. MRI of the brain showed ' thinning of the posterior body and splenium of the corpus callosum'.

Clinically, the patient did not present a clear ADHD picture, but more of a Mood disorder with psychomotor slowing, inattention and some impulsivity. His methylphenidate was discontinued and he was started on liquid fluoxetine 1 cc (4 mgs) initially, He showed good response to this medication and his schoolwork improved. He also became more verbal and was encouraged to use art and clay work to express his feelings. His growth parameters are beginning to show an upward slope and he is being followed by a paediatric endocrinologist. He had marked orthodontic problems seen in prenatal alcohol exposure as ARBD

2. JC is a 17 year old Polish teenager with ARND who lives with his birth mother in a two room inner city apartment. His mother was a 6 beer binge drinker every week-end throughout his pregnancy. She had a long history of Bipolar Disorder, but no sustained Psychiatric follow-up care , and had taken no psychotropic medications during the pregnancy. Currently JC and his mother were living on welfare with little health care insurance. JC has always been a loner and has never fitted into the school environment. He has been bullied and teased for many years and avoids school for varying periods. JC has problems expressing his feelings and many of his absences from school have been for psychosomatic pains and aches with no organic etiology discovered. His school attendance has affected his academic record. He is bright and a WISC III at 15 years gave him a verbal IQ of 129 and a Performance IQ of 120 with Full scale 126. Subtests showed Mathematics at 5th percentile and marked problems in Spelling. His Ht was 25th percentile, Wt 50th percentile and Head circumference at the 98th percentile. He had no FAS dysmorphic features. He presented a mixed clinical picture of

ADHD, inattention type with co morbid mood disorder. The patient has not responded to methylphenidate but has responded to l-tryptophan at night. He now sleeps better and has more energy for school and concentrates better. The school are now aiding JC in planning a work experience programme as they understand from his VABS testing that his functional ability is quite a bit lower than his cognitive ability and he needs practical, 'hands on' experience for his next stage in life .His profile is not unlike a patient with high functioning Autism or Aspergers Disorder.

Table 7. Questions Used to elicit BARC Score

Estimate the following (write 0 if it never happened	Month or so before pregnancy	During this pregnancy
Number of times per month that you drank 5 or more drinks on one occasion		
Number of times per month that you consumed 3-4 drinks on an occasion		
Number of times per month that you consumed just 1-2 drinks on an occasion		
Did you drink alcohol almost every day, even if only a small quantity? (circle answer)	Yes No	Yes No

Note: The fourth question is redundant, but is suggested as a check on the first three questions, and seems to reflect the tone of many of the respondents.

1. Fetal Alcohol Syndrome (FAS) (adapted Stratton et al 1996)

A. Confirmed maternal alcohol exposure

B. Evidence of a characteristic pattern of facial anomalies that includes features such as short palpebral fissures (2 SD or greater below mean), and abnormalities in the premaxillary zone (i.e. flat upper lip, flattened philtrum and flat midface)

C. Evidence of Growth retardation, as in at least one of the following:
- low birth weight
- decelerating weight over time not due to nutrition (less than 3rd percentile for height and weight),
- disproportional low weight to height.

D. Evidence of CNS neurodevelopmental abnormalities, such as:
- structural brain abnormalities, i.e.decreased cranial size at birth, microcephaly (head circumference less than 3 rd percentile), partial or complete agenesis of the corpus callosum, cerebellar hypoplasia,
- neurophysiological abnormalities, complex partial seizure disorder, absence seizure, other seizure,
- neurological hard or soft signs(as age appropriate):
    - motor:
        - gross motor function; poor tandem gait, positive romberg test, balance problems,

- fine motor function, fine motor problems with evidence of constructional apraxia, poor hand-eye co-ordination motorically disorganized in the under 5 year age group,
    - sensory:
        - abnormal sensation upper or lower limbs,
        - neurosensory hearing loss,
        - abnormal visual, auditory, gustatatory, olfactory or tactile sensations, including hallucinations, includes craving touch and can make the patient a victim of false accusation of sexually inappropriate behavior
        - Regulatory disorder, type 1, 11 or 111, in under 5 year age (see table 1).

2. Alcohol Related Neurodevelopmental Disorder (ARND)

A. Confirmed maternal alcohol exposure

B. No characteristic pattern of facial anomalies

C. No or little growth retardation

D. Evidence of CNS neurodevelopmental abnormalities, such as:

- structural brain abnormalities i.e. decreased cranial size at birth
- microcephaly, partial or complete agenesis of the corpus callosum, cerebellar hypoplasia, decreased hippocampal size
- neurophysiological abnormalities i.e. complex partial seizure disorder, absence seizure, or other seizure
- neurological hard or soft signs (as age appropriate),
    - motor:
        - gross motor problems, poor tandem gait, positive romberg sign, balance problems
        - fine motor problems, poor eye-hand co-ordination, intentional tremor, motorically –disorganized in the under 5 year age group
    - sensory:
        - abnormal sensation upper or lower limbs,
        - neurosensory hearing loss,
        - Abnormal auditory, visual, gustatatory, olfactory, or tactile sensations,(including hallucinations), including craving touch and can make the patient a victim of false accusation of sexually inappropriate behavior
        - Regulatory Disorder, Hypersensitive or Hyposensitive, in the under 5-year age group
- and/or evidence of complex pattern of behavior, cognitive or language abnormalities that are inconsistent with developmental level and cannot be explained by familial background or environment alone:
    - Behavioral:
        - attentional problems, visual and auditory
        - poor impulse control
        - working memory problems

- poor adaptive functioning
    - Cognitive:
        - complex learning disorder with inability to link cause and effect
        - specific deficits in mathematical skills
        - marked split between verbal and performance IQ, over 12-15 points
        - poor capacity for abstraction and metacognition
        - deficits in school performance
        - poor insight
        - impaired judgment
    - Language:
        - deficits in higher level receptive and expressive language i.e. the patient does not fully comprehend the "gist" of a social situation
        - impairment in social interaction
        - problems in social perception, cognition and communication
        - problems in expressing emotions, Alexithymia, where the patient does not have the words to express feelings and acts them out ,or expresses them, physically (see Table 1)

REFERENCES

Anway MD (2005) Epigenetic transgenerational actions of endocrine disruptors and male fertility. *Science*, 308: 1466-1469

*Astley SJ and Clarren SK (1997) *Diagnostic Guide for Fetal Alcohol Syndrome and Related Conditions*. Seattle, WA: University of Washington.

Baer, JS ,Barr, HM, Bookstein, FL, Sampson, PD, Streissguth, AP (1998) Prenatal alcohol exposure and family history of alcoholism in the etiology of adolescent alcohol problems. *Journal of Studies on Alcohol*, Vol. 59, No. 5, 533-543

Baer JS, Sampson PD, Barr HM, Connor PD and Streissguth AP (2003) A 21- year longitudinal analysis of the effects of prenatal alcohol exposure on young adult drinking. *Arch Gen Psychiatry*, Vol. 60, April 377-385.

Barr, AM, Hofman, CE, Phillips, AG, Weinberg, J, Honer, WG (2005) Prenatal ethanol exposure in rats decreases levels of complexin proteins in the frontal cortex, *Alcohol Clin Exp Res* , Vol 29, No. 11, 1915-1920

Barr HM and Streissguth AP (2001) Identifying maternal self- reported alcohol use associated with fetal alcohol spectrum disorders. *Alcohol Clin Exp Res*, Vol 25, No. 2, 283-287.

Bonthius, DJ, Woodhouse, J, Bonthius, NE, Taggard, DA, and Lothman, EW (2001) Reduced seizure threshold and hippocampal cell loss in rats exposed to alcohol during the brain growth spurt. *Alcohol Clin Exp Res*, Vol. 25, No. 1, 70-82

Bookstein FL, Sampson PD, Streissguth AP, Connor PL (2001) Geometric morphometrics of corpus callosum and subcortical structures in fetal alcohol effected brain. *Tetratology*, 4, 4-32.

Brown, Hilary J (1993) Sexuality and intellectual disability: The new realism. *Current Opinion in Psychiatry*, 6, 623-628.

Coggins TE, Olswang LB, Carmichael Olson H and Timler GR (2003) On becoming socially competent communicators: The challenge for children with fetal alcohol exposure, *International review of research in mental retardation*, Vol. 27, 121-150.

**DC:0-3R (2005) Diagnostic classification of mental health and developmental disorders of infancy and early childhood: Revised Edition, Zero to Three Press, Washington, DC

Famy, C Streissguth, AP & Unis, A (1998) Mental illness in adults with fetal alcohol syndrome or fetal alcohol effects. American Journal of Psychiatry, 155, 552-554

*Gardner H (1993) *Multiple Intelligence. The Theory in Practice*. Harper Collins, New York.

Guerri, C, Renau-Piqueras, J (1997) Alcohol, astroglia and brain development. Mol Neurobiol 15 (1), 65-81

*Grant TM, Ernst CC, and Streissguth AP (1999) Intervention with high-risk alcohol and drug abusing mothers: 1.Administrative strategies of the Seattle model of paraprofessional advocacy. *Journal of Community Psychology*, 27, 1-18.

Hagerman RJ (1999) *Neurodevelopmental Disorders. Diagnosis and Treatment. Fetal Alcohol Syndrome*, 3-59, Oxford University Press, New York, Oxford.

Huggins, J & O'Malley KD (2006) Suicidal risk in fetal alcohol spectrum disorders, Letter to the Editor, Can J Psychiatry

Ikonomidou, C, Bittigau, P, Ishimaru, MJ, Wozniak, DF, Koch, C, Genz, K, Price, MT, Stefovska, V, Horster, F, Tenkova, T, Dikranian, K, Olney, JW (2000) Ethanol- induced apoptotic neurodegeneration and fetal alcohol syndrome. *Science*, Vol. 287, 1056-1059

Jones KL, Smith DW, Ulleland CN and Streissguth A P (1973a) Pattern of malformations in offspring of chronic alcoholic mothers *Lancet,* June, 1267-1270.

Jones KL and Smith DW (1973b) Recognition of the fetal alcohol syndrome in early infancy. *Lancet*, 2, 999-1101.

**Kapp FME and O'Malley KD (2001) *Watch for the Rainbows. True stories for educators and caregivers of children with fetal alcohol spectrum disorders*; 64-83, Publisher Frances Kapp Education, Calgary, Canada.

King BH, State MW, Bhavik S, Davanzo P, Dykens (1998) Mental Retardation: A review of the past 10 years. Part I, in *Reviews in Child and Adolescent Psychiatry, AACAP*, 126-133.

Koren G, Nulman I, Chudley AE, Loocke C (2003) Fetal Alcohol Spectrum Disorder. *CMAJ*, 169 (11) 1181-1185.

Lemay J-F, Herbert AR, Dewey DM, Innes AM (2003) A rational approach to the child with mental retardation for the paediatrician. *Paediat Child Health*, vol. 8, No. 6, 345-356.

Lemoine P, Harousseau H and Borteyru JP (1968) Les enfants de parents alcoholiques: Anomalies observees a propos de 127 cas. *Quest Med*, 21, 476- 482.

Li TK (2000) Pharmacogenetics of response to alcohol and genes that influence alcohol drinking. *J Stud Alcohol*. 61, 5-12.

Mattson, SN, Riley, EP, Jernigan, TL, Garcia, A, Kaneko, WM, Ehlers, CL, Jones, KL (1994) A decrease in the size of the basal ganglia following prenatal alcohol exposure: a preliminary report. *Neurotoxicol Teratol*, 16: 283-289

Nanson, J, Hiscock, M (1990) Attention deficits in children exposed to alcohol prenatally. Alcoh Clin Exp Res : 14: 656-661

**Nowicki S and Duke MP (1992) *Helping the Child Who Doesn't Fit In*. Peachtree Publishers. Atlanta, Georgia.

Olney, JW, Farber, NB, Woziak, DF, Jevtovic, -Todorovic,V , Ikonomidou, C (2000) Environmental agents that have the potential to trigger massive neurodegeneration in the developing brain. *Environ Health Project*, 108(Suppl.3), 383-388

*O'Malley KD, Hagerman RJ (1998) Developing Clinical Practice Guidelines for Pharmacological Interventions with Alcohol-affected Children. *Proceedings of a special focus session of the Interagency Co-ordinating Committee on Fetal Alcohol Syndrome*. Chevy Chase Ma, Sept 10TH and 11th, Centers for Disease Control and National Institute of Alcohol Abuse and Alcoholism (Eds.), USA, 145-177.

O'Malley, KD (2001) The National FAS Conference, CDC, Medication in FASD . Uses in primary, secondary and tertiary prevention, Invited Paper April 25-28th, Atlanta

*O'Malley KD and Streissguth AP (2003) Clinical intervention and support for children aged zero to five years with fetal alcohol spectrum disorder and their parents / caregivers. In: Tremblay RE, Barr RG, Peters RdeV, eds. *Encyclopedia on Early Childhood Development (online)*, Montreal, Quebec: Centre for Excellence for Early Childhood development: 1-9 Available at, http://www/excellence-earlychildhood.ca/documents/ OMalley-StreissguthANGxp.pdf.

*O'Malley KD and Storoz L (2003) Fetal alcohol spectrum disorder and ADHD: diagnostic implications and therapeutic consequences. *Expert Review of Neurotherapeutics*, July, Vol. 3. No. 4, 477-489.

O'Malley, KD (2003) Youth with Comorbid Disorders. Chapter 13, 276- 315, in *The Handbook of Child and Adolescent Systems of Care*, Pumariega AJ and Winters NC (eds.) Jossey- Bass, San Francisco.

*O'Malley, KD (2005) *Behavioural Phenotype of Fetal Alcohol Syndrome , Alcohol related neurodevelopmental disorder*. 9th International Symposium, Society for Study of Behavioural Phenotypes, Cairns, Australia, October 6th to 8th , 36-37

O'Malley, KD, Barr, HM, Connor, PD and Streissguth, AP (2006) *The frequency of psychiatric problems in children with fetal alcohol spectrum disorders (FASD)*, Submitted Pediatrics

Pembrey , ME (2002) Time to take epigenetic inheritance seriously. *European Journal of Human Genetics*, 10: 669-671

Phillips, DE (1994) *Effects of alcohol on glial cell development in vivo: morphological studies*, In FE Lancaster (Ed.) , Alcohol and glial cells (Vol. 27) Bethesda: NIH: NIAAA

Riley, EP, Mattson, SN, Sowell, ER, Jernigan, TL, Sobel, DF,Jones, KL (1995) Abnormalities of the corpus callosum in children prenatally exposed to alcohol. *Alcohol Clin Exp Res*, 19 (5), 1198-1202

Sampson, PD, Streissguth AP, Bookstein FL, Little RE, Clarren SK, Dehaene P, Hanson Jr. JW (1997) Incidence of fetal alcohol syndrome and prevalence of alcohol-related neurodevelopmental disorder. *Teratology*, 56 (6): 317-326.

Sawada, K, Young, CE, Barr, AM, Longworth, K, Takahashi, S, Arango, v, Mann, JJ, Dwork, AJ, Falkai, P, Phillips, AG, Honer, WG (2002) Altered immunoreactivity of complexin proteins in prefrontal cortex in severe mental illness. *Mol Psychiatry*, 7:484-492

Sawaka, K, Barr, AM, Nakamura, M, Arima, K, Young, CE, Dwork, AJ, Falkai, P, Phillips, AG, Honer, WG (2005) Hippocampal complexin proteins and cognitive dysfunction in schizophrenia. *Arch Gen Psychiatry*, 62:263-272

Sher, L. (2003) Developmental alcohol exposure, circadian rhythms, and mood disorders. *Can J. Psychiatry*, vol. 48, No. 6, 428

Song, J et al (2003) Association of GABA (A) receptors and alcohol dependence and the effects of genetic imprinting. *Am J Med* Genet B Neuropsychiatry Genet,117 (1): 39-45

Sowell, ER, Jernigan, TL, Mattson, SN, Riley, EP, Sobel, DF, Jones, KL (1996) Abnormal development of the cerebellar vermis in children prenatally exposed to alcohol: size reduction in lobules I-V, *Alcohol Clin Exp Res*, 20, 31-34

*Stratton KR, Rowe CJ and Battaglia FC (1996) *Fetal Alcohol Syndrome: Diagnosis, epidemiology, prevention and treatment in medicine* . National Academy Press, Washington DC.

Streissguth , A.P and Little, R.E (1994) "Unit 5: Alcohol , Pregnancy, and the Fetal Alcohol Syndrome": *Second Edition of the Project Cork Institute Medical School Curriculum (slide projection series) on Biomedical Education*: Alcohol Use and Its Medical Consequences, produced by Dartmouth Medical School.

*Streissguth, A.P., Barr, H.M., Kogan, J. and Bookstein, F.L. (1996). Understanding the occurrence of secondary disabilities in clients with fetal alcohol syndrome (FAS) and fetal alcohol effects (FAE). *Final Report, August, C.D.C. Grant R04*.

**Streissguth AP (1997) *Fetal alcohol syndrome. A guide for families and communities.* Brookes Publishing, Baltimore.

*Streissguth AP and O'Malley KD (2000) Neuropsychiatric implications and long-term consequences of fetal alcohol spectrum disorders. *Seminars in Clinical Neuropsychiatry*, 5, 177-190.

*Streissguth, AP, Bookstein, FL, Barr, HM, Sampson, PD, O'Malley KD, Kogan Young (2004) Risk factors for adverse risk outcomes in fetal alcohol syndrome and fetal alcohol effects. *Developmental and Behavioral Pediatrics*, Vol. 25. No. 4, 228-238

Sutherland, RJ, Mc Donald, RJ, Savage, DD (1997) *Prenatal exposure to moderate levels of ethanol can have long–lasting effects on synaptic plasticity in adult offspring.* Hippocampus. 7: 232-238

Swayze, VW, Johnson, VP, Hanson, JW, Piven, J, Sato, Y, Giedd, JN, Mosnick, D, Moore, L (1997) Magnetic resonance imaging of brain abnormalities in fetal alcohol syndrome. *Pediatrics*, 99(2), 232-240

Tchurikov, NA (2005) Molecular mechanisms of epigenetics. *Biochemistry (Moscow)*, 70: 406- 423

Waterland, RA, Jirtle, RA (2003) Transposable elements: targets for early nutritional effects on epigenetic gene variation, *Mol Cell Biol*, 23: 5293-5300

* Recommended for primary care physicians or psychologists
** Recommended for families

In: ADHD and Fetal Alcohol Spectrum Disorders (FASD)   ISBN: 1-59454-573-1
Editor: Kieran D. O'Malley, pp.25-38   © 2008 Nova Science Publishers, Inc.

Chapter 2

INFANT, TODDLER AND YOUNG CHILD SYSTEMS OF CARE FOR PATIENTS WITH FETAL ALCOHOL SPECTRUM DISORDERS (FASD) AND THEIR FAMILIES

Kieran D. O'Malley[*]

INTRODUCTION

Alcohol is a true teratogen which disrupts the embryological development of the fetus throughout the three trimesters of pregnancy. It does not just cause a dysmorphic disorder but causes a chronic developmental and neuropsychiatric disorder which can be diagnosed in infancy and early childhood (Hagerman 1999, Streisgguth and O'Malley 2000, O'Malley and Streissguth 2003). Recently the United States Surgeon General commented in the Children's Section of his report on Mental Health that,"it seems likely that the roots of most mental disorders lie in some combination of genetic and environmental factors," and that the environmental factors could be biological or psychosocial (Rutter et al., 1999; U.S. Surgeon General, 1999). Prenatal alcohol exposure offers an example of a common biological environmental factor. However recent evidence is beginning to suggest that it may also have an effect on genetic transcription.Therefore, prenatal alcohol may actually show the synergistic effect of an environmental teratogen coupled with epigenetic effects Fetal Alcohol Spectrum Disorders (FASD) refers to the range of clinical disorders that result from a variety of prenatal exposures to alcohol, in combination with individual differences in the mother and child's susceptibility to the adverse effects of alcohol. FASD is an umbrella term that includes several descriptive terms that have previously been used. There are three primary subtypes, which were described in 1996 by the Institute of Medicine, and initially documented as a

---

[*] Kieran D. O'Malley M.B. D.A.B.P.N.(P), Lecturer /Adjunct Faculty, Department of Psychiatry and Behavioral Sciences and Henry M. Jackson School of International Studies, University of Washington, Fetal Alcohol and Drug Unit, Seattle, WA. Phone: (206) 543-7155; Fax: (206) 685-2903; CORRESPONDENCE: Kieran D. O'Malley. E-mail: omalley.kieran@gmail.com

'spectrum' by O'Malley and Hagerman in 1998. They are Full Fetal Alcohol Syndrome (FAS), Partial Fetal Alcohol Syndrome (PFAS) and Alcohol Related Neurodevelopmental Disorder (ARND) (Stratton et al 1996,O'Malley and Hagerman, 1998). These subtypes are primarily differentiated by the presence or absence of pathognomonic facial features, as were the previous-used terms FAS and FAE, the latter referring to children who had been examined for FAS, but who lacked the full features of FAS although exposed to significant alcohol prenatally (Jones and Smith 1973,Clarren and Smith 1978). Central Nervous System characteristics through the lifespan include: neurodevelopmental abnormalities in attention, distractibility, working memory, complex learning problems (including language), fine and gross motor skills and general adaptive functioning especially judgement (Harris 1995, Steinhausen 1996, Streissguth 1997a, Hagerman 1999, Streissguth and O'Malley 2000).

Infants, toddlers and young children with prenatal alcohol exposure can present with immediate physical, developmental, social-emotional and behavioral problems (Streissguth et al 1983, Jacobson et al 1994b, Harris 1995, Streissguth at al 1996a, Hagerman 1999).These symptoms and signs are not just related to alcohol withdrawal as postulated by earlier research (Robe et al 1981, Coles et al 1984) but are associated with the direct alcohol effect on developing body organ systems (i.e. cardiac, renal, eye, ear, skeletal), as well as specific central nervous system irritability and dysregulation due to the neurotoxic effect of alcohol on autonomic dysfunction, neurotransmitter development, sleep architecture, muscle tone and seizure threshold to name a few (Clarren and Smith 1978, Day 1992, Streissguth 1997a, Hagerman 1999).

At the moment no infant psychiatry or paediatric developmental clinics are routinely assessing infants or toddlers who have a history of prenatal alcohol exposure and possibly one of the Fetal Alcohol Spectrum Disorders (FASD). In the more specialized FAS dysmorphology screening clinics these clinical issues are not infrequently over-looked because patients in this age group are deemed too young to show the required classical facial dysmorpholgy (Astley and Clarren 1997). Finally, infants and toddlers with Fetal Alcohol Spectrum Disorders (FASD) are rarely holistically assessed because they fail to demonstrate general developmental delay on standardized psychological and paediatric tests of mental and motor function.

Many professionals, from medicine to psychology, still regard FASDs as mental retardation conditions although the epidemiology and science has shown that 70- 75% of these patients are not mentally retarded (Streissguth et al 1996b, Streissguth et al 2004).

CLINICAL PROBLEMS IN INFANT AND TODDLER SYSTEMS OF CARE FOR FASD

1. The developmental and neuropsychiatric problems in infants , toddlers and young children from zero to 5 years of age with FASD have not been systematically studied.
2. There are almost no science-based intervention studies performed on the zero to 5-year-old population of infants, toddlers and young children with FASD.
3. Fetal Alcohol Spectrum Disorders need to be conceptualized as *transgenerational conditions* . Only when this transgenerational conceptual frame is incorporated will

general (paediatric and adult) medical health and mental health care systems begin to co-operate and stop treating the patient with a FASD in isolation (O'Malley and Streissguth 2003).

PREVIOUS ANIMAL AND HUMAN STUDIES

There are 3 main susceptible periods of embryological fetal growth that are effected by alcohol.

1. Pre-Differentiation Period. This is the interval between fertilization of the oocyte and its implantation in the endometrium. It is during this period that the ovum undergoes a series of mitiotic divisions changing from an unicellular zygote to a multi-cellular blastocyst. Previous animal studies of alcohol exposure in this period have shown conflicting results (Stratton et al 1996).

2. Period of the Embryo: This is the time of early germ cell layer differentiation and the completion of major organ formation (i.e. organogenesis). The classical FAS cranio-facial dysmorphological features are created in this period, and the prenatal effects on other organ systems such as the heart, kidney, eye, skeletal system and brain are occurring, these teratogenic effects of the prenatal alcohol are collectively called Alcohol Related Birth Defects (ARBD). They include atrial septal defects, ventricular septal defects, aplastic or hypoplastic kidneys, strabismus and clinodactyly (Clarren and Smith 1978, Driscoll et al 1991, Harris 1995)

3. Period of the Fetus. This is the time from the end of organogenesis until parturition (approximately 9 to 40 weeks of the human pregnancy). This is where prenatal alcohol produces histological changes in tissues, inhibits growth and produces more subtle changes to the central nervous system. (Majewski 1993, Harris 1995, Steinhausen 1996, Hagerman 1999). For example, dendritic changes, later correlated with decreased learning ability, were demonstrated in animals prenatally exposed to alcohol (Abel et al 1983). CNS development can be affected by alcohol throughout the intra-uterine period. Alcohol interferes with neurogenesis, neuronal differentiation and migration, arborization and synaptogenesis, functional synaptic organization, myelination, gliogenesis, glial migration and glial differentiation and neurotransmitter development (Hagerrman 1999, Streissguth and O'Malley 2000)

Animal studies going back at least 20- 25 years have shown the neurocognitive and neurodevelopmental effects of prenatal alcohol on young animals without dysmorphic or growth features (Means 1989). One classic study of alcohol-exposed chicks demonstrated their working memory impairment in locating food after being taught where the food was placed.

Further animal studies have also shown the transgenerational challenges to FASD management as they have analysed the problems in pup retrieval and nest building in alcohol-exposed female rat mothers. This showed the organizational and memory problems in these rat mothers which obviously impaired their basic nurturing skills.(Hard et al 1985, Baron et al 1985).

IDENTIFICATION OF INFANTS AT RISK FOR FASD

1. Biomarkers for FASD

Research has revealed promising haematological markers for detecting alcohol consumption and abuse in adults including pregnant mothers. They include gamma glutamyl transferase (GGT), aspartate aminotransferase (AST), alanine aminotransferase (ALT), alkaline phosphatase (AP), mean corpuscular volume (MCV) acetaldehyde adducts, and carbohydrate-deficient transferrin (CDT) (Stratton et al., 1996). Haemoglobin acetaldehyde adduct (HbAA) levels were studied in 19 alcohol abusing pregnant women and the levels were elevated in 68% of the women with alcohol- affected infants (8 infants diagnosed as having fetal alcohol effects), whereas only 28% of the alcohol abusing pregnant women had elevated HbAA levels when they had non-affected infants (Niemala, 1991).

Blood and Meconium analysis. More recent work has focused on Fatty Acid Ethyl Esters (FAEE), which have been detected in many animal tissues, including fetuses and placentas following maternal ethanol consumption (Bearer et al. 1992a, b). The FAEE has also been detected in both cord blood and meconium in humans (Bearer et al. 1996).

Other research on biomarkers has explored the usage of ultrasound studies of the brain of developing fetuses , prenatally, with particular attention to the developing frontal cortex.(Wass et al. 2001). This ultrasound technique is being extended, postnatally, to analyse the development of the corpus callosum which has already shown to be effected by prenatal alcohol exposure (Bookstein et al 2001).It may be that a neonatal ultrasound could become a standard screening practice to assess for corpus callosum damage in infants prenatally exposed to alcohol, especially if of a binge drinking variety.

Furthermore, McLeod and colleagues in 1983 found that drinking alcohol for 15 minutes abolished fetal breathing movements. As well research from Queens University in Belfast has analysed the effect of prenatal alcohol on fetal movement and post natal startle response. (Hepper et al 2006).

Thus, this technique may be utilized as a biomarker in obstetric practice, as an indirect way of assessing alcohol use in the current pregnancy.(O'Malley and Streissguth 2003, O'Malley and Streissguth 2005)

2. Clinical Presentation of Infants and Toddlers with FASD

Physical, developmental, social- emotional and behavioral disorders in infants and toddlers with FASD has not been scientifically determined. However, a number of empirical studies have documented offspring effects during the first 5 years of life that relate to prenatal alcohol exposure.

(i) Physical effects. Certain studies have analyzed the physical growth; infant size, dysmorphology and Alcohol Related Birth Defects (ARBD). The physical problems include; low apgar scores, failure to thrive, cardiac and renal problems, eye problems, otitis media and skeletal problems (Streissguth et al. 1982, Barr et al. 1984; Day, 1992; Jacobson & Jacobson 1994a; Harris 1995, Stratton et al. 1996).

(ii) Developmental and cognitive effects. CNS neurodevelopmental abnormalities has been documented, with decreased cranial size at birth, structural brain abnormalities (e.g., microcephaly, partial or complete agenesis of the corpus callosum, cerebellar hypoplasia) Also neurological hard or soft signs, such as, E.E.G abnormalities, impaired fine motor skills with hypotonia, poor tandem gait, poor eye-hand coordination , neurosensory hearing loss, (Aronson et al 1985; Majewski 1993; Streissguth 1997a, Hagerman 1999).

Electroencephalogram (EEG) abnormalities have been demonstrated in infants prenatally exposed to alcohol. These abnormalities were shown to persist for at least 6 weeks. They included more EEG activity during REM sleep and quiet sleep which has been shown to correlate with poor motor and mental development at 10 months (Ioffe and Chernick 1990). Animal studies in rats have demonstrated that prenatal exposure to alcohol during rat brain development can permanently alter the physiology of hippocampal formation.This physiological change can enhance kindling and facilitate spreading depression thereby promoting epileptic activity (Bonthius et al 2001)

There is a wide variation in IQ scores in children affected by prenatal alcohol exposure (Nanson and Hiscock 1990; Streissguth 1986).

(iii) Social, emotional and behavioral effects. It has been postulated that some of the behavioral patterns seen in infants with FASD can be associated with withdrawal from alcohol as a CNS depressant. Thus these infants may show excessive arousal, disturbed sleep patterns, gastrointestinal symptoms and hyperactive reflexes if exposed to high amounts of alcohol in the pregnancy, especially just prior to delivery (Coles and Platzman 1993). The excessive arousal and disturbed sleep patterns may persist over the first month of life or longer (Coles and Platzman 1993; Rosett et al. 1979; Stratton et al., 1996). However, clinical observations by a number of varied clinicians and researchers have described continuing problems with sleep disturbance, and sucking and eating from infancy to early childhood. Moreover, the sleep problems in FASD patients clearly persist through childhood to adulthood, which belies the simple alcohol withdrawal hypothesis as the sole aetiology (Steinhausen 1996, O'Malley and Hagerman 1998, O'Malley and Storoz 2003). The Seattle 500 longitudinal study showed that neonates prenatally exposed to alcohol showed some distinct clinical signs and symptoms. They included poor suck reflex, long latency to suck, poor habituation and poor state control.The problems with sucking had obvious negative effects on maternal bonding, especially if the birth mother was breast feeding. Habituation was more subtle and complicated, but this has been long recognized as a basic CNS function of an infant which protects it from being overwhelmed by new stimuli in it's envirionment. Infants with prenatal alcohol exposure are often unable to filter out these new and changing environmental stimuli and become quite aggitated and anxious.(Streissguth et al 1983).

The Seattle Prospective Longitudinal Study of Alcohol and Pregnancy found a number of outcomes in the infant and toddler age groups. All groups that were tested for prenatal alcohol exposure even after co-variate effects were taken into account. In neonates on day 1 and 2 these included poor state regulation, poor habituation, weak suck reflex and long latency to suck. At 4 years of age this same study described hyperactivity, poor attention and impulsivity (Streissguth et al.1993,1994, 1996a). Other studies have described early onset hyperactivity (Aronson et al. 1985; Carmichael Olson et al 1992; Driscoll et al.1990; Olegård et al.1979; Shaywitz et al.1979; Steinhausen 1996). As well,other researchers have examined the threshold of prenatal alcohol exposure and neurobehavioral development (Jacobson & Jacobson 1994b).

The neurobehavioral presentation of a toddler or young child with FASD can be compounded by the added effect of psychosocial environmental stressors such as physical abuse or neglect, sexual abuse and multiple foster home placements. These can create an overlapping Post Traumatic Stress Disorder (PTSD) and /or Reactive Attachment Disorder of Childhood, which can obscure the neurobehavioral presentation of the CNS dysfunction due to the prenatal alcohol exposure (O'Connor et al. 2000; Wolff 1987, O'Malley 2004).

THE UTILISATION OF EARLY INTERVENTION IN FASD INFANT AND TODDLER SYSTEM OF CARE

The studies in infants and toddlers with FASD include a number of techniques for the infants, for the parents and for the infant / parent dyad. Two key times of Intervention will be discussed.

a. Pre-conception Period. This intervention time acknowledges the **intergenerational aspect** to the FASD condition by using interventions to discourage alcohol consumption in the current generation of pregnant women and decreasing the occurrence of FASD in the coming generation. The Centers for Disease Control (CDC) reported that, although drinking by women of child-bearing age decreased in the 1980's, it has unfortunately steadily increased in the 1990's (CDC 1997) This was especially true for binger drinking i.e. 5 or more drinks per occasion. Furethermorew, a recent study of 44 adult women with FASD's showed that 49% were drinking during a pregnancy (Streissguth et al 2001)

This time of intervention should also include greater recognition of the co-morbid psychiatric disorders, such as bipolar disorder, depressive disorder or post traumatic stress disorder, in pregnant women who drink heavily (Astley et al, 2000; Zickler 2002, O'Malley 2003). Some of these women may also have a co-morbid developmental disorder, not uncommonly FASD itself. The developmental disability component of FASD in an adolescent or young adult female can affect her organizational skills, attention, distractiblity, imulsivity and judgement.: all essential skills for parenting an infant or toddler.

The Parent Child Assistance Program (PCAP) is an intervention for substance abusing mothers and their children aged zero to 3 years. It involves the addition of a paraprofessional advocate for each mother whether or not the child remains with the mother. The goal is to prevent future alcohol-affected pregnancies. This intervention model uses the concept of intensive, relational and long-term advocacy. This program has had success decreasing the mother's alcohol and substance abuse, increasing her active birth control and increasing health visits for her infant. It has been replicated in 4 centres in Washington State and in Canada (Alberta and Manitoba) (Ernst et al.1999, Grant et al.1999; Streissguth and Kanter 1997b). This programme as well serves to protect the infants and toddlers from the child abuse and neglect that can often occur in the sometimes chaotic homes of alcoholic mothers.

b. Prenatal Period. This includes:

1. Management of the pregnant woman's addictive, psychiatric, or developmental (i.e. FASD). disorders.
2. Neuroprotective agents to protect the developing fetus.

3. Identification of infants at risk from maternal alcohol consumption during pregnancy.

1. There are a number of *clinical treatment programmes for pregnant alcohol-dependent women* (Humphrey 1991,Finkelstein 1993).These programmes are generally broad- based with multimodal interventions, incorporating medical and obstetric services, and are intended to address the complex problems of this specific patient population (Stratton et al 1996).The presence of FASD in a pregnant or new mother has obvious effects on her organizational skills and emotional reactivity , and this makes parenting a greater challenge. This has already been demonstrated previous animal studies. (Abel et al 1983, Baron et al 1983, Hard et al 1985), and in the 21 year follow-up of the Seattle Longitudinal Study of Alcohol in Pregnancy (Streissguth et al 2002).

2. *Neuroprotective agents,* such as folic acid, taken by the alcohol abusing woman have been shown to have a ameliorating influence on the developing fetus.(Bower et al 1993). Also, ASA and indomethicin, which inhibit the alcohol- induced high prostaglandin levels in uterine and embryonic tissue. These agents have been shown to reduce perinatal mortality and decrease the incidence of Alcohol Related Birth Defects (ARBD) (Randall et al.1991a, b; Stratton et al 1996).

As well, some nutrients including; thiamin, folate, pyridoxine, vitamin A, vitamin D, magnesium and zinc have been identified as decreased due to excessive consumption of alcohol in pregnancy (Randels and Streissguth 1992,Dreosti1993).Supplementation of these nutrients have been proposed as a probable neuroprotective agents. Already,zinc supplementation has been studied as a neuroprotective agent during an alcohol exposed pregnancy (Jameson, 1993).

Lastly, a long-chain fatty acid diet has been introduced in animal studies to offset the toxic effect of alcohol on phospholipid development in the brain (Wainwright et al.1990, Peet et al 1999).

3.The *identification of "at risk" infants* should be pursued using certain maternal alcohol use self report screening tools such as the T-ACE (tolerance, annoyed, cut down, eye opener) and TWEAK (tolerance, worried, eye opener, amnesia, cut down) (Russell 1994). There is a 10 question drinking history questionnaire which has also proven to be useful (Rosset et al 1983).Some recent research has suggested that the Binge Alcohol Rating Criteria (BARC) and The Frequency–Binge Aggregate Score (F–BAS) may offer better specificity in identifying maternal alcohol use and "at risk" infants than other instruments (Barr and Streissguth 2001).

Vignette: The age, ethnicity and/ or gender of this patient has been altered to protect their identity. A 3 year old native American boy, VB, who is in the custody of his maternal grandparents since he was 1 month of age. His birth mother, Tracy, is native American and had FAS herself with Borderline intellectual functioning. The birth mother drank alcohol daily in the last trimester of pregnancy, and was unable to cope with the daily duties of raising her infant.the maternal grandparents applied for interim guardianship of the infant boy and now have full parental custodial rights.

There were no problems in the pregnancy except thast the mother had a mild amaemia. This was her first pregnancy. Tracy was followed by an advocate for the early pregnancy period, but lost this support in late pregnancy due to moving to a different city with her

Native American boyfriend (Michael).This boyfriend , and the birth father of VB, has since left the mother.

VB was born at term. His birth weight was 7 lbs 4 ozs.His apgar scores were 6 and 8. He was irritable and hard to settle from birth.Although Tracy stopped drinking after his birth she was unable to breast feed him, had no health care accewsss, and lived in an apartment that did not allow children.the maternal grandparents applied for guardianship at the same time that the social services worker had been called in to apprehend the baby because of neglect.there had been no history of physical abuse.

Clinically, VB was delayed in motor milestones sitting, standing and walking. He still did not speak at 2 years but showed receptive language understanding of simple one or two stage commands. His weight and height were at the 25th to 50th percentile from 1 year to 3 years old and his head circumference was at the 50th percentile. He had no FAS dysmorphological features when examined at 1, 2 or 3 years of age. Since infancy and increasing in toddler age he had displayed features of a Regulatory Disorder, Type I, Hypersensitive, Fearful and Cautious. He is closely attached to both grandparents, especially the grandfather. A recent sensory-motor history showed that VB had many problems in tactile, auditory, oral and visual sensations.

He is closely attached to both grandparents, especially the grandfather . A recent sensory-motor history showed that VB had many problems in tactile, auditory, oral and visual sensations which included:

- disliking his hair being washed because water scares him
- overly sensitive to all sounds, in house or out of house
- avoids foods with certain textures such as rice, potato(only takes corn)
- easily distracted by visual stimuli

His grandparents have managed to obtain Head Start financing through a State grant and with the help of VB's Native tribe. He has been enrolled 3 days a week in Montessori school for over 6 months.theer he receives speech/language therapy and OT for sensory integration. Also his careproviders, the maternal grandparents, are able to avail of respite care one week-end a month.

VB is progressing slowly but steadily, and in the last 3 months his birth mother, Tracy (who is now in recovery) has been visiting him weekly.The grandparents are involved in monthly instrumental family therapy with a community child psychiatrist. He is taking no medication.

CONCLUSION

There are few sustained, co-ordinated interventions for infants and toddlers with FASD and their families, be they birth, foster or adoptive parents. However, the general recognition of social-emotional, behavioral and developmental disorders has been greatly enhanced in the last 10 years by the publication of the Zero to Three-classification system (Wittenberg 2001; Zero to Three 1994).Axis I Disorders such as Regulatory Disorder, Type I Hypersensitive, either Fearful and Cautious or Negative and Defiant ; Type II Under-reactive, either

Withdrawal and Difficult to Engage or Self-Absorbed; and Type III Motorically Disoganized, Impulsive, need to be quantified in infants and toddlers prenatally exposed to alcohol. As well as that the Axis II disorders of Zero to Three classification quantify the all important interaction (including attachment) between the infant/ toddler and the parent or care-provider.The general prevalence of social-emotional and behavioral problems has previously been studied in toddlers and preschool children (Lavigne et al 1995, Mathieson et al 2000, Briggs-Gowan et al 2001), and needs to be compared with the FASD population of infants and toddlers.

There needs to be a more coordinated "system of care" for these alcohol or substance abusing pregnant women. At the moment there is little recognition of the connection between psychiatric or developmental disorders and the pregnant women's addictive disorder (O'Malley 2003).The obstetric, psychiatric, addiction and adult developmental services are historically disconnected and so unable to intervene properly to prevent, or treat, the next infant with FASD. For example drug treatment programmes often refuse to accept pregnant women and addiction centres often exclude patients with a developmental disability (Chavkin et al 1990; O'Malley 2002).

Only when there is a marriage of infant, child and adult providers dealing with evelopmental disorders will there be a hope of preventing the occurrence of this pervasive Dual Diagnosis (i.e. developmental and neuropsychiatric disorder) condition in the next generation , or at least decreasing its clinical impact on the current generation of infants and toddlers. This must take into consideration the need for an early diagnosis of the FASD. Already research has shown that the odds of escaping adverse life outcomes, such as disrupted school experience, trouble with the law or confinement, are increased 2 to 4 fold by receiving the diagnosis of FAS or FAE (ARND) under 6 years of age and being raised in a good stable environment (Streissguth et al 2004).

Finally, to end on a positive note, the American Academy of Child and Adolescent Psychiatry (AACAP)Work Group on Community Systems of Care are putting the finishing touches to a new instrument ECSII (Early Childhood Service Intensity Instrument), which will be utilized in infants and children under five years. This instrument will be used to quantify the medical and psychiatric needs of the infant/toddler, the careproviding environment, and will as suggest an appropriate intensity of intervention for infants, toddlers and their families(AACAP 2000, 2004). This has obvious utility for the zero to 5 year population of patients with FASD and their respective families.

ACKNOWLEDGEMENTS

First Draft of this Paper was initially presented at " The Truth and Consequences of Fetal Alcohol Syndrome", 30th Anniversary Conference, October 27th and 28th 2003, Atlantic City Convention Center, Atlantic City, NJ.

Kieran D. O'Malley M.B, D.A.B.P.N. (P),
Consultant Adolescent Psychiatrist, South & East Belfast Trust, Belfast.
Previously, Department of Psychiatry & Behavioral Sciences and Henry M. Jackson School of International Studies,University of Washington, Fetal Alcohol and Drug Unit,Seattle, WA.
CORRESPONDENCE: Kieran D. O'Malley. E-mail: omalley.kieran@gmail.com

REFERENCES

AACAP (2000) *Best Principles For Early Childhood Systems Of Care*.(2000) Washington, DC.: American Academy of Child and Adolescent Psychiatry

AACAP (2004) *Early Childhood Service Intensity Instrumene for Infants, Toddlers and Preschool-aged Children (ECSII)*,Work Group on Community Systems of Care, Nancy Winters and Mark Chenven , co-chairs,Washington DC (in final preparation)

Abel, EL, Jacobson, S and Sherwin, BT (1983) In- utero alcohol exposure: functional and structural brain damage. *Neurobehavioral Toxicology and Teratology*, 5: 363-366

Aronson M, Kyllerman M, Sabel KG, Sandin B, Olegård R.(1985) Children of alcoholic mothers: Developmental, perceptual and behavioral characteristics as compared to normal controls. *Acta Paediatr.* ; 74(1): 27–35.

Astley, SJ, and Clarren, SK (1997) *Diagnostic guide for FAS and related conditions.* University of Washington, Seattle

Astley SJ, Bailey D, Talbot C, Clarren SK(2000). Fetal Alcohol Syndrome (FAS) primary prevention through FAS diagnosis: 11. A comprehensive profile of 80 birth mothers of children with FAS. *Alcohol Alcohol.*; 35(5): 509–519.

Baer JS, Sampson PD, Barr HM, Connor PD, Streissguth AP(2003) A 21- Year longitudinal analysis of the effects of prenatal alcohol exposure on young adult drinking, *Arch Gen Psychiatry*, 60: 377-385.

Baron S and Riley EP (1985) Pup-induced maternal behavior in adult and juvenile rats exposed to alcohol prenatally. *Alc Clin and Exp Res*, 9: 360-365

Barr HM. Streissguth AP, Martin DC, Herman CS.(1984) Infant size at 8 months of age: Relationship to maternal use of alcohol, nicotine, and caffeine during pregnancy. *Pediatrics.* ; 74(3): 336–341.

Barr HM, Streissguth AP(2001). Identifying maternal self-reported alcohol use associated with fetal alcohol spectrum disorders. *Alcohol Clin Exp Res.* ; 25(2): 283–287.

Bearer CF, Gould S, Emerson R, Kinnunen P, Cook CS.(1992a) Fetal alcohol syndrome and fatty acid ethyl esters. *Pediatr Res.*; 31: 492–495.

Bearer C.F, Emerson R, Harm L(1992b). Fatty acid ethyl esters in peripheral blood. Pediatr Res. *31: 68A.*

Bearer C.F. Swick A, Singer L(1996). FAEE: Biomarker for prenatal alcohol use. *Alcohol Clin Exp Res.*; 20: 139A.

Bonthius, DJ, Woodhouse, J, Bonthius, NE, Taggard DA & Lothman EW (2001) Reduced seizure threshold and hippocampal cell loss in rats exposed to alcohol during the brain growth spurt. Alcoh Clin Exp Res, Vol 25, No. 1, 70-82

Bookstein FL, Sampson PD, Streissguth AP, Connor PD (2001) Geometric morphometrics of corpus callosum and subcortical structures in fetal alcohol affected brain. *Teratology,* 4, 4-32

Bower C. Stanley FJ, Nicol DJ. Maternal folate status and the risk for neural tube defects. The role of dietary folate. In: Keen CL, Bendich A, Willhite CC, eds. Maternal nutrition and pregnancy outcome. *Ann NY Acac Sci.* 1993; 678: 146–155.

Briggs-Gowan MJ, Carter AS, Moye Skuban E, McCue Horowitz S.(2001) Prevalence of social-emotional and behavioral problems in a community sample of 1- and 2- year old children. *J Am Acad Child Adolesc Psychiatry* ; 40(7): 811–819.

Carmichael Olson H, Burgess DM, Streissguth AP(1992). Fetal alcohol syndrome (FAS) and fetal alcohol effects (FAE): A lifespan view, with implications for early intervention.*Zero to Three*.; 13(1): 24–29.

Centers for Disease Control and Prevention (CDC) (1997) Alcohol consumption among pregnant and childbearing- aged women United States, 1991-1996, *MMWR*, 46:349-350

Chavkin W, Kendall SR.(1990) Between a 'rock' and a hard place. *Pediatrics* ; 85: 223–225.

Clarren SK, Smith DW(1978). The fetal alcohol syndrome. *N Engl J Med.*; 298: 1063–1067.

Coles, CD, Smith IE,Fernhoff, PM, Falek, A (1984) Neonatal ethanol withdrawal: Characteristics in clinically normal, nondysmorphic neonates. *Journal of Pediatrics,* 105 (3): 445-451

Coles CD, Platzman KA.(1993) Behavioral development in children prenatally exposed to drugs and alcohol. *Int J Addict.,* 28: 1393–1433.

Day NL.(1992) Effects of Prenatal Alcohol Exposure. In: Zagon IS, Slotkin TA, eds. *Maternal Substance Use and The Developing Nervous System*. San Diego: Academic Press, 27–43.

Driscoll CD, Streissguth AP, Riley EP(1991). Prenatal alcohol exposure: Comparability of effects in humans and animal models. *Neurotoxical Teratol.*; 12: 231–237.

Dreosti IE.(1993) Nutritional factors underlying the expression of the fetal alcohol syndrome. In: Keen CL, Bendich A, Willhite CC, eds. Maternal nutrition and pregnancy outcome. *Ann NY Acac Sci* ; 678: 193–204.

Ernst CC, Grant TM, Streissguth AP, Sampson PD (1999). Intervention with high risk alcohol and drug abusing mothers: II Three year findings from the Seattle Model of Paraprofessional Advocacy. *J Community Psychol* ; 27(1): 19–38.

Finkelstein N.(1993) Treatment programming for alcohol and drug-dependent pregnant women. *Int J Addict.*; 28: 1275–1309.

Grant TM, Ernst CC, Streissguth AP(1999). Intervention with high- risk alcohol and drug abusing mothers: 1. Administrative strategies of the Seattle Model of Paraprofessional Advocacy. *J Community Psychol.*; 27(1): 1–18.

Hagerman RJ (1999*) Neurodevelopmental Disorders.Diagnosis and Treatment.*Oxford University Press, 3-47, New York, Oxford

Hard E, Musi B, Dahlgren IL, Engel J, Larsson K, Liljequist S, Lindh AS (1985) Impaired maternal behavior and altered central serotonergic activity in the adult offspring of chronically treated dams. *Acta Pharmacol et Toxicol*, 56, 347-353et al (1985)

Harris JC (1995)*Developmental Neuropsychiatry ,Volume II, Assessment, Diagnosis, and Treatment of Developmental Disorders*, 361-365, Oxford University Press, New York, Oxford

Hepper, PG, Dorman, JL, Little, JF (2005) Maternal alcohol consumptiom during pregnancy may delay the development of spontaneous fetal startle behaviour. Physiology & Behavior, 83, 711-714

Humphrey K, Marvis B, Stofflemavr B(1991)). Factors predicting attendance at self-help after substance abuse treatment. Preliminary findings. *J Consult Clin Psychol,* 59: 591–593.

Ioffe S, Chernick V.(1990) Prediction of subsequent motor and mental reatardation in newborn infants exposed to alcohol in uterro by computerized EEG analysis. *Neuropediatrics,* 21 (1) 11-17.

Jacobson JL, Jacobson SW(1994a). Prenatal exposure and neurobehavioral development; Where is the threshold? *Alcohol Health Res World.*; 18: 30–36.

Jacobson,SW, Jacobson, JL, Sokol, RJ (1994b) Effects of fetal alcohol exposure on infant reaction time. *Alcoholism: Clinical and Experimental Research*, 18 (5): 1125-1132

Jameson S.(1993) Zinc status in pregnancy: The effect of zinc therapy on perinatal mortality, prematurity, and placental ablation. In: Keen CL, Bendich A, Willhite CC, eds. Maternal nutrition and pregnancy outcome. *Ann NY Acac Sci* ; 678: 178–192.

Jones KL, Smith DW.(1973) Recognition of fetal alcohol syndrome in early infancy. *Lancet.* 2(836):999–1101.

Lavigne JV, Gibbons RD, Christoffel KK(1995). Prevalence rates and correlates of psychiatric disorders among preschool children. *J Am Acad Child Adolesc Psychiatry* ; 35: 204–214.

Majewski F.(1993) Alcohol embryopathy: Experience with 200 patients. *Dev Brain Dysfunct*; 6: 248–265.

Mathieson KS, Sanson A.(2000) Dimensions of early childhood behavior problems: stability and predictors of change from 18 to 30 months. *J Abnorm Psychol* ;28: 15–31.

McLeod N, Brien J, Loomis C, Carmichael L, Probert C, Patrick J (1983). Effect of maternal ethanol ingestion on fetal breathing movements, gross body movements, and heart rate at 37 to 40 weeks gestational age. *Am J Obstet Gynecol.*; 145: 251–257.

Means LW, Mc Daniel K, Pennington SN (1989)Embryonic ethanol exposure impairs detour learning in chicks. *Alcohol,* 6: 327-330

Nanson J, Hiscock M.(1990) Attention deficits in children exposed to alcohol prenatally. *Alcohol Clin Exp Res.*; 14: 656–661.

Niemela O, Halmemake E, Jlirorkala O.(1991) Hemoglobin–acetaldehyde adducts are elevated in women carrying alcohol-damaged fetuses. *Alcohol Clin Exp Res* ; 15: 1007–1010.

Olegård R, Abel KG, Aronsson M, Sandin B, Johansson PR, Carlson C, Kyllerman M, Iversen K, Hrbek A(1979). Effects on the child of alcohol abuse during pregnancy. *Acta Paediatr Scand.*; 275(suppl): 112–121.

O'Connor MJ, Kasari C(2000). Prenatal alcohol exposure and depressive features in children. *Alcohol Clin Exp Res.*; 24(7): 1084–1092.

O'Malley KD, Hagerman RJ (1998) Developing clinical practice guidelines for pharmacological interventions with alcohol-affected children. *Proceedings of a Special Focus Session of the Interagency Coordinating Committee on Fetal Alcohol Syndrome.*Chevy Chase, MD, September 10-11,National Institute of Alcohol Abuse and Alcoholism (NIAAA),145–177.

O'Malley KD(2002). Examining Canada's community support to young adults with FASD. *Iceberg.*;12(3): 6–7.

O'Malley KD (2003) Youth with Comorbid Disorders,Chapter 13, In *The Handbook of Child and Adolescent Systems of Care. The New Community Psychiatry.*Eds. Andres J Pumariega and Nancy C. Winters, 276- 315

O'Malley KD and Storoz L (2003) Fetal Alcohol Spectrum Disorder and ADHD: diagnostic implications and therapeutic consequences. *Expert Rev Neurotherapeutics* 3 (4), 477- 489

O'Malley KD and Streissguth AP (2003) Clinical Intervention and support for children aged zero to five years with fetal alcohol spectrum disorder and their parents/caregivers. In :

Encyclopaedia on Early Childhood Development. Center of Excellence for Early Childhood Development Website, *www.excellence-earlychildhood.ca*

O'Malley KD & Streissguth AP (2006) Clinical Intervention and support for children aged zero to five years with fetal alcohol spectrum disorders and their parents/caregivers. An Update.In Encyclopaedia on Early Childhood Development. Center of Excellence for Early Childhood Ddevelopment Website, www.excellence-earlychildhood.ca

Peet M, Gilen I and Horrobin DF (1999) *Phospholipid Spectrum Disorder in Psychiatry* , Marius Press, Lanchashire, UK

Randal CL. Anton RF, Becker HC, Hale RL, Ekblad U. Aspirin dose-dependency reduces alcohol induced birth defects and prostaglandin E levels in mice. *Teratology.* 1991a; 44: 521–529.

Randall CL. Becker HC, Anton RF (1991b). Effect of ibuprofen on alcohol- induced teratogenesis in mice. *Alcohol Clin Exp Res.*; 15: 673–677.

Randels SP, Streissguth AP(1992) Fetal alcohol syndrome and nutrition issues. *Nutrition Focus.* 7(3): 1–6.

Robe, LB , Gromish, DS, Iosub, S(1981) Symptoms of neonatal ethanol withdrawal. *Currents in Alcoholism* , 8: 485-493

Rosett HL, Synder P, Sander S, Lee A, Cook P, Weiner L, Gould J(1979). Effects of maternal drinking on neonatal state regulation. *Dev Med Child Neurol.*; 21(4): 464–473.

Rosett HL, Weiner L, Edelin KC(1983). Treatment experience with pregnant problem drinkers. *JAMA* ; 248: 2092–3033.

Russell M.(1994) New Assessment Tools for Risk Drinking During Pregnancy, T-ACE, TWEAK and Others. *Alcohol Health Res World*; 18(1)

Rutter M, Silberg J, O'Connor T, Simonoff E. Genetics and Child Psychiatry (1999): 1. Advances in quantitative and molecular genetics. *J Child Psychol Psychiatry*; 40: 3–18.

Shaywitz BA, Griffith GG, Warshaw JB.(1979) Hyperactivity and cognitive deficits in developing rat pups born to alcoholic mothers. An experimental model of the expanded fetal alcohol syndrome (EFAS). *Neurobehavioral Toxicol.* 1: 113–122.

Steinhausen HC(1996) Psychopathology and cognitive function in children with fetal alcohol syndrome. In: Spohr HL, Steinhausen HC, eds. *Alcohol, pregnancy and the developing child.* New York:Cambridge University Press, 227–249.

Stratton KR,Howe CJ,Battaglia FC (1996) *Fetal Alcohol Syndrome: Diagnosis, Epidemiology, Prevention and Treatment,* Institute of Medicine, National Academy Press,Washington DC

Streissguth AP. Barr HM, Martin DC (1982). Offspring effects and pregnancy complications related to self- reported maternal alcohol use. *Dev Pharmacol Ther.*5, 21–32.

Streissguth, AP, (1983) A lcohol and pregnancy: An overview and an update. Substance ansd Alcohol Actions?Misuse, 4 (2-3): 149-173

Streissguth AP, (1986) The behavioral teratology of alcohol: Performance, behavioral and intellectual deficits in prenatally exposed children. In: West J, ed. *Alcohol and brain development.* New York: Oxford University Press

Streissguth , AP, Bookstein, FL, Sampson, PD, & Barr, HM (1993) *The enduring effects of prenatal alcohol exposure : Birth through 7 years: A partial least squares solution.* Ann Arbor, University of Michigan Press

Streissguth AP, Barr HM, Sampson PD, Bookstein FL (1994). Prenatal alcohol and offspring development: The first fourteen years. *Drug Alcohol Depend.* 36: 89–99.

Streissguth AP, Bookstein FL, Barr HM.(1996a) A dose-response study of the enduring effects of prenatal alcohol exposure; Birth to 14 years. In: Spohr HL, Steinhausen HC eds. *Alcohol, pregnancy and the developing child.* New York: Cambridge University Press, 141–168.

Streissguth AP, Barr HM, Kogan J, Bookstein FL(1996b). *Understanding the occurrence of secondary disabilities in clients with fetal alcohol syndrome (FAS) and fetal alcohol effects (FAE). Final report to Centers for Disease Control and Prevention.* Seattle, WA: University of Washington, Fetal Alcohol and Drug Unit, Tech. Rpt. No. 96-0.

Streissguth AP.(1997a) *Fetal alcohol syndrome. a guide for families and communities.* Baltimore, London, Toronto, Sydney: Paul H. Brookes Publishing.

Streissguth AP, Kanter J.(1997b) *The challenge of fetal alcohol syndrome; overcoming secondary disabilities.* Seattle, WA: University of Washington Press.

Streissguth AP, O'Malley KD.(2000) Neuropsychiatric Implications and Long term Consequences of Fetal Alcohol Spectrum Disorders. *Semiars in Clin Neuropsychiatry,* 5(3) 177–190.

Streissguth ,AP, Porter, JK and barr, HM (2001)A study of patients with fetal alcohol spectrum disorders (FASD) who became parents. *Alcoholism: Clinical and Experimental Research,* 25 (Supplement), 123

Streissguth AP, Sampson PD, Bookstein FL, Connor PD, Barr HM (2002) 21- year dose response effects of prenatal alcohol exposure on cognition. *Alcoholism: Clinical and Exp Research,* Supplement,Vol. 26, No. 5, 93A

Streissguth, AP,Bookstein, FL,Barr, HM, Sampson, PD, O'Malley, KD, Kogan Young, J (2004) Risk factors for adverse life outcomes in fetal alcohol syndrome and fetal alcohol effects. *Developmental and Behavioral Pediatrics,* vol. 25, No. 4, august, 228-238

U.S. Surgeon General. *Mental Health: A Report of the Surgeon General.*(1999) Department of Human and Health Services, Substance Abuse and Mental Health Services Administration, Center for Mental Health Services, National Institutes of Health, National Institute of Mental Health.

Waas TS, Persutte WH, Hobbins JC(2001) The impact of prenatal alcohol exposure on frontal cortex development in utero. *Am J Obstet Gynecol* ; 185: 737–742

Wainwright PE, Hsuang YS, Simmons V, Wared RP, Ward GR, Winfield D.(1990) Effects of prenatal ethanol and long chain n-e fatty acid supplementation on development in mice. 2. Fatty acid composition of brain membrane phospholipids. *Alcohol Clin Exp Res.* 14: 413–420.

Wittenberg JV(2001). Regulatory Disorders: a new diagnostic classification for difficult infants and toddlers. *Can J Diagn.*; (September): 111–123.

Wolff P.(1987) *The development of behavioral states and the expression of emotion in early infancy; New proposals for investigation.* Chicago; University of Chicago Press.

ZERO TO THREE classification(1994). *Diagnostic Classification of Mental Health and Developmental Disorders of Infancy and Early Childhood.* National Center for Infants, Toddlers and Families. Washington, DC.

Zickler P(2002). Childhood Sex Abuse Increases Risk for Drug Dependence in Adult Women. *NIDA Notes.*; 17(1): 5 and10.

In: ADHD and Fetal Alcohol Spectrum Disorders (FASD)   ISBN: 1-59454-573-1
Editor: Kieran D. O'Malley, pp. 39-49   © 2008 Nova Science Publishers, Inc.

Chapter 3

SENSORY INTEGRATION AND SENSORY PROCESSING DISORDERS[*]

Tracy Jirikowic

Poor sensory processing is associated with a wide range of behavioral and developmental difficulties, many of which also have been reported in children with FASD. Occupational therapists may use a sensory integration framework to observe, understand, and develop interventions for challenging behaviors and decreased functional abilities that stem from neurological impairments related to sensory processing disorders. This chapter provides an overview of sensory integration as a model for understanding behavioral responses to sensation and related developmental problems and as a framework to guide parents and professionals seeking support for children with FASD.

Sensory processing is a general term that refers to the brain's ability to process, organize and use information from the sensory systems involving vision, hearing, smell, taste, and touch, vestibular (movement) and proprioception (muscle and body position in space) (Ayers, 1979). Efficient sensory proceesing is assumed to underlie the ability to manage many "automatic" behavioral responses to stimuli and changes in the environment. With efficient sensory processing the brain automatically modulates or balances incoming sensory information as it filters out irrelevant stimuli and helps us organize and respond adaptively to important stimuli. This facilitates our attention to new, interesting, and possibly dangerous stimuli; allows us to discriminate important details about what we see, feel, hear, etc.; or helps us get used to or ignore certain types of sensations.

Sensory integration is considered an important developmental foundation for higher-level social, cognitive, and motor learning (Ayres, 1979). When the ability to process and modulate sensory input is efficient and accurate, individuals can respond adaptively to the multitude of sensory information from the environment and function more optimally in their surroundings. They are more readily able to adapt to changes in the environment and self-regulate behavior to meet their needs. In contrast, when sensory processing is poor, individuals cannot respond

---

[*] Tracy Jirikowic, PhD, Occupational Therapist, University of Washington Fetal Alcohol Syndrome Diagnostic and Prevention Network, Seattle, WA 98195

in accordance to the task or environmental demands due to disorganized or inaccurate information, which may result in stressful, disorganized or maladaptive behavior (Dunn, 1997).

How do sensory processing and sensory integration relate to children with FASD? Prenatal alcohol exposure clearly has wide-ranging and persistent effects on the developing brain and nervous system. A large body of literature from both human and animal studies describes numerous neurobehavioral deficits that can result from prenatal alcohol exposure (see Harris et al, 1993 and Mattson and Riley, 1998 for review). Sensory-motor deficits such as decreased coordination and balance, motor immaturities and motor delays are among those included within the broad and variable spectrum of neurobehavioral problems reported in this population. Further, numerous adaptive deficits and maladaptive behavioral problems, many of which are theoretically linked to sensory integration dysfunction are reported to occur in children affected by prenatal alcohol exposure. Finally, clinical and anecdotal reports of abnormal responses to sensory information, along with preliminary studies specifically investigating sensory processing behaviors, indeed suggest children with FASD experience impairments in this neurobehavioral domain. Such evidence, points towards the importance of understanding and examining sensory-motor and related functional problems from a sensory integration perspective.

Further, sensory-motor experiences play a critical role in early development. When early development is disrupted by factors such as exposure to stressful environments (e.g., too much or aversive sensory stimulation), or environments that lack sensory stimulation there are clearly negative and persistent developmental consequences on both brain and behavior (Cermak, 2001). Since many children with FASD also experience other prenatal and postnatal risk factors early in life, it is important to acknowledge that such risk factors may further disrupt the ongoing and dynamic development of early sensory integrative functions. Thus, while the mechanism and magnitude of sensory processing problems in children with FASD are not fully understood at this time, the wide-ranging and often diffuse effects of prenatal alcohol exposure on the central nervous system coupled with early environmental and biological risk factors suggest that this area of development should not be overlooked.

Poor sensory processing and integration may contribute to many challenging behaviors that are common among those diagnosed with FASD. Although it is important to acknowledge that sensory processing differences may be only one of several underlying causes of such observable behaviors, it is the unique notion that an individual's sensory "threshold" (e.g., tendency to be hyper or hyposensivity to "normal" amounts of sensation) drives a continuum of behavioral responses that sets this framework apart from other interpretations of behavior. Some common behavioral symptoms of sensory processing problems include:

- inattention/distractibility
- hyperactivity
- emotional dysregulation or lability
- clumsiness
- behavioral and motoric disorganization

Deficits in sensory processing are not unique to individuals with FASD. They have also been described in children with attention deficit disorders (Mangeot et al, 2001 Mulligan,

1996), as well as learning disabilities (Parham, 1997), developmental disabilities and autism (Miller, et al., 1999), and motor incoordination disorders (Dahl Reeves and Cermak, 2001). While some children with FASD have additional diagnoses such as ADHD or learning disabilities, symptoms of sensory integration dysfunction can present with or without these additional diagnoses. In children with FASD it is especially important to consider the multiple etiologies of challenging behaviors. There may be language, cognitive or other environmental factors that are collectively impacting the individual's behavior and ability to function.

The theory of sensory integration (SI) is based on information from child development, neurobiology, psychology, and education (Ayers, 1979). Sensory integration (SI) as a theory and framework for understanding behavior and CNS dysfunction continues to evolve and undergo refinement as the research-based evidence regarding sensory processing disorders continues to grow (Schaaf and Miller, 2005). The diagnoses and treatment of sensory processing problems is most commonly done by occupational therapists (OTs) with specialized training. It is one of several frameworks that OTs or other professionals (such as physical therapists or speech language pathologists), may use to help children with neurological dysfunction improve their ability to function in daily life. Sensory integration has been considered a particularly useful framework for understanding and reframing children's learning and behavioral difficulties because it considers a neurological basis for difficult behaviors.

As historically described by Ayers, sensory integrative dysfunction, more recently labeled as sensory processing disorders, refers to a heterogeneous group of symptoms that reflect subtle, primarily subcortical, neural dysfunction involving multisensory systems (Miller and Lane, 2000; Parham and Mailloux, 2005). The theory of sensory integration and associated dysfunction has its roots in nonspecific forms of brain deficiency (Ayres, 1979; Parham and Mailloux, 2005). No specific neural mechanism has been identified as the cause of sensory integrative dysfunction or sensory processing disorders. The theory assumes normal sensory reception at the peripheral level, with the breakdown of function occurring centrally, where the information must be interpreted, integrated, and organized for efficient use in learning and functional behavior.

Children with sensory processing problems have difficulty clearly perceiving and/or organizing information from their senses. They process sensation from their bodies or environment in an inaccurate or disorganized way. This results in a diminished ability to respond and interact effectively and efficiently with their surroundings and meet the day-to-day expectations of others. They may demonstrate poor sensory modulation (e.g. hypo (under) or hyper (over) sensitivity to stimuli or a combination of these responses), poor sensory discrimination, or postural and motor problems. Difficulties managing and interpreting sensory information can be expressed through behavior in several ways. Poor sensory processing have been associated with maladaptive behaviors such as emotional reactivity and aggression, disorganized, withdrawn, and avoidant behaviors (Hanft, Miller, and Lane, 2000; Wilbarger and Wilbarger, 1991).

Although each child's responses to different types and even the same kind of sensation can vary, children with sensory processing disorders, including children with FASD may show the following tendencies:

1. POOR SENSORY MODULATION

A. Sensory Seeking

Children who are **sensory seeking** have nervous systems that do not always clearly process that sensory input is coming to the brain. They are considered under-responsive to sensation. As a result, they demonstrate slow or diminished responses to sensation, and/or seek out sensory experiences that are more intense or of longer duration. They may appear both withdrawn and avoidant, or overactive and disorganized Dunn (1999). It takes a higher intensity or increased duration of the input to elicit a response (Dunn 1999). Children with under responsive tendencies may seek intense sensory experiences (e.g., high intensity movement activities, touch or mouth objects constantly), or demonstrate flattened responses to sensation (e.g. show less awareness of details, appear clumsy and bump into objects or other children) (Hanft et al., 2000).

A child who is under responsive to touch or proprioception may appear less responsive to pain or appear clumsy and bump into things frequently. In order to get a more clear signal regarding where they bodies are in space or to maintain a certain level of alertness children who are hypo-responsive may fidget and move excessively and appear hyperactive. They may appear impulsive as they crave intense stimulation, touching objects and people more often and harder than most children, and engage in unsafe behaviors such as jumping from places that are too high or "crashing" their bodies into objects or furniture.

B. Sensory Avoiding

Children who are **sensory avoiding** have nervous systems that feel sensation more intensely than others. They are overly responsive to sensation. As a result they feel some sensations too easily or interpret them as painful or irritating which can be stressful and trigger a "flight or fight" response. This is also known as sensory defensiveness (Wilbarger and Wilbarger, 1991). They may appear aggressive in response to sensation that is overwhelming to their nervous systems, or they may withdraw or avoid certain sensations they perceive as uncomfortable.

Children who are sensory avoiding often respond to unexpected touch with aggression or withdrawal (e.g., when getting bumped by another child while standing in line at school). They may feel uncomfortable or irritable in highly stimulating environments such as malls, school gyms or auditoriums. Additionally, they may seem very sensitive to touch and textures, appear to be "picky" eaters, wear only certain types of clothing or demonstrate "inflexible" preferences.

C. Fluctuating Responses

Children who demonstrate **fluctuating responses** to sensation may shift rapidly from being over sensitive to under sensitive to different types of sensory input throughout the day. Their nervous systems have a difficult time maintaining a balance between "not enough" and "too much" sensory input. They may demonstrate a combination of the behaviors listed above, but may particularly labile in their emotion, attention, and activity level.

2. POOR SENSORY DISCRIMINATION

Individuals with **poor sensory discrimination** have problems interpreting the temporal and spatial characteristics of sensory stimuli so that the ability to perceive qualities of sensory stimuli is impaired (Lane et al., 2000). Accurate discrimination of sensory input is essential for the development of skilled movements and function (Spitzer and Smith Roley, 2001). Various behavioral and performance difficulties have been described and associated with dysfunction in sensory discrimination (Hanft et al., 2000).

Individuals with poor tactile discrimination may have difficulty differentiating or manipulating objects without close visual monitoring and/or difficulty localizing touch on their body. An individual with poor auditory discrimination may have problems locating the source of sounds, or judging the distance and location of a sound. Poor visual discrimination may result in problems recognizing or categorizing colors, shapes, and textures; changing visual focus rapidly; scanning sequential images, or differentiating foreground from background images. Poor vestibular-proprioceptive discrimination may result in problems with dynamic balance, maintaining an upright posture, as well as gauging the correct amount of force to use when interacting with people or objects (such as when writing with a pencil or giving a hug).

3. SENSORY-BASED MOTOR DIOSRDERS

Children with **sensory-based motor disorders** also known as dyspraxia, or motor planning problems, may appear clumsy and awkward. They have particular difficulty with postural abilities and/or learning new motor skills. Children with dyspraxia do not efficiently process sensory information about their bodies and movement, relative to their physical environment, in a manner that contributes to efficient motor learning and skilled motor actions (Dahl Reeves and Cermak, 2002). Children with developmental dyspraxia may appear poorly coordinated, demonstrate difficulty learning and sequencing new movements, as well as appear disorganized or lack initiative within their environments. Children with dyspraxia may present with poor hand skills such as handwriting, or using a scissor, poor large motor skills (difficulty learning how to ride a bike, pump a swing) and difficulty "knowing" how to move or play with new toys.

As with other areas of development, it is important to understand that there are a wide range of "normal" behavioral responses within this continuum and that differences in sensory processing and integration represent one way to interpret some maladaptive behaviors or poor functional abilities (Hanft et al., 2000). Responses between and within individuals vary greatly, in most cases contributing to individual differences in areas such as arousal, adaptation to stress, motivational and adaptive behavior (Dahl-Reeves, 2001).

There is an emerging body of anecdotal and research evidence that children with FASD differ from typically developing children in their responses to sensory information, and sensory-motor function (Jirikowic, 2003; Morse and Cermak, 1994; Morse, Miller, and Cermak 1995). In individuals with FASD, symptoms of poor sensory processing manifest in different ways throughout the lifespan and may be observed in infancy and throughout childhood. Infants may have difficulty handling bright lights or multiple types of stimulation (being rocked, talked to and fed all at once). These infants may seem irritable and difficult to soothe unless just the right amount or combination or sensory information is provided. Some infants with touch sensitivity may have difficulty tolerating solid foods or food textures which can contribute to feeding difficulties.

Irritability, a weak suck, poor habituation, sleep problems, lower levels of arousal, and failure to thrive have also been reported in infants with FASD (Harris et al., 1993; Elyer and Behnke, 1999). These symptoms suggest that neonates with prenatal alcohol exposure may have poorly modulated responses to sensory stimuli (i.e., they are less responsive to stimuli or are more likely to "shut down" in response to over stimulation) and are possible early indicators of poor sensory processing and integration.

Toddlers and preschool children may demonstrate high activity levels and impulsivity with poor regard for safety because they crave high intensity movement or proprioceptive input (i.e., crashing, jumping) to meet the needs of an underesponsive nervous systems that needs extra or more intense stimulation. They may break toys easily, appear clumsy, destructive or aggressive towards other children because they do not get clear internal feedback about where their bodies are in space, how hard to touch or hug a person, or push or pull a toy. As a result of poor sensory modulation, they may get wound up very easily and have difficulty calming down.

School-aged children with FASD and sensory processing difficulties may have difficulty filtering auditory information and/or demonstrate hypersensitivities to loud sounds. As a result, they may appear uncooperative or fearful if they avoid or refuse to participate in school activities (such as assemblies or fire drills). They may also appear disorganized, distractible and even "out of control" as the intensity of the stimulation increases or becomes more prolonged. As the stimulation stresses their nervous systems they have difficulty calming down because they are overstimulated and can no longer effectively regulate their behavior.

Children who are sensitive to touch may be particular about certain types of clothing or foods they eat. They may be irritated by tags or seams of refuse to wear certain textures. They may also respond defensively and strike out aggressively (as we respond to a bug crawling on our skin, or startle when someone approaches us from behind) when accidentally pushed or touched by another child. Older children who crave movement may seem distractible, fidgety, and hyperactive in the classroom as they try to meet the needs of their nervous system to help maintain their attention and alertness.

Assessment of Sensory Processing

Sensory processing is typically assessed by using a combination of standardized tests, caregiver interviews, behavioral checklists, and formal and informal observations of the child's movement, play, and social interactions (Parham and Mailloux, 2005). Such tools and observations provide a range of data from which to hypothesize about the child's neurobiological processing of sensation and its impact on behavior and performance. From a

SI perspective, behavioral problems and performance difficulties are thus, reframed by analyzing motor performance and sensory processing behaviors (Ayres, 1979).

There are standardized tests that measure sensory functions in infants, preschoolers and school-aged children. Standardized tests provide a reliable and systematic method to assess development and behavior. The Sensory Integration and Praxis Test (SIPT) (Ayres, 1989) provide the most in-depth evaluation of sensory integrative functions primarily related to praxis (Bundy, 2002). The SIPT consists of subtests that evaluate somatosensory processing, praxis, visuo-motor function and motor free visual perception. Additionally, several standardized assessments of neuropsychological, motor, and sensory-motor development include items or subtests from which inferences about the child's sensory processing and related behaviors can be drawn (Bundy, 2002; Parham and Mailloux, 2005).

Formal and informal observations of a child's interaction with the physical and social environment are also key components of an evaluation of sensory processing. Formal clinical observations of neurological soft signs and postural functions (e.g., integration of reflexes, postural responses to movement, and muscle tone) have historically been used to supplement standardized assessments (Ayres, 1979; Bundy, 2002). Informal observations of a child's movement, play and social interaction skills across different environments can also provide important insights about how the child responds to and organizes sensation, and how this affects their behavior, adaptation and skill performance. Such observations provide important contexts for interpreting and applying standardized test results, but are widely variable based on the individual child and his or her physical and social environments.

Sensory-motor histories, checklists and interviews also have been used to document sensory processing behaviors (Dunn, 1999; Parham and Mailloux, 2005). Such tools typically involve caregiver ratings of a child's behavioral responses to various types of sensation across different environments. Information from these tools provide a systematic format for caregivers to report their observations and perceptions of the child's behaviors which can further contribute to an understanding of how poor sensory processing may be impacting children in their daily lives and routines (Dunn, 1997). The Sensory Profile (Dunn, 1999) is one example of a recently standardized sensory history checklist that has been useful in documenting sensory processing differences, primarily related to sensory modulation, in children with various disabilities (Dunn, 1997). A separate version for infants and toddlers as well as self-report version for adolescents and adults provide opportunities to examine sensory processing behaviors across the lifespan.

NB. ADD PART OF SENSORY PROFILE

Intervention Strategies

A variety of intervention strategies are available to help children with FASD with sensory processing problems. Occupational therapists are specially trained and skilled in the use of therapeutic activities that involve the careful application of somatosensory input (movement, tactile, and proprioceptive) to help children respond more adaptively to sensation and improve their capacity to function in their environment. Environmental accommodations which might include a "diet " of sensory activities to increase or reduce sensory stimuli to meet the child's needs at home or school may also be recommended. Additionally, simply learning about sensory integration is powerful strategy that can help caregivers, teachers, and other professionals working with children with FASD reframe difficult behaviors associated with poor sensory processing and integration.

Direct intervention involves the therapeutic use of somatosensory (tactile, movement , proprioceptive) input to facilitate and enhance adaptive responses and behavior. Therapists use these modalities and therapeutic activities to help individuals improve their adaptive responses to the environment to enhance functional skills and behavioral regulation. Therapeutic intervention involves careful consideration of the child's sensory thresholds, attention to behavioral cues and the anticipation of behavioral responses. By understanding how the child typically responds to sensory events and stimuli, therapists and caregivers can use sensory input and modify environments to prevent challenging behaviors and as a means for helping the child regulate his/her behavior.

Three important things parents and professionals can do to help children with sensory processing difficulties include:

1. Recognize how sensory processing differences can impact behavior and observe the ways each child responds to or experiences various types of sensation. Since we cannot see how the brain processes sensation, we can only make guesses about how the brain is responding to and organizing input by watching a child's behavior. Becoming good observers and thinking about how different types of sensory input can impact a child's attention, emotions, and adaptive behavior are important steps to reframing some difficult behaviors from a sensory integration perspective. Consider how a child's need for more sensation or the need to avoid sensations can affect his or her actions and behavior. Also remember that every child is an individual with unique interests, responses, and needs. There is no "cookbook" that can tell you all the right sensory activities for a specific child's development.

2. Change the environment to match the child's surroundings with his or her sensory needs and preferences. This might involve decreasing sights and sounds in the immediate environment (e.g., home, child's bedroom), keeping things in the environment well organized, and being aware of the sensory demands of different tasks or environments (going to the mall or roughhouse play are highly stimulating; taking a warm bath or rocking a child can be calming and are less stimulating). It might also involve rethinking daily routines and changing expectations (it may be better to go to the mall on a different evening if it's been a stressful day at school, or avoiding such an environment if at all possible). For a child who is under responsive to sensory information finding structured ways to provide sensory input or cues from his/her environment may also be helpful.

3. Use sensation in play and daily routines to help meet a child's sensory needs. Sensory input can have a powerful impact on a child's nervous system. It can wind us up and increase our alertness and activity level, or it can calm us down and facilitate attention or relaxation. For example, children who are sensory seeking like movement because their nervous systems need more stimulation to stay alert and pay attention. Finding ways for the child to move, or providing them with a number of "fidgets" (e.g., toys or objects they can squeeze or manipulate) more may be more fruitful than making a child sit still. At times we may want children to calm down so using activities with sensory qualities that soothe or relax (rocking, soft music, weighted blanket, a quiet space to cool down) may help them "switch gears" and get focused.

Conclusion

Children's behavior is complex and constantly changing from day to day, and within different environments. A sensory integration framework provides one perspective for understanding challenging behaviors exhibited by children with FASD (as well as many not so challenging behaviors) by considering how a child's nervous system takes in, makes sense, and uses information from the sensory world. By understanding a child's "sensory reactivity" it may be possible to change ones perceptions of and reactions to some difficult behaviors and implement creative and caring strategies to create "just right" environments and expectations to help children cope with complex world around them. Several of these ideas and strategies have been useful when addressing some of the challenging behaviors children with FASD may demonstrate. These strategies combined with other educational, developmental and behavioral interventions may help children with FASD function better in their home, schools, and communities.

References

Ayres, A. J. (1979). *Sensory integration and the child.* Los Angeles: Western Psychological Services.

Bundy, A.C. (2002). Assessing sensory integrative dysfunction, in *Sensory Integration Theory and Practice.* 2nd ed. (Bundy AC, Lane SJ, Murray EA eds), pp 169-198. FA Davis, Philadelphia.

Cermak, S. (2001). The effects of deprivation on processing, play and praxis. In S. Smith Roley, E. I. Blanche, and R. C. Schaaf, (Eds.). *Understanding the nature of sensory integration with diverse populations* (pp. 385-408). San Antonio, TX: Therapy Skill Builders.

Dahl-Reeves, G., Cermak, S.A. (2002). Disorders of praxis, in *Sensory Integration Theory and Practice.* 2nd ed (Bundy AC, Lane SJ, Murray, EA eds), pp 71-100. FA Davis, Philadelphia.

Dunn, W. (1999). *Sensory Profile manual.* San Antonio, TX: Psychological Corporation.

Dunn, W. (1997). The impact of sensory processing abilities on the daily lives of young children and their families: A conceptual model. *Infants and Young Children, 9*(4), 23-35.

Hanft, B. E., Miller, L. J., and Lane, S. J., (2000). Toward a consensus in terminology in sensory integration theory and practice: Part three: Observable behaviors: sensory integration dysfunction. *Sensory Integration Special Interest Section Quarterly, 23*(2), 1-4.

Harris, S.R., Osborn, J.A., Weinberg, J., Loock, C., Junald, K. (1993). Effects of prenatal alcohol exposure on neuromotor and cognitive development during early childhood: A series of case reports. Physical Therapy 73:608-617.

Jirikowic, T, (2003) *Sensory processing and integration and children with alcohol-related diagnoses: An explanatory analysis.* Unpublished doctoral dissertation. University of Washington

Kimball, J. G. (1999). Sensory integration frame of reference: Theoretical base, function/dysfunction continua and guide to evaluation. In P. Kramer and J. Hinojosa,

(Eds.), *Frames of reference for pediatric occupational therapy* (2nd ed.). (pp. 119-168), Baltimore, MD: Lippincott, Williams, and Wilkins.

Lane, S. J. and Miller, L. J. (2000). Toward a consensus in terminology in sensory integration theory and practice: Part Two: Sensory integration patterns of function and dysfunction. *Sensory Integration Special Interest Section Quarterly, 23*(2), 1-4.

Mangeot, S. D., Miller, L. J., McIntosh, D. N, McGrath-Clarke, J, Simon, J, Hagerman, R. J., Goldson, E.. (2001). Sensory modulation dysfunction in children with attention-deficit-hyperactivity disorder. *Developmental Medicine and Child Neurology*;43(6):399-406

McIntosh, D. N. Miller, L. J., Shyu, V., Dunn, W. (1999). In *Sensory Profile test manual,* (pp. 59-73). San Antonio, TX: Psychological Corporation.

Miller, L. J., Lane, S.J. and Hanft, B. (2000, March). Toward a consensus in terminology in sensory integration theory and practice: Part one: Taxonomy of neurophysiological process. *Sensory Integration Special Interest Section Quarterly 23*(1), 1-4.

Morse, B.A., & Cermak, S. A. (1994). Sensory integration in children with fetal alcohol syndrome. *Alcoholism: Clinical and Experimental Research, 18(2)*, 502 (abstr).

Morse, B.A., Miller, P.T., & Cermack, S.A. (1995). Sensory processing in children with fetal alcohol syndrome. *Alcoholism: Clinical and Experimental Research, 19(2)*, 588 (abstr).

Mulligan, S. (1996). An analysis of score patterns of children with attention disorders on the Sensory Integration and Praxis Tests. *American Journal of Occupational Therapy, 50*(8), 647-654.

Osborn, J. A., Harris, S. R., Weinberg, J. (1993) Fetal alcohol syndrome: review of the literature with implications for physical therapists. *Physical Therapy*, 73:99-607..

Parham, L. D. (1998). The relationship of sensory integrative development to achievement in elementary students: Four-year longitudinal patterns. *Occupational Therapy Journal of Research, 18*(3), 105-127.

Parham L. D. Mailloux, Z. (2005). Sensory integration. In *Occupational Therapy for Children.* 5th ed. (Case-Smith J, Allen AS, Pratt PN eds), pp 356-405 Mosby, St. Louis.

Schaaf, R.C., & Miller, L. J. (2005). Occupational therapy using a sensory integrative approach for children with developmental disabilities. *Mental Retardation and Developmental Disabilities Research Reviews, 11*, 143-148.

Spitzer and Smith Roley, S, (2001). Sensory integration revisited: A philosophy of practice. In S. Smith Roley, E. I. Blanche, and R. C. Schaaf, (Eds.). *Understanding the nature of sensory integration with diverse populations* (pp. 3-28). San Antonio, TX: Therapy Skill Builders.

Wilbarger, P. and Wilbarger, J. (1991). *Sensory defensiveness in children ages 2-12: An intervention guide for parents and other caretakers.* Santa Barbara, CA: Avanti Educational Programs.

Additional Resources

Kranowitz, C. S. (1998). *The out of sync child.* New York: Skylight Press.

Schwab, D .(1999). Reframing perceptions: How children with FAS/FAE sense the world. In Lorna Mayer (ed.) Living and Working with FAS/ FAS/FAE

Sensory Processing Disorder Network *http://www.sinetwork.org/*

Questions

1. Children with sensory processing problems typically present with dysfunction in one specific sensory modaility (e.g. touch, vision)

True/False-False

2. Children with poor sensory processing demonstrate which of the following behavioral response patterns to sensation:

a. hypersensitive
b. hyposensitive
c. fluctuating
d. all of the above

3. Observation of behavioral responses to sensation is an important assessment strategy to determine if a sensory processing problem exists.

True/False- True

4. An important sensory-based intervention strategy involves modifying the environment and/or daily routines based on the sensory needs of each individual child.

True/False-True

In: ADHD and Fetal Alcohol Spectrum Disorders (FASD)   ISBN: 1-59454-573-1
Editor: Kieran D. O'Malley, pp. 51-67   © 2008 Nova Science Publishers, Inc.

Chapter 4

PATHOPHYSIOLOGY OF ADHD IN PATIENTS WITH ADHD AND FETAL ALCOHOL SPECTRUM DISORDERS. THE ROLE OF MEDICATION

Kieran D.O'Malley[*]

INTRODUCTION

There is long standing and newly emerging clinical, neuropsychological and neurochemical evidence in animal and human research for a link between FASD and ADHD (Driscoll, et al 1990). The evidence of the link between these two conditions has implications for clinical medication management.

The clinical quality of ADHD in children with FASD is often quite distinct. It is more likely that the ADHD is earlier onset, presenting as a regulatory disorder in the infancy and toddler years (O'Malley, 1994, Mayes, 2000, DC 0-3R, 2005, O'Malley and Streissguth, 2006).This includes temperament profiles in the infants which are skewed to the difficult to settle or slow to warm types. The temperamental and regulatory problems in the infant or toddler frequently create interaction issues between the parent and the infant. Thus a secondary ambivalent / resistant, ambivalent / avoidant or disorganized attachment disorder may develop which compounds the emerging ADHD features.

The ADHD symptomatology is more commonly encountered with co-morbid psychiatric disorders, such as mood disorder, anxiety disorder, or intermittent explosive disorder (conduct disorder).Co-morbid medical conditions; such as cardiac, renal or eye problems are frequently present. As these children and adolescents are brain-injured and have a disturbance in brain neurophysiology i.e. brain wave development, neurochemistry (i.e. adrenergic or

---

[*] Kieran D. O'Malley M.B., D.A.B.P.N. (P) Lecturer, University of Washington, Department of Psychiatry and Behavioral Sciences and Adjunct Faculty Henry M. Jackson School of International Studies, Fetal Alcohol and Drug Unit, Seattle, WA (He formerly started the Edmonton FAS clinic at Glenrose Hospital, Canada, 1991-1996); (Address correspondence to Kieran D.O' Malley at above address or e mail address: omalley.kieran@gmail.com)

dopaminergic neurotransmitter development), or even brain structure (i.e. corpus callosum, hippocampus or cerebellum size and morphology) as a result of prenatal alcohol exposure, their response to standard psychostimulant medication can be quite unpredictable.

Only 25 -30% of these children and adolescents with FASD have mental retardation. Nevertheless, the majority of them invariably demonstrate complex learning disorders, i.e. mathematics disorder, disorder of written expression or reading disorder. As well as a mixed receptive / expressive language disorder with deficits in social cognition and communication. The language disorder is reminiscent of sensory aphasia and apraxia and is often not seen with the standard school language proficiency screening tests, but is only detected with secondary level tests such as a formal narrative discourse analysis (Thomas and Chess 1977, Coggins et al 1998, Lishman 1998, Kapp and O'Malley, 2001, O'Malley and Nanson 2002, O'Malley and Storoz 2003, Barr et al 2005, DC: 0 to 3R 2005).

The Seattle Longitudinal Prospective Study on Alcohol and Pregnancy examinations of neonates at day 1 and day 2 showed possible evidence of an infant regulatory disorder and temperamental disturbance which predated the ADHD diagnosis. The clinical features described include; weak suck reflex and long latency to suck, state regulation and habituation problems. (Streissguth et al 1984a, 1984b, Streissguth 1997, Thomas and Chess 1997, Wittenberg 2001). Many clinical descriptions give a picture of the natural history of prenatal alcohol C.N.S. dysfunction and highlight the prevalence of inattention hyperactive and impulsive symptomatology (Olegard et al 1979, Streissguth et al 1985, Barr et al 1990, Coles et al 1997). ADHD symtomatology, memory and executive function deficits persist through the lifespan. (Streissguth et al 1984a, Connor et al 1997, Hagerman 1999) The recent hypothesis that prenatal alcohol exposure may have an effect on genetic imprinting makes the careful assessment of familial history of ADHD, and exploration of the non-shared environment, important considerations When unraveling the ADHD in children and adolescents with FASD (Pike et al, 1996, Weinberg, 1997, Eisenhower, et al 2005). For example maternal stress, negativity or depression as well as the child or adolescent's exposure to abuse may have separate as well as cumulative effects on childhood or adolescent psychopathology including the type of ADHD presentation (Pike, et al 1996, Kendler, et al 2000, Diego, et al 2001, Eisenhower, et al 2005). Also genetic studies have revealed an association between dopamine transporter gene (DAT) and ADHD, Predominantly Hyperactive- Impulsive Type, and dopamine 4 receptor gene and ADHD, Predominantly Inattention Type (Cantwell 1975, Stevenson 1992, Cook et al 1995, Lacoste 1996, Eaves et al 1997, Waldman 1997, Thapar, et al, 1999) 1999).is may help differentiate familial ADHD from acquired ADHD.

Coles and other researchers has reported a "qualitative difference" in the ADHD in children with FASD. Coles analyzed the Continuous Performance Task (CPT) as well as a four factor model of attention developed by Mirsky (Mirksy et al 1991). The results suggested that ADHD patients had more significant problems in the "focus" and "sustain" factors, whereas patients with FASD, FAS subtype, had more problems with the factors of "encode" and "shift"(Coles 1997). Numerous other studies and authors have demonstrated and described the complex learning disorders with ADHD in FASD patients. They include problems in working memory, executive function and social use of language (Abel 1984, Harris 1995, Streissguth 1997, Connor et al 1997, Coggins et al 1998, Oesterheld and O'Malley 1999, Hagerman 1999).

Using the DSM –TR classification it is possible to describe children and adolescents with FASD as having ADHD, Combined Type (314.01), Predominantly Inattention Type (314.00), Predominantly Hyperactive-Impulsive Type (314.01).

FASD AND ADHD LINK

The clinical link between ADHD and FASD is consistent with the concept of acute and long term clinical sequelae of organic brain damage (Lishman, 1998), and of Developmental Neuropsychiatry described in the UK by Michael Rutter, 1977, 1984, and expanded on in the USA by James Harris in 1995 and Judith Rapapport in 2000. Rapapport discussed the association between prenatal and perinatal adverse events or stressors and adult psychiatric outcomes. At the same David Skuse in the UK (2000) integrated models from behavioral neuroscience and linked them with child psychopathology .We are in an era where the 'developmental origins of health and disease' are becoming a modern template for research and clinical understanding (Gillman, 2005).The embryogenesis of prenatal alcohol effect was captured in early work by Kathy Sulik in 1981, but current scientific knowledge of Epigenetic/neurotoxic environments is bringing FASD into the arena of classical developmental neuropsychiatry.

Ironically, over 50 years ago, the public health physicians and paediatricians had postulated, and studied, the link between birth and delivery causing central nervous system trauma and the later development of the patient. These researchers formed the concept "continuum of reproductive wastage" and described a range of effects due to this early trauma. They were: lethal i.e. abortion, neonatal death or stillbirth sublethal i.e. cerebral palsy, epilepsy or hemiplegia, and subtle i.e. minimal brain dysfunction, learning disability and hyperactivity.

Subsequently the researchers developed the term "continuum of reproductive casualty" which elaborated on the range of subtle effects. They now included minor motor gross and fine abnormalities, perceptual disturbances, and behavioral problems (Lilienfeld and Parkhurst 1951, Pasamanick et al 1956, Pasamanick and Knoblock 1966).

Finally, 53,000 infants were studied in the Collaborative Perinatal Project of the National Institute of Neurological Diseases and Stroke during the six year period 1959-1965. The study involved pregnancy, birth, neonatal, four month, eight month, early childhood and elementary school assessments. The study found maternal level of education and socio-economic factors to be the most consistent predictors of later cognitive competence in the growing child. It highlighted the importance of the interaction between high- risk pregnancies, poverty and the adverse environmental rearing conditions of infants. This critical interaction was instrumental in the appearance and severity of long-term developmental problems of the child and later adolescent. As well, the study documented the influence of early brain abnormality and early developmental delay on later cognitive development and functioning (Niswander et al 1972, Broman et al 1975).

ADHD has now become the most common psychiatric disorder of childhood, affecting 3% to 11% of children and often continues into adulthood (Barkley, 1990, Biederman, et al, 1991, Arnold and Jensen, 1995). It is not a unitary condition and overlapping symptoms are often present (i.e. mood disorder, anxiety disorder, conduct disorder) (Biederman et al 1991,

Jensen 1995, Milberger, et al 1995). The prevalence of co-morbid psychiatric
been variously estimated as conduct or oppositional defiant disorder 50%,
depression 25% to 33% anxiety 25%, and the prevalence of co-morbid cognitive issues such
as learning disorder 25%.

NEUROCHEMISTRY CHANGES IN ADHD AND FASD

There is a common aetiological cause of both FASD with ADHD symptoms and ADHD
without FASD, and the ADHD resulting from prenatal alcohol exposure is an 'acquired' form
of ADHD primarily related to its affect on the developing dopamine and/ or noradrenergic
neurotransmitter systems (Hagerman 1999, O'Malley and Nanson 2002).

1. There are two main theories on the neurochemistry of ADHD:
   a) The condition is related to a dysregulation in the frontal-nigrostriatal dopamine
      system, manifesting itself as varying states of arousal (Cyr 1998, Cooper at
      2003)
   b) The condition is due to a dysregulation of the noradrenergic system
      (norepinephrine) (Arnold and Jensen 1995, Pliska et al 1996, Cooper et al 2003).
      Numerous animal and human studies involving a variety of body fluids e.g.
      urine, blood and cerebrospinal fluid have implicated catecholamine
      abnormalities but with inconsistent results (Castellanos et al 1997).
2. The neurochemistry of FASD has been informed by 25 years of animal research.
   Deficits have been found in most systems, including dopaminergic, noradrenergic,
   serotonergic, cholinergic, glutamatergic, GABAergic, and histaminergic systems
   (Ferrer 1987, Druse 1992, Maneuffel 1995, Harris 1995, Hannigan et al 1996,
   O'Malley and Hagerman 1998, Hagerman 1999). The deficits in dopamine and
   noradrenergic systems most likely relate to the 'hyperactive' symptoms seen in
   animals with prenatal alcohol exposure. Rat research has shown the D1 receptors of
   the mesolimbic dopamine system are more impacted by alcohol exposure than
   nigrostriatal or tegmental dopamine system (Hannigan et al 1996). Animal studies on
   rats and mice prenatally exposed to alcohol have shown that the physical
   hyperactivity tends to diminish with increasing age and to be worse in males than
   females, which appears to parallel the situation in humans with prenatal alcohol
   exposure (Abel 1984, Riley 1990)

The years of animal and human research have demonstrated a group of symptoms (e.g..
increased activity, exploration and reactivity, decreased attention, inhibition deficits and
impaired habituation) all of which are consistent with ADHD symptomatology and linked to
dopamine and noradrenaline neurotransmitter disturbance (Driscoll et al 1990, Hannigan et al
1996, Streissguth 1997, O'Malley and Hagerman 1998, O'Malley and Nanson 2002,
O'Malley and Storoz 2003). These studies dovetail with other research studies which have
analyzed critical embryological periods of vulnerability for the developing central nervous
system, as well as the role played by the effect of alcohol on the developing neurotransmitters
(Rice, et al 2000, Tomkins, et al 2001).

GENERAL GUIDELINES WHEN PRESCRIBING MEDICATION IN FASD

1. There needs to be an acknowledgement of the *possible negative effect of the psychotropic medication of the developing brain.* This has been best described in the previous work on the chronic use of Phenobarbital in children with a risk of recurrent febrile seizures (Farwell 1990, see O'Malley & Hagerman 1998).It was shown that 2 years of chronic usage of the Phenobarbital resulted in lower I.Q. in the children, and furthermore, this cognitive impairment was still present at least 6 months after the drug was discontinued. The developing brain of a child prenatally exposed to alcohol already has experienced neurotoxic damage to the developing CNS neurotransmitter, neurophysiology and/or brain structure. Thus it is very likely such a child with 'acquired brain injury' from prenatal alcohol exposure will show atypical response to standard medications, including psychostimulants. The atypical clinical response may be intolerance, hypersensitivity, paradoxical reaction, over-sedation, as well as blunted cognitive ability, or the unmasking of a primary psychiatric familial disorder, such as Bipolar disorder or marked Hyperactivity and Impulsivity precipitated in a child with ARND by the usage of a SSRI.

2. The severe ADHD symptomatolgy in children and adolescents with FASD can be *a mixture of familial / inherited and acquired* from prenatal alcohol exposure.

3. The ADHD symptomatology in a child or adolescent with a FASD may be *coloured and/or exacerbated by living in a chaotic or abusive home environment.* This may include the ADHD symptomatology having a protective effect in a toxic or violent home environment. Here, the ADHD is coupled with a self-protective 'hypervigilance'.

4. *Co-morbid psychiatric conditions* commonly are part of the ADHD presentation in FASD. These include autistic spectrum disorder, affective (mood) instability, generalized anxiety disorder with or without panic attacks, and intermittent explosive disorder.

5. *Co-morbid medical or neurological conditions* are also present in children or adolescents with ADHD and FASD. These include, seizure disorder, cardiac disorder, (structural or pulse irregularity), renal disorder (structural), thyroid disorder or diabetes.

6. *Co-morbid cognitive disorders* are also present with the ADHD in FASD children and adolescents. They include low, moderate or severe mental retardation, or a complex learning disorder.

7. The classical ADHD symptomatolgy in children and adolescents with FASD is *commonly preceded by a presentation of a Regulatory Disorder in infancy and toddler ages* (O'Malley and Hagerman 1998).

Psychostimulant Response

Animal researchers have demonstrated that animals prenatally exposed to alcohol tend to show an exaggerated response to psychostimulant (Ulug et al 1983, Means et al 1984,

Hannigan et al 1996). This medication response was influenced by age, gender and drug dosage.

Pychostimulants have been used in normal IQ patients for a long time but also with developmental disability, mental retardation and ADHD with controlled efficacy studies documenting their benefit (Bradley, 1937, Gadow 1992, Aman 1993a, 1993b, Handen et al 1990, 1992, Mayes 1994, King et al 1998). Different studies have analyzed the neurochemical and metabolic impact of stimulants in ADHD (Matochik, et al 1993, Volkow, et al 1997). O'Malley and Hagerman (1998) reviewed the action of the stimulants and their usage in FAS, PFAS and ARND. Clinical response to stimulants varied. In Denver, patients with ARND had an 80% response rate, whereas patients with FAS had a 48% response rate (Hagerman 1999). In the UW Secondary Disabilities study, 32% of 415 patients with FAS or FAE [ARND] were given methylphenidate for ADHD, and had a response rate of 47%. (Streissguth et al 1996). Another study by O'Malley et al found a higher response rate to dextroamphetamine (79%) than methylphenidate (22%) in a retrospective case series of 30 children and adolescents with FAS, PFAS or FAE (ARND) who were followed by 3 psychiatrists in Canada and U.S.A. (O'Malley et al 2000).

Only two controlled studies have been published regarding psychostimulant intervention for ADHD symptomatology in FASD Synder et al. studied 11 children, known positive responders to stimulants, and used different drug dosages on a mg. per kg.basis Three different types of psychostimulant were studied e.g. methylphenidate, dextroamphetamine and pemoline. The results showed no significant effect on sustained attention but as expected, significant effects on parent rating scales (Synder et al 1997). Oesterheld's study analysed 4 patients (all Native Americans) using a randomized double blind, crossover study design, lasting only 5 days, with two placebos and a fixed dose of methylphenidate. Using daily Conners Parent Rating Scales and Conners Teacher Rating Scales methylphenidate significantly improved scores of the Hyperactivity Index Scale on both measures, but not the Daydreaming -Attention score on the Conners Teacher Rating Scale (Oesterheld et al 1998).

Research has shown the impact of prenatal alcohol on causing structural brain defects (Mattson, et al 1996, Bookstein, et al 2001).Generally, patients with neurochemical or structural changes in the CNS, including those with FASD are often overly sensitive to the effects of medication, including the side effects (Means, et al 1984, Ulug, et al 1985, Van Groll, 1992, O'Malley and Hagerman 1998, Hagerman 1999). The response to psychostimulants, may improve with age; so a negative response may occur in a child under 5 years, but a subsequent positive response may be seen when the child is 6 or 7 years of age (Hales et al 1994, Aman et al 1998). There may be ethnic differences in clinical response to stimulants, and certain clinicians have suggested that methylphenidate should not be used in treating the ADHD symptoms of Native American children with FASD because of their possible lack of effectiveness, or growth retarding effect (Weinberg 1997, Oesterheld et al 1998).

Attention should be given to possible medical complications, called Alcohol Related Birth Defects (ARBD), which may occur in individuals with FASD related to cardiac, renal, eye or nutritional problems. This also includes currently unstudied effects on the developing liver (Stratton et al 1996, Streissguth 1997, Kapp and O'Malley 2001).

DISCUSSION

It is important to remember that there may be no link between FASD and ADHD because ADHD is a common condition, and Adults with ADHD are more likely to drink and so pass on the ADHD to their infants through genetic transmission. The ADHD resulting from prenatal alcohol exposure is an acquired form of brain injury. This type of ADHD is suggested by the early onset CNS dysfunction, complex learning disorders and co-morbid psychiatric and medical disorders, and atypical medication response. Thus, the medication may sometimes increase a patient's impulsivity or aggressiveness and an increase in the dosage may actually worsen the clinical situation rather than alleviating it (O'Malley and Hagerman 1998). This is especially a concern if polypharmacology is used. At the current time researchers are commenting on the unproven benefit of adding fluoxetine to stimulants for ADHD with co-morbid Anxiety (Abikoff, et al 2005). No scientific research on combined drug therapy has been performed on children or adolescents with FASD who present ADHD symptoms. There also have been some general concerns about the lack of empirical support for the rationale in utilizing combined psychotropic medication in the first place, let alone the safety and efficacy of this clinical approach (McClellan and Werry, 2003).

These patients often present early onset ADHD, frequently as an infant or toddler Regulatory Disorder, Type I, II or III resulting from the prenatal brain neurotoxic damage. The clinical presentation of ADHD in children with FASD is commonly seen with *co-morbid psychiatric* and medical issues such as mood disorder, anxiety disorder (with or without panic attacks) and intermittent explosiveness features.

The ADHD may present with *co-morbid medical conditions* and cardiac, renal, eye or orthodontic problems. Sometimes there may also be a complex partial seizure disorder (Stratton, et al, 1996, O'Malley and Hagerman 1998, O'Malley and Storoz, 2003).

Dextroamphetamine may be the more effective 'first line stimulant ' in treatment of ADHD associated with FASD This is consistent with the animal work of Hannigan and Randall (1991) which showed the impact of prenatal alcohol exposure on the D1 receptors of the mesolimbic dopamine system, the area where dextroamphretamine has been shown to act. A negative response to methylphenidate has been reported in animals and humans with ADHD who have a history of prenatal alcohol exposure, suggesting that the frontal-nigrostriatal dopamine pathway might not be the mechanism involved in patients with FASD with ADHD (Means, et al 1984, Ulug, et al 1985, Hannigan, et al 1996, 0'Malley and Hagerman , 1998).

FASD is a chronic developmental neuropsychiatric disorder and proper treatment of FASD with ADHD symptomatology offers an opportunity to decrease the documented destructive secondary disabilities (Streissguth, et al 1996, Streissguth, and O'Malley, 2000, Streissguth, et al 2004). Nevertheless, it is important to be aware of the long term effects of stimulants in the adult ADHD population (Schacher, et al 1993, Matochik, et al 1993, Schachter, et al 2001). Clinical experience has already shown a probable negative effect on growth hormone from many years of stimulant medication in FASD with the subsequent challenges for endocrinological management.

Stimulant medication for children with FASD and ADHD should be considered as part of a multi-modal treatment array, with careful attention given to the possible impact of Tran generational stress or trauma on the individual and/or the family (O'Malley, 1997,

Cummings, et al 2000, Horowitz, 2003). This is especially valid for birth families dealing with the legacy of FASD in both parents and children. The present context of psychotropic medication utility includes no medium or large scale study trials of even one drug therapy in children or adolescents with FASD and ADHD. It therefore makes it impossible for a clinician to obtain proper informed consent or assent from a child or adolescent for the use of psychotropic medication as there is no current literature available on the risks and benefits in patients with FASD who present with ADHD (AACAP 2005). Ideally, management would include a variety of treatment modalities such sensory integration, language therapy, special schooling, non- verbal play therapy, medication therapy, parent education and very importantly supportive family therapy (Sprenger et al 1998). Multi-modal treatment has been recommended by the MTA Cooperative Group and American Academy of Pediatrics in the management of childhood ADHD (MTA 1999, APA). Benedetto Vitiello (2001) from NIMH has posed an interesting reflective question which resonates very much with the FASD population who present ADHD symptoms. He provocatively questions 'whether the reduction of the ADHD symptoms , achieved through pharmacological or behavioral intervention, will ultimately translate into a better prognosis with respect to improved educational and occupational achievement, and decreased risk of accidental trauma, anti-social behaviors and substance abuse'. In the current climate of NO scientific pharmacological intervention research in children or adolescents with FASD this is an important horizon far, far away. Only recently have researchers begun to acknowledge the complexity of adaptive functioning and psycho-social outcomes in young adults with ADHD (Barkley, et al, 2006).His group highlighted sexual activity and early parenthood as important domains of functioning. Both these areas are of recurring importance in FASD and lead to the need for early intervention, under 5 years of age, when there is a greater possibility of working with the birth mother, and interrupting this transgenerational condition.

Furthermore, we cannot comment on the animal research which postulated that prenatal exposure to alcohol alters drug sensitivity in adulthood (Abel, et al, 1981). This is, of course, a critical area in the clinical management of young adults with FASD. We understand the liver drug is enzyme pathways in which psychotropic drugs are metabolized by the cytochrome **P450** system, but we have no basic science knowledge about how these liver pathways are effected in embryological development by exposure to alcohol in utero. So we are unable to determine any safety or efficacy levels for medication in patients born with FASD and present ADHD symptoms.

Within the constraints mentioned above it is worth acknowledging that stimulant medication can have a profound, and sustained, positive effect on children or adolescents with FASD (and thereby decrease parent stress) who present ADHD symptoms. The secret is to carefully re-evaluate the patient's clinical symptomatology and clarify if the symptoms could be medication related either a hypersensitivity or hyperreponsiveness in the first 48 hours, or a subtle unmasking of other neuropsychiatric conditions such as a bipolar disorder or affective instability after 3 to 4 weeks usage. It does appear, however, that the dopaminergic pathways are one of the areas most effected by prenatal alcohol and their disruption is commonly expressed in the neuropsychiatric disorder ADHD (Figure 1).

The Four Dopamine Pathways in the Brain

(i) The **nigrostriatal dopamine pathway** projects from the substantia nigra to the basal ganglia, and is part of the extrapyramidal nervous system which controls muscle movements. It has been implicated in the origins of ADHD behaviors.

(ii) The second is the **mesolimbic dopamine pathway** which projects from the midbrain ventral tegmental area to the nucleus accumbens (NA). The NA is part of the limbic system and is thought to be involved in many pleasurable sensations and behaviors, as in the powerful craving and euphoria of street drugs, but also psychotic delusions and hallucinations. This pathway is most affected by prenatal alcohol in animal studies.

(iii) The third pathway is related to the mesolimbic dopamine pathway and it is called the **mesocortical dopamine pathway**. It also projects from the midbrain ventral tegmental area, but sends its axons to the limbic cortex. Controversary surrounds the proposal that it may have a role in mediating the cognitive negative symptoms of schizophrenia.

(iv) The fourth dopamine pathway is called the **tuberoinfundibular dopamine pathway** and it controls prolactin secretion. It projects from the hypothalamus to the anterior pituitary gland. No clear clinical role has been defined.

Figure 1. The Four Dopamine Pathways in the Brain. Adapted from Hannigan, 1996, Stahl, 2002.

PROPOSED DRUG ALGORITHM

The psychostimulant which appears to be the best 1st choice is Dextraoamphetamine. Initially short acting, then in long acting spansule form(less than 1mg/kg/day).

2nd choice would be methtylphenidate. Initially short acting, then long acting preparation (less than 1 mg/kg/day).

3rd choice would be 2nd generation bi-modal long acting preparations such as Concerta (start with 18mgs).

THE FUTURE: We are in an era of rapidly expanding neurobiological knowledge. Now researchers have isolated critical CNS functions such as memory and activation to the synapse rather than just gross anatomical structural regions i.e. in the hippocampus different biological markers for memory and seizure kindling are being identified.

The road ahead offers some fascinating areas of continued research all of which have potential implications for management of neuropsychiatric disorders such as the ADHD presentation of FASD.

They include:

1. Genetic Testing As it becomes more sophisticated and specific it may begin to help separate familial ADHD, with a clear genetic component, from acquired ADHD, which would include the ADHD seen in patients with FASD. This will then begin to inform medication management as scientific studies will be able to incorporate genetic data establishing a genetic pharmacology of ADHD. It may be shown that common psychostimulants such as methylphenidate are more efficacious with ADHD patients with a genetic component than with the acquired ADHD patients. However, the new research on the epigenetic effect of prenatal alcohol will have to be taken into consideration. This will place FASD within the framework of the expanding knowledge in the evolution of developmental

regulatory pathways. The dynamic equilibrium between genes and environment will continue to show how both these components are inextricably intertwined (Pollard 2002).

2. Glutamate. The amino acid glutamate or glutaminic acid is a neurotransmitter as well as an essential building block need for protein synthesis. The neurotransmitter role of glutamate is created by the conversion of glutamine to glutamate by the enzymatic action of glutaminase which is found in the cell mitochondria. Subsequently it is stored in synaptic vesicles for release during neurotransmission. (Glutamine can be obtained from glial cells adjacent to neurons.) There are a number of glutamate receptors. One receptor, N-methyl-d-aspartate (NMDA) is reputed to mediate normal excitatory neurotransmission as well as excitatory excitotoxicity. Excess excitotoxicity has been hypothesized to cause various forms of neurodegeneration. Animal neurotoxic studies have shown that prenatal alcohol can kindle this excess excitatory response. Future approaches to management of FASD may incorporate glutaminergic agents.

3. N-acetylaspartate (NAA) which is found primarily in neurons and axons, and is seen as a marker of neuronal integrity, specifically neuronal degeneration. Current studies are analyzing the psychiatric significance of decreased levels in the prefrontal and frontal lobes.

4. Choline is a precursor of acetylcholine and has been identified as an important component of cell membranes. The clinical significance of increased or decreased levels in areas of the brain such as the frontal, temporal and basal ganglion are still being debated. Already animal researchers are studying the effect of neonatal choline supplementation in decreasing the neurotoxic effects of prenatal alcohol (Thomas, et al 2000)

5. Calcium. It has been shown that changes in intracellular calcium are closely involved in neurotransmitter synthesis and release. The postulated action of the intracellular calcium is through the intracellular proteins. Calcium may have a role as an adjunct to standard psychotropic medication or even as a neuroprotective agent in pregnant alcohol-abusing women.

6. 3-Methoxy-4-hydroxyphenylglycol. (MHPG). This has been identified as the main metabolite of adrenaline in the human brain. Furthermore, levels of MHPG in peripheral body fluids such as CSF, blood and urine are believed to be related to MHPG levels in the brain. At the moment the most value of these measurements would be in ADHD with co-morbid mood disorder.

7. Protein Kinase C. This has been shown to be a major intracellular mediator of signals which occur following the binding of noradrenaline, and serotonin, agonists to their receptors. Thus it is involved in the regulation of both pre- and post synaptic neurotransmission. This may have potential as a biomarker of neurotoxic brain damage from prenatal alcohol (Hagerman 1999, Stahl, 2002, Cooper et al 2003).

REFERENCES

AACAP (American Academy of Child and Adolescent Psychiatry)(Draft July 2005) Practice parameters on the use of psychotropic medication in children and adolescents , in press, Washington DC

Abel, EL, Bush, R, Dintcheff, BA (1981) Exposure of rats to alcohol in utero alters drug sensitivity in adulthood, *Science,* 212, 1531

Abel E.L (1984) Fetal alcohol syndrome and fetal alcohol effects. Plenum Press, New York 54,

Abikoff, H, Mc Gough, J, Vitiello, B, Mc Cracken, J, Davies, M, Walkup, J, Riddle, M, Oatis, M, Greenhill, L, Skrobola, a, March, J, Gammon, P, Robinson, J, Lazell, R, McMahon, DJ, Ritz, L & The RUPP ADHD/ ANXIETY Study group,(2005) Ssequential pharmacotherapy for children with co morbid Attention- Deficit/ hyperactivity and Anxiety disorders, J Amer Acad Child adolesc. Psychiatry, 44: 5, 418-427

Aman MG, Kern RA, McGhee DE, Arnold LE (1993 a) Fenfluramine and methylphenidate in children with mental retardation and ADHD: Clinical and side effects. *J Am Acad Child and Adolesc Psychiatry,* 32:851-859.

Aman, MG, Kern RA, McGhee DE, Arnold LE.(1993b) Fenfluramine and methylphenidate in children with mental retardation and ADHD: Laboratory effects. *Journal of autism and developmental disorders*, 23:491-506.

American Academy of Pediatrics,(2001) Subcommittee on Attention-Deficit /Hyperactivity disorder, Committee on Quality Improvement, Clinical Practice Guideline: Treatment of the School-Aged Child With Attention –Deficit /Hyperactivity Disorder, *Pediatrics, Vol.* 108, No. 4, 1033-1044.

Arnold LE, Jensen PS.(1995) Attention-Deficit Disorders, In: Sadock and Yudofsky editors. *Comprehensive Textbook of Psychiatry,* 6th Ed , 2295-2310.

Aronson M, Hagberg B, Gilberg C (1997) Attention deficits and autistic spectrum problems in children exposed to alcohol during gestation: A follow-up study. *Dev Med Child Neurol;* 39:583-587

Barkley RA.(1990) Attention deficit hyperactivity disorder: A handbook for diagnosis and treatment. New York: The Guilford Press. .

Barkley, RA, Fischer, M, Smallish, L, and Fletcher, K (2006)Young adult outcome of hyperactive children: Adaptive functioning in major life activities. *J Am Acad Child Adolesc Psychiatry*, 45, 2, 192-202

Barr HM, Streissguth AP, Darby BL, Sampson PD.(1990) Prenatal exposure to alcohol, caffeine, tobacco and aspirin: Effects on fine motor and gross motor performance in 4 year old children. *Developmental Psychology;* 26:339-348.

Barr, HM, Bookstein, FL, O'Malley, KD, Connor, PD, Huggins, JE, Sampson, PD, Streissguth, AP (2006) Binge drinking during pregnancy doubles the odds of psychiatric disorders and traits on the structured clinical interview for DSM-IV in young adult offspring. *Amer. J.Psychiatry*, June.

Biederman J, Newcorn J, Sprich S.(1991) Co-morbidity of attention deficit hyperactivity disorder with conduct, depression, anxiety and other disorders. *Am. J Psychiatry;* 148:564.

Biederman J, Wilens T, Mick E, Farone SV, Weber W, Curtis S, et al. (1997) Is ADHD a risk factor for psychoactive substance use disorders? Findings from a four-year prospective follow-up study. *J Amer Acad Child Adolesc Psychiatry;* 36:21-28

Bierich JR, Majewski F, Michaelis R.(1975) The Fetal Alcohol Syndrome. *Paedatric Research*; 9:864.

Bookstein F.L., Sampson P.L., Streissguth A.P., Connor P.L (2001). Geometric Morphometrics of Corpus Callosum and Subcortical Structures in the Fetal Alcohol Affected- Brain, Teratology, 64: 4 –32

Bradley C(1937) The behavior of children receiving benzedrine. *Amer.J. of Psychiatry* ; 94: pp 577-585.

Broman. SH, Nichols, PL, Kennedy, WA(1975) Preschool IQ: Prenatal and early developmental correlates. Hillsdale. NJ. Erlbaum

Buitelaar JK, Van der Gaag RJ, Swaab-Barneveld H, Kuiper M. Prediction of clinical response to methylphenidate in children with attention deficit hyperactivity disorder(1995). *J Amer Acad Child Adolesc Psychiatry*; 34:1025-1032.

Cantwell DP.(1975) Genetics of hyperactivity. *J Child Psychol Psychiatry*; 16:261-264

Castellanos FX. (1997) Toward a pathophysiology of attention deficit/hyperactivity disorder. *Clin Paediatr* ; 3:381-193.

Clarren SK, Astley SJ, Bowden DM, Lai H, Milam AH, Rudeen PK, Shoemaker WJ.(1990) Neuroanatomic and neurochemical abnormalities in nonhuman primate infants exposed to weekly doses of ethanol during gestation. *Alcoholism, Clin & Exp. Res*; 14:674-8.

Coggins T.E., Friet T., & Morgan T.(1998) Analyzing narrative productions in older school – age children and adolescents with fetal alcohol syndrome; an experimental tool for clinical applications, *Clinical Linguistics & Phonetics* , Vol. 12, No. 3, 221-236

Coles CD, Platzman KA, Raskind-Hood CL, Brown RT, Falek A, Smith IE.(1997) A comparison of children affected by prenatal alcohol exposure and attention deficit hyperactivity disorder. *Alcohol Clin Exp Res* ; 1:150-161.

Connor P.D., Sampson P.D., Bookstein F.L., Barr H.M., Streissguth A.P.(1997) Direct and Indirect Effects of Prenatal Alcohol Damage on Executive Function. *Developmental Neuropsychology*, 18, (3), 331- 354.

Cook EH, Stein MA, Krasowski MD.(1995) Association of attention deficit disorder and the dopamine transporter gene. *Am J Hum Genet*, 56:993-998.

Cooper, JR, Bloom, FE, Roth, RH (2003)The biochemical basis of neuropharmacology. 8th edition, Oxford University Press, Oxford, New York

Cummings, EM, Davies, PT, Campbell, SB(2000) Developmental psychopathology and family process, The Guilford Press, New York, London

Cyr M, Brown CS.(1998) Current drug therapy recommendations for the treatment of ADHD. Drug ; 56:215-222.

DC: 0 to 3R(2005) Diagnostic classification of mental health and developmental disorders of infancy and early childhood: Revised Edition, *Zero to Three Press*, Washington DC

Diego, MA, Field, T, Hernandez-Reif M (2001) BIS/BAS scores are correlated with frontal EEG asymmetry in intrusive and withdrawn depressed mothers. *Infant Mental Health Journal*, 22 (6), 665-675

Driscoll C.D., Streissguth A.P., & Riley E.P.(1990) Prenatal alcohol exposure: comparability of effects in humans and animal models, *Neurotoxicity & Teratology* 12, (3), 231- 237.

Druse MJ.(1992) Effects of maternal alcohol consumption on the developing nervous system. In: Watson RR, Editor. Alcohol and neurobiology: Brain development and hormone regulation. Boca Raton: CRC Press;

Eaves LG, Silberg JL, Meyer JM et al.(1997) Genetics and deverlopmental psychopathology, 2; The main effects of genes and environment on behavioral problems in the virginia twin study of adolescent behavioral development. *J Child Psychol Psychiatry*; 38; 965-980.

Eisenhower, AS, Baker, BL, Blacher, J (2005)   Preschool children with intellectual disability: syndrome specificity, behaviour problems, and maternal well–being, *Journal of Intellectual Disability Research,* Vol. 49, Part 9, 657-671

Elia J, Borcherding BG, Rapoport JL, Keysor CS.(1991) Methylphenidate and dextroamphetamine treatments of hyperactivity: Are there true nonresponders? *Psychiatry Res* ; 36:141-155

Ferrer I, Galofre E.(1987) Dendritic spine anomalies in fetal alcohol syndrome. *Neuropediatrics*; 18: 161-163.

Gadow KD, Pomeroy JC, Nolan EE.(1992) A procedure for monitoring stimulant medication in hyperactive mentally retarded school children. *J Child and Adolesc Psychopharm*; 2:131-143

Gillman, MW(2005) Developmental origins of health and disease. *N Engl J Med,* 353, 17, 1848-1849

Hagerman R.J.(1999) Neurodevelopmental Disorders. Diagnosis and treatment. New York: Oxford University Press, 3-59.

Hales RE, Yudofsky SC.(1994) Synopsis of psychiatry 2nd Edition. *American Psychiatric Press,* 837-946 & 1127-1167,

Handen BL, Breaux AM, Gosling A, Ploof DL, Feldman H.(1990) Efficacy of methylphenidate among mentally retarded children with attention deficit hyperactivity disorder. *Ped*; 86:922-930.

Handen BL, Breaux AM, Janosky J, McAuliffe S, Feldman H, Gosling A.(1992) Effects and noneffects of methylphenidate in children with mental retardation and ADHD. *J Am Acad Child and Adolesc Psychiatry*; 31:455-461.

Hannigan, JH, Pilati, ML(1991) The effects of chronic postweaning amphetamine on rats exposed to alcohol in utero.: weight gain and behavior. Neurotoxicol Teratol, 13, 649-656

Hannigan, JH, Randall, S.(1996) Behavioral pharmacology in animals exposed prenatally to alcohol. In: Abel, E.L. editor. Fetal alcohol syndrome: From mechanism to prevention. New York: CRC Press; 191-213.

Harris JC.(1995) *Developmental Neuropsychiatry, Vol II. Assessment, Diagnosis and Treatment of Developmental Disorders,* Oxford University Press , Ch. 5, 8,12, 20.and 386-388.

Horowitz, MJ (2003) Treatment of stress response syndromes , American Psychiatric Press, Washington DC

Jones KL, Smith DW.(1976) Recognition of the fetal alcohol syndrome in early infancy. Lancet ; 2:999-1001

Kapp F.M.E., O'Malley K.D.(2001) Watch for The Rainbows. True Stories for Educators and Other Caregivers of Children with Fetal Alcohol Spectrum Disorders, Frances Kapp Education Publisher, Calgary, Canada

Kendler, KS, Myers, JM, Neale, MC (2000) A multidimensional twin study of mental health in women. Am J Psychiatry,157: 506-513

Lahoste G, Swanson JM, Wigal SB(1996). Dopamine D4 receptor gene polymorphism is associated with attention deficit hyperactivity disorder. *Mol Psychiatry* :121-124.

Lilienfeld, AM & Parkhurst, E (1951) A study of the association of factors of pregnancy and parturition with the development of cerebral palsy. *Amer Journal of Hygiene,* 53, 262-282

Lishman, WA (1998) Organic psychiatry. The psychological consequences of cerebral disorder, 3rd Edition, Blackwell Science, Oxford, London

Lou HC, Henriksen L, Bruhn P, Borner H, Nielsen JB(1989). Striatal dysfunction in attention deficit and hyperkinetic disorder. *Archives of Neurology* ; 46:48.

Mattson SN, Riley EP.(1995) Prenatal exposure to alcohol what the images reveal. Alcohol health research world ; 19:273-278.

Manteuffel MD (1996). Neurotransmitter function: Changes associated with in utero alcohol exposure. In: Abel EL, editor. Fetal alcohol syndrome: From mechanism to prevention. New York: CRC Press; 171-189

Matochik JA, Nordahl TE, Gross M, Semple WE, King AC, Cohen RM, Zametkin AJ. (1993) Effects of acute stimulant medication on cerebral metabolism in adults with hyperactivity. *Neuropsychopharmacology*, 8:377-86.

Mattson SN, Riley EP, Sowell ER, Jernigan TL, Sobel DF, Jones KL.(1996) A decrease in the size of the basal ganglia in children with fetal alcohol syndrome. *Alc. Clin. & Exp. Res*; 20:1088-93.

Mayes SD, Crites DL, Bixler EO, Humphrey FJ, Mattison RE.(1994) Methylphenidate and ADHD: Influence of age, IQ and neurodevelopmental status. *Dev Med Child Neurol*; 36:1099-1.

Mayes, LC (2000) A developmental perspective on the regulation of arousal states. Seminars in Perinatology, Vol. 24, No.4, 267-279

Mc Clellan, J, Werry, J (2003)Evidence -based treatments in child and adolescent psychiatry: an inventory. *J Amer Acad Child Adolesc Psychiatry*, 42: 1388-1400

Means LW, Medlin CW, Hughes VD, Gray SL.(1984) Rats exposed in utero to ethanol are hyperresponsive to methylphenidate when tested as neonates or adults. *Neurobehav Toxicol Teratol*; 6:18.

Milberger S, Biederman J, Farone SV, Murphy J, Tsuang MT.(1995) Attention deficit hyperactivity disorders: Issues of overlapping syndromes. *Am J. Psychiatry*; 152:1793-1799.

Mirsky AF, Anthony BJ, Duncan CC, Ahern MB, Kellam SG.(1991) Analysis of the elements of atttention: A neuropsychological approach. *Neuropsychological Review*; 2:75- 88.

The MTA Co-Operative Group.(1999) Moderators and mediators of treatment response for children with ADHD: The multi-modal treatment study of children with ADHD. *Arch Gen Psy* ; 56:1088-1096.

Nanson JL, Hiscock (1990) M. Attention deficits in children exposed to alcohol prenatally. *Alcohol Clin Exp Res* ; 5:656-661.

Niswander, KR, Gordon, M (1972) The women and their pregnancies; The collaborative perinatal study of the National Institute of Neurological Diseases and Stroke., Saunders, Philadelphia,

Oesterheld JR, Kofoed L, Tervo R, Fogas B, Wilson A, Fiechtner H.(1998) Effectiveness of methylphenidate in native american children with fetal alcohol syndrome and attention deficit /hyperactivity disorder: A controlled pilot study. *Journal of Child and Adolescent Psychopharmacology*; 8:39-48.

Oesterheld J, O'Malley K.D(1999). Are ADHD and FAS really that similar? Iceberg, Vol.9, 1,7.

Olegard R, Sabel KG, Aronson M, Sanding B, Johansson PR, Carlsson C, Kyllerman M, Iversen K, Hrbek A (1979). Effects on the child of alcohol abuse during pregnancy-retrospective and prospective studies. Acta Paediatrica Scandinavia ; 275; suppl. 112-21.

O'Malley KD.(1994) Fetal alcohol effect and ADHD *J Amer Acad Child Adolesc Psychiatry*; 33:1059-1060.

O'Malley KD(1997). Medication therapy's role for FAS. Iceberg ; 7:1,3-4

O'Malley KD, Hagerman RJ.(1998) Developing clinical practice guidelines for pharmacological interventions with alcohol-affected children. In: Centres for Disease Control and Prevention, Editors. Intervening with children affected by prenatal alcohol exposure: Proceedings of a special focus session of the interagency coordinating committee on fetal alcohol syndrome. Chevy Chase, MD: National Institute on Alcohol Abuse and Alcoholism; 145-177.

O'Malley K.D, Koplin B, Dohner VA(2000). Psychostimulant response in Fetal Alcohol Syndrome. *Can J of Psychiatry*; 45; 90-91.

O'Malley, KD & Nanson, J (2002) Clinical implications of a link between fetal alcohol spectrum disorder and ADHD, *Can J Psychiatry*, 47; 349-354

O'Malley, KD & Storoz, L(2003) Fetal alcohol spectrum disorder and ADHD: diagnostic implications and therapeutic consequences Expert Review of Neurotherapeutics, Vol. 3, No. 4, 477-489

O'Malley, KD & Streissguth, AP (2006) Clinical intervention and support for children aged zero to five years with fetal alcohol spectrum disorders and their parents/caregivers, Revised, 2006, In Tremblay RE, Barr RG, Peters, RDeV, eds. Encyclopedia on early childhood development (on line) Montreal, Quebec, Centre of Excellence for Early Childhood Development, available at http://www.excellence-earlychildhood.ca/documents/OMalley-StreissguthANGnp.rev.pdf

Pasamanick B, Knoblock, H & Lilienfeld, AM (1956) Socioeconomic status and some precursors of neuropsychiatric disorders. *Amer J Orthopsychiatry*, 26, 594-601

Pasamanick, B & Knoblock, H(1966) Retrospective studies on the epidemiology of reproductive casuality; Old and new. Merrill-Palmer Quarterly of Behavior and Development, 12, 7-26

Pike A, Plomin, R(1996) Importance of nonshared environmental factors for childhood and adolescent psychopathology, J Amer Acad Child Adolesc. Psychiatry, 35(5): 560-570

Pliszka SR, McCracken JT, Maas JW (1996). Catecholamines in attention deficit hyperactivity disorder current perspectives. *J Am Acad Child Adolesc Psychiatry*; 35:264-272.

Pollard, TD (2002) The future of biomedical research. From the inventory of genes to understanding physiology and the molecular basis of disease *JAMA*, Vol. 287, No. 13, 1725,1727

Rapoport J.L.(2000) The Development of Neurodevelopmental Psychiatry, *Am. J. Psychiatry*, 157, 2, 159 -161

Reiss S, Aman MG.(1998) Psychotropic medication and developmental disabilities: The international consensus handbook. In: Reiss S, Aman MG, editors. Columbus, OH: The Ohio State University Nisonger Center;

Rice, D, Barone, S(2000) critical periods of vulnerability for the developing nervous system: evidence from humans and animal models. *Environmental Health Perspectives*, Vol.108, Supplement 3, 511-533

Riley, E.P (1990). The long-term behavioral effects of prenatal alcohol exposure in rats. *Alcoholism, Clinical & Experimental Research*; 14: 670-3.

Rutter M.(1977) Brain damage syndromes in childhood: Concepts and findings. *Journal of Child Psychology and Psychiatry*; 18:1-21.

Rutter, M(1983) Developmental Neuropsychiatry, Churchill Livingstone, London/Edinburgh, UK

Sampson PD, Streissguth AP, Bookstein FL, Little RE, Clarren SK, Dehaene P, Hanson J, W, Graham JM.(1997) Incidence of Fetal Alcohol Syndrome and the Prevalence of Alcohol-Related Neurodevelopmental Disorder. Teratology ; 56:317-326

Schacher R, Tannich R.(1993) Childhood hyperactivity and psychostimulants. A review of extended treatment studies. *J Amer Child Adol Psychopharmacol*; 3:81.

Schachter, HM, Pham, B, King, J, Langford, S, Moher, D,(2001) How efficacious and safe is short -acting methylphenidate for the treatment of attention-deficit disorder in children and adolescents? A meta-analysis. *CMAJ*, 165 (11), 1475-1488

Skuse, DH (2000) Behavioral neuroscience and child psychopathology: insights from model systems. *Child Psychol Psychiat*, Vol. 41, No. 1,3-31

Snyder J, Nanson J, Snyder, RE, Block GW.(1997) Stimulant efficacy in children with FAS. In: Streissguth A., Kanter J. editors. The challenge of fetal alcohol syndrome: Overcoming secondary disabilities. Seattle, WA: University of Washington Press; 64-77

Sprenger DL, Josephson AM.(1998) Integration of pharmacotherapy and family therapy in the treatment of children and adolescents. *J Am Child Adolesc Psychiatry*; 37:887-889.

Stevenson J.(1992) Evidence for a genetic etiology in hyperactivity in children. Beh Genet; 22:337-343.

Stahl, SM(2002) Essential Psychopharmacology, Cambridge University Press, UK

Stratton KR, Howe CJ, Battaglia FC(1996). Fetal alcohol syndrome: Diagnosis, Epidemiology, Prevention and Treatment. In: Institute of Medicine, editors. Washington (DC): National Academy Press; .

Streissguth AP.(1997) Fetal alcohol syndrome: A guide for families and communities. Baltimore: Brooks Publishing Co..

Streissguth AP, Barr HM, Martin DC.(1984a) Alcohol exposure in utero and functional deficits in children during the first four years of life. In: Mechanisms of alcohol damage in utero, Ciba Foundation Symposium, Pitman, London; 176-196.

Streissguth AP, Martin DC, Barr HM, MacGregor Sandman B, Kircher GL, Darby BL (1984b) Intrauterine alcohol and nicotine exposure: Attention and reaction time in 4 year old children. *Developmental Psychology*; 20: 553-541.

Streissguth AP, Clarren SK, Jones KL(1985). Natural History of the Fetal Alcohol Syndrome: A 10-year follow-up of eleven patients. Lancet , 85-91.

Streissguth AP, Barr HM, Kogan J, Bookstein FL.(1996) Understanding the Occurrence of Secondary Disabilities in Clients with Fetal Alcohol Syndrome (FAS) Fetal Alcohol Effect (FAE) (Technical report 96-0). Final Report to the Centers for Disease Control and Prevention. August . Seattle: University of Washington, Fetal Alcohol and Drug Unit.

Streissguth AP, O'Malley KD(2000). Neuropsychiatric implications and long term consequences of fetal alcohol spectrum disorders. Seminars in Clinical Neuropsychiatry, 5:177-189

Streissguth, AP, Bookstein, FL, Barr HM, Sampson, PD, O'Malley, KD, Kogan Young J(2004) Risk factors for adverse risk outcomes in fetal alcohol syndrome and fetal alcohol effects. *Developmental and Behavioral Pediatrics*, Vol. 25, No. 4, 228-238

Sulik KK, Johnston MC, Webb MA.(1981) Fetal alcohol syndrome: embryogenesis in a mouse model. *Science;* 214:936-8.

Thapar, A, Holmes, J, Poulton, K, Harrington, R (1999) Genetic basis of attention deficit and hyperactivity, *Brit. J Psychiatry*, 174, 105-111

Thomas A. & Chess S.(1977) Temperament and Development. New York: Brunner /Mazel,

Thomas, JD La Fiette, MH, Quinn VR, Riley, EP(2002) Neonatal choline supplementation ameliorates the effects of prenatal alcohol exposure on a discrimination learning task in rats. *Neurotoxicology and Teratology*, 22 (5), 703-711

Tomkins, DM, Sellers, EM(2001) Addiction and the brain: the role of neurotransmitters in the cause and treatment of drug dependence. *CMAJ*, 164(6), 817-821

Ulug S, Riley EP(1983). The effect of methylphenidate on overactivity in rats prenatally exposed to alcohol. *Neurobehav Toxicol Teratol,* 5:35-39.

Van Groll BJ, Appel JB.(1992) Stimulant effects of D-amphetamine 1; DA mechanisms. *Pharmacol Biochem Behav*; 43:967-973.

Vitiello, B*(2001)* Methylphenidate in the treatment of children with attention-deficit hyperactivity disorder, *CMAJ*, 165, (11) 1505-1506

Volkow N, Wang GJ, Fowler JL, Angrist B, Hitzemann R, Lieberman J, Pappas N.(1997) Effects of methylphenidate on regional brain glucose metabolism in humans: Relationship to dopamine D2 receptors. *American Journal of Psychiatry;* 154:50-55.

Waldman I. (1997) Transmission disequilibrium tests of the association of DRD4 and DAT to symptoms of ADHD. presented at World Congress of Psychiatric Genetics, Santa Fe, NM

Weinberg NZ(1997). Cognitive and behavioral deficits associated with parental alcohol use. *J Am Acad Child Adolesc Psychiatry*; 36:1177-1186.

Wittenberg J.V.(2001) Regulatory Disorders: A New Diagnostic Classification for Diffficult Infants and Toddlers, *The Canadian Journal of Diagnosis*, September; 111 – 123

In: ADHD and Fetal Alcohol Spectrum Disorders (FASD)   ISBN: 1-59454-573-1
Editor: Kieran D. O'Malley, pp. 69-93   © 2007 Nova Science Publishers, Inc.

Chapter 5

THE ROLE OF THERAPEUTIC INTERVENTION WITH SUBSTANCE ABUSING MOTHERS: PREVENTING FASD IN THE NEXT GENERATION

Therese Grant[*], Julie Youngblood Pedersen,
Nancy Whitney and Cara Ernst

INTRODUCTION

Maternal alcohol and drug abuse during pregnancy is a serious public health problem that incurs risk for both mother and child. For the mother, substance abuse is associated with increased risk of prenatal complications, sexually transmitted diseases, depression, and domestic violence. For the child, prenatal exposure carries the potential for neonatal complications, lifelong neurodevelopmental damage, and the likelihood of a compromised home environment.

Alcohol is legal and widely available, so it is not surprising that among pregnant women alcohol drinking is more prevalent than illicit drug use. In population-based studies, approximately 10.1% of pregnant women reported drinking any alcohol during the previous month (Centers for Disease Control and Prevention [CDC], 2004), compared to 3.7% reporting drug use (Substance Abuse and Mental Health Services Administration [SAMHSA], 2002). The irony is that alcohol is a known teratogen whose neurobehavioral effects are more harmful than cocaine and other illicit substances of abuse (Jacobsen, Jacobson, and Sokol, 1994; Jacobson, Jacobsen, and Sokol, 1994; Coles, Platzman, Smith, James, and Falek, 1992; Institute of Medicine [IOM], 1996). Prenatal alcohol exposure puts children at risk for fetal alcohol syndrome (FAS), a permanent birth defect and a leading cause of mental retardation and neurodevelopmental disorders. FAS and related fetal alcohol

[*] For more information about the Parent-Child Assistance Program (PCAP) contact: Therese Grant, Ph.D. Director, Washington State Parent-Child Assistance Program; University of Washington; Department of Psychiatry and Behavioral Sciences; 180 Nickerson, Suite 309; Seattle, WA 98109; Phone: 206-543-7155 Fax: 206-685-2903; E-mail: granttm@u.washington.edu; http://depts.washington.edu/pcapuw/inhouse/index.html

spectrum disorders (FASD) are tragedies that know no socioeconomic, race, or age boundaries.

FAS and FASD are entirely preventable, a fact that was a compelling impetus for us as we developed the Parent-Child Assistance Program (PCAP). The purpose of this chapter is to describe the PCAP intervention, and examine how PCAP therapeutic strategies help prevent births of alcohol and drug exposed children in the next generation.

BACKGROUND

PCAP began in 1991 at the University of Washington as a federally-funded research demonstration designed to test the efficacy of an intensive, 3-year advocacy/case management model with high-risk mothers and their children. The primary aim of the model was to prevent subsequent alcohol and drug exposed births among birth mothers who abused alcohol and/or drugs during an index pregnancy. Research findings demonstrated the model's efficacy (Ernst, Grant, Streissguth, and Sampson, 1999; Grant, Ernst, and Pagalilauan, 2003), and the Washington State legislature subsequently funded PCAP to develop sites in seven counties, creating a capacity to serve over 500 families statewide. The model has been replicated at numerous other sites in the United States and Canada.

In 1999 PCAP broadened eligibility criteria to enroll a limited number of women who themselves have FASD, and who have surprisingly poor access to even the most basic community amenities. Access to services is critical because individuals with FASD are at risk for a host of adverse life outcomes (including homelessness, untreated mental illness, physical/sexual abuse, domestic violence) unless environmental risk factors are decreased and protective factors enhanced (Streissguth et al., 2004). Women with FASD who become pregnant have a high likelihood of drinking during pregnancy and delivering a next generation of children with this same birth defect, particularly if their lives are impaired by these kinds of dire life circumstances (Grant, Ernst, Streissguth, and Porter, 1997; Streissguth, Porter, and Barr, 2001).

A PROFILE OF THE MOTHERS

Women are eligible to enroll in PCAP who: 1) are pregnant or up to six months postpartum; 2) abused alcohol and/or drugs heavily during the pregnancy; and 3) are ineffectively engaged with community service providers. Enrollment in PCAP does not require that a woman have confirmed or suspected FASD.

At enrollment, most PCAP clients' lives are characterized not only by substance abuse, but by problems that result from a dysfunctional upbringing and chaotic lifestyle (Table 1) (Grant, Ernst, Streissguth, Stark, 2005). The typical PCAP client was born to substance abusing parents. She was physically and/or sexually abused as a child, she did not complete high school and began to use alcohol and drugs herself as a teenager. She is now in her late 20s, has been in jail more than once, and has been through drug treatment and relapsed. She does not use birth control or plan her pregnancies, and now has three or more children, with at least one in the foster care system. She is abused by her current partner, her housing situation is unstable, and her main source of income is welfare.

Table 1. Baseline Demographics and Characteristics of Participants in the Original Demonstration (1991-1995) and the Seattle and Tacoma PCAP Replications (1996-2003)

	Original Demonstration (N=60) *mean or n (%)*		Seattle Replication (N=76) *mean or n (%)*		Tacoma Replication (N=80) *mean or n (%)*		Replications Combined (N=156) *mean or n (%)*	
Age (mean yrs)	27.6		28.7		28.4		28.6	
Education (mean yrs)	11.5		10.7		10.8		10.8	
High school diploma/GED	31/60	(52)	32/75	(43)	38/80	(48)	70/155	(45)
Race								
White	18/60	(30)	29/76	(38)	45/80	(56)	74/156	(47)
African American	27/60	(45)	32/76	(42)	25/80	(31)	57/156	(37)
Native American	10/60	(17)	7/76	(9)	7/80	(9)	14/156	(9)
Other (Hispanic, Asian)	5/60	(8)	8/76	(11)	3/80	(4)	11/156	(7)
Married	2/60	(3)	12/76	(16)	11/80	(14)	23/156	(15)
Number prior children	2.1		2.1		2.3		2.2	
Living with mother (mean)	0.8		0.5		0.8		0.7	
Primary income source								
Public Assistance	50/60	(83)	60/76	(79)	50/80	(63)	110/156	(71)
Stable housing	28/60	(47)	34/76	(45)	42/80	(53)	76/156	(49)
Childhood risk indicators								
Parent(s) abused alcohol/drugs	40/53	(75)	56/67	(84)	61/71	(86)	117/138	(85)
Physical/sexual abuse	40/62	(65)	61/76	(80)	59/79	(75)	120/155	(77)
Adult risk indicators								
Domestic violence, current partner	10/57	(18)	29/54	(54)	22/70	(31)	51/124	(41)
Ever incarcerated	47/59	(80)	62/75	(83)	66/79	(84)	128/154	(83)

Women who fit this bleak description have been vilified in a social and political climate suggesting that alcohol/drug-addicted mothers are responsible for a variety of social ills (Greenhouse, 2000; Nelson and Marshall, 1998; Paltrow, Cohen, and Carey, 2000; Will, 1999). They have been labeled unmotivated and difficult to reach, and many professionals have come to view them as a hopeless population. Not surprisingly, chronic substance-abusing women become distrustful of "helping" agencies. Yet alienation from community resources only exacerbates the problem. The result is that those women at highest risk for delivering children with serious medical, developmental and behavioral problems are the least likely to seek and receive prenatal care and other assistance from community resources designed to help them.

Some suggest the real victims of maternal substance abuse are the children, and question the wisdom of investing scarce resources on mothers who are unlikely to change. The PCAP model was developed because we understand that these mothers *were themselves* the abused and neglected children of just a decade or two ago. They were born into troubled families, and grew into young women who used alcohol and drugs and delivered babies born into the same circumstances as their mothers had been. Social welfare, medical, and educational systems, if available, were not able to break this ongoing cycle of deprivation. Turning our backs on mothers because they are difficult to work with does not make their problems go away. It does ensure that these women will continue to experience a host of problems associated with intergenerational substance abuse, and continue to bear children who suffer in turn. PCAP undertook the challenge to find a way to connect with this population.

Co-Occurring Disorders Among Birth Mothers

Substance abuse among American women co-occurs with mental disorders at high rates. In 2002, almost 6 percent of adult women (6.4 million) were estimated to have a substance use disorder in the past year. Of these, approximately 30% (almost 2 million) had both a substance use disorder and a serious mental disorder as defined by DSM-IV (SAMHSA, 2004). The most common psychiatric conditions co-morbid with substance abuse are anxiety and affective disorders, primarily major depression (Kessler et al., 1997). Substance abusing pregnant women similarly have a high incidence of co-occurring psychological distress (Miles, Svikis, Kulstad, and Haug, 2001) and depressive symptoms (Burns, Melamed, Burns, Chasnoff, and Hatcher, 1985; Marcenko and Spence, 1995). The burden of mental health problems coupled with substance abuse makes the treatment prognosis worse than for either problem alone (Bobo, McIlvain, and Leed-Kelly, 1998; Greenfield et al., 1998; Driessen et al., 2001).

Among people who have FASD or suspected FASD there is an even higher prevalence of mental health problems (Famy, Streissguth, and Unis, 1998; Streissguth et al., 2004). Among PCAP clients statewide, 129/445 (29%) reported that their mothers were heavy drinkers during their pregnancy with them (11 had an actual FASD diagnosis). Among the 129, all had a substance abuse disorder (the condition that made them eligible for PCAP), and 61/129 (47%) reported having received a diagnosis of a co-occurring mental health disorder in the past. The eleven young women with diagnoses of FASD had a mean IQ of 82. Ten had been sexually abused and seven physically abused. Six reported having a formal psychiatric diagnosis: bipolar disorder (4), depression (1), or schizophrenia (1). The clients were assessed by the Brief Symptom Inventory (BSI), a screening for psychiatric illness. Mean BSI scores for the group were greater than 1.0 SD above standardized means on six of nine primary symptom dimensions, and six of the women had a total score suggesting the need for more extensive psychiatric assessment (Grant, Huggins, Connor, and Streissguth, 2005).

The PCAP Intervention

PCAP is an advocacy/case management model that offers personalized support over three years, a period of time long enough for the process of gradual and realistic change to occur. The primary aim of the intervention is to prevent future alcohol and drug exposed births among high-risk mothers who have already delivered at least one exposed child. To achieve this aim, trained and supervised PCAP case managers with a caseload of 15 to 20 families each, work with clients for 3 years beginning during pregnancy or within six months after the birth of an index child.

PCAP case management is not delivered according to a specific model of behavioral intervention. Instead, case managers develop a positive, empathic relationship with their clients, offer regular home visitation, and help the women address a wide range of environmental problems. A foremost task is to assist clients in obtaining alcohol and drug treatment and staying in recovery. Case managers connect women and their families with existing community services and teach them how to access those services themselves, coordinate services among this multidisciplinary network, assist clients in following through with provider recommendations, and assure that the children are in safe home environments and receiving appropriate health care.

When we ask former clients what made the program work for them, we consistently hear "persistence": "My case manager never gave up on me. She kept believing in me until I finally started to believe in myself."

PCAP Outcomes and Cost Effectiveness

Future alcohol and drug exposed births can be prevented in one of two ways: by helping women avoid alcohol and drug use during pregnancy, or by helping them avoid becoming pregnant if they are using alcohol or drugs. We compared PCAP intervention findings from two different cohort experiences in Washington State: the original demonstration (OD) (1991-1995) and the Seattle/Tacoma replications (1996-2003) (Grant, Ernst, Streissguth and Stark, 2005). Compared to the OD, outcomes at the replication sites were either improved (alcohol/drug treatment completed; abstinence from alcohol/drugs; subsequent delivery unexposed to alcohol or drugs) or maintained (regular use of contraception and use of a reliable method; number of subsequent deliveries during the program) (Table 2) (Grant, Ernst, Streissguth, Stark, 2005).

On program exit, at PCAP replication sites we found that 65% of the 78 prenatal binge drinkers were no longer at present risk of having another alcohol or drug exposed pregnancy, either because they were using a reliable contraceptive method (31%), or had been abstinent from alcohol/drugs for at least 6 months (23%), or both (12%). Based on state subsequent birth rates and the estimated incidence of FAS among heavy drinkers, we estimate that PCAP prevented at least one and up to 3 new cases of FAS. The cost of the PCAP program is approximately $15,000 per client for the 3-year program including intervention, administration and evaluation. The estimated average lifetime cost for an individual with FAS is $1.5 million (Harwood, Fountain, and Livermore, 1998; Rice, 1993). If PCAP prevented just one new case of FAS, the estimated lifetime cost savings is equivalent to the cost of the PCAP intervention for 102 women. A 2004 independent economic analysis by the Washington State Institute for Public Policy found an average net benefit of $6197 per client among selected well researched home visiting programs, including PCAP, for at-risk families in the U.S. (Aos, Lieb, Mayfield, Miller, and Pennucci, 2004).

**Table 2. Exit Outcomes at 3 Sites: Original Demonstration (1991–1995)
and the Seattle and Tacoma Replication Sites (1996–2003)**

	Original Demonstration (N=60) n (%)	Seattle Replication (N=76) n (%)	Tacoma Replication (N=80) n (%)	Replications Combined (N=156) n (%)
Alcohol/drug treatment				
Inpatient or outpatient	31/60 (52)	58/76 (76)	58/80 (73)	116/156 (74)
Inpatient	28/60 (47)	41/76 (54)	49/80 (61)	90/156 (58)
Outpatient	21/60 (35)	45/76 (59)	34/80 (43)	79/156 (51)
Other (e.g, AA, counseling)	27/60 (45)	55/76 (72)	39/80 (49)	94/156 (60)
Abstinence from alcohol/drugs				
≥ 6 mo at program exit	17/60 (28)	33/76 (43)	31/80 (39)	64/156 (41)
≥ 1 year at program exit	10/60 (17)	26/76 (34)	26/80 (33)	52/156 (33)
Abstinence ≥ 1 yr during program	22/60 (37)	45/76 (59)	37/80 (46)	82/156 (53)
Family planning and subsequent birth				
Regular contraceptive use	44/60 (73)	56/76 (74)	57/80 (71)	113/156 (72)
Reliable method	26/60 (43)	37/76 (49)	42/80 (53)	79/156 (51)
Subsequent birth during program	17/60 (28)	22/76 (29)	20/80 (25)	42/156 (27)
Unexposed to alcohol/drugs	3/17 (18)	7/22 (32)	8/20 (40)	15/42 (36)
Primary income source				
Public Assistance	30/60 (50)	20/76 (26)	21/80 (26)	41/156 (26)
Employment	7/60 (12)	22/76 (29)	23/80 (29)	45/156 (29)
Index child Custody at 3 years				
Biological mother	28/54 (52)	43/76 (57)	45/79 (57)	88/155 (57)
Other family	10/54 (19)	10/76 (13)	16/79 (20)	26/155 (17)
Adopted	2/54 (4)	10/76 (13)	11/79 (14)	21/155 (14)
State foster care	14/54 (26)	13/76 (17)	7/79 (9)	20/155 (13)
Regular well-child care	35/38 (92)	51/53 (96)	58/61 (95)	109/114 (96)

THEORETICAL FOUNDATIONS AND CORRESPONDING INTERVENTION STRATEGIES

Relational Theory

The PCAP model draws on the concept of relational theory, which emphasizes the importance of positive interpersonal relationships in women's growth, development, and definition of self (Miller, 1991), and in their addiction, treatment, and recovery (Finkelstein, 1993). The relationship aspect of intensive intervention—"having a person to talk to who really cared"—may be more critical to improvement than the concrete services received (Pharis and Levin, 1991).

Building on this concept, PCAP hires ethnically diverse case managers with shared history and cultural experiences, who understand clients in a way that allows them to gain access and build rapport with women who might otherwise be unapproachable. PCAP case managers have each faced at least one significant obstacle to well-being, for example, domestic violence, poverty, single parenting, an alcoholic parent, or personal alcohol or drug abuse. More importantly, each has overcome the obstacle and achieved significant success, for example, by going back to school or maintaining steady and meaningful employment. When a PCAP clinical supervisor assigns a new client to a case manager, she does not necessarily make the assignment based on race or ethnicity in common. Instead, it is the case managers' life struggles and successes that enable them to be positive and credible role models, offering their clients hope and motivation grounded in reality. For example, among the statewide PCAP staff, approximately 60% formerly used or abused alcohol or drugs, but all had been clean and sober for at least 6 years at the time they were hired.

PCAP case managers are paraprofessionals in the sense that they are uncredentialed in helping professions such as nursing or social work. However, the model requires more of its case managers than most programs that use paraprofessionals. Prior to hire, PCAP case managers must have at least four years of community-based experience related to prenatal substance abuse or associated problems, or the equivalent combination of education and experience.

> "I know what it's like to be a single parent, homeless, and on welfare. I share a common ground with my clients as far as those things go. The difference is that I saw what the obstacles were, and overcame them. I just kept moving ahead and learned that where there's a will, there's a way". — PCAP Case Manager

Stages of Change

PCAP incorporates stages-of-change paradigms and motivational interviewing strategies. The approach recognizes that clients will be at different stages of readiness for change at different times, and that ambivalence about changing addictive behavior is normal (Miller and Rollnick, 1991).

The constructs of stages-of-change and self-efficacy dovetail (Olds, Kitzman, Cole and Robinson, 1997; Sherman, Sanders and Yearde, 1998). Self-efficacy is the belief in one's ability to perform in ways that will produce desired outcomes, and expectations about self-efficacy are influenced most powerfully by an individual's own past accomplishments (Bandura, 1977). A client's self-efficacy determines whether she will begin a behavior, put the required effort into it, and maintain her efforts.

PCAP case managers understand that for clients who have never experienced competence and accomplishment, each small step toward rebuilding her life is a risk the woman takes deserving of attention and encouragement. Case managers have a positive influence on clients' efficacy expectations, motivational states, and, ultimately, behavior by:

- providing clients with concrete, practical opportunities to accomplish goals of abstinence, recovery, and social adjustment;
- helping clients recognize and celebrate each step toward performance achievements;
- offering ongoing verbal and emotional encouragement regardless of temporary setbacks or relapse;
- role-modeling, as someone who has achieved personal goals similar to those the client may be aiming toward; and

- helping clients learn daily coping strategies, including compliance with mental health recommendations and medication regimens in order to avoid negative emotional mood states.

    "You wait for that tiny indication that the client sees the way and is ready to change. Then you reach out at the right time to help her move along. I have hope and faith in people. I really believe they want to change if they say they do." — PCAP Case Manager

Harm Reduction

The framework of the PCAP intervention was influenced by harm reduction theory. Harm reduction is based on the assumption that alcohol and drug addiction and the associated risks can be placed along a continuum, with the goal being to help a client move along this continuum from excess to moderation, and ultimately to abstinence, in order to reduce the harmful consequences of the habit (Marlatt and Tapert, 1993). In this view, "any steps toward decreased risk are steps in the right direction" (Marlatt, Somers and Tapert, 1993, p. 148).

In practice, case managers focus attention not simply on reducing alcohol and drug use, but on reducing other risk behaviors and addressing the health and social well-being of the clients and their children. For example, an important PCAP goal is to reduce the incidence of future drug and alcohol-exposed births. While not every client will be able to become abstinent from alcohol and drugs, harm can be reduced by encouraging the woman to use effective family planning methods to avoid becoming pregnant if she is still using.

Case Manager Training

Comprehensive ongoing training is essential to a successful paraprofessional program. Formal training sessions on relevant topics are conducted by professionals at the beginning of the project and throughout the program (Grant, Ernst, and Streissguth, 1999). PCAP supervisors arrange training sessions with representatives from key provider agencies (e.g., Child Protective Services, Planned Parenthood) so case managers can learn the dynamics of the agencies and work more effectively with them, and for agency staff to be introduced to the role of the case managers. Their familiarity with the PCAP model and with individual staff members enhances our ability to address specific service barriers encountered by clients and resolve them more quickly. Case managers attend community trainings offered by health and social services agencies in the area in order to increase their knowledge-base and to establish contacts and share strategies with providers who encounter similar issues working with a substance-abusing population.

Therapeutic Aspects of the Intervention

The PCAP intervention is a therapeutic process between case managers and their clients that develops and grows over the course of the program. The process allows for a client's gradual transition from initial dependence on the case manager's assistance and support, to interdependence as they work together to accomplish steps toward goals, to independence as the client begins to trust in herself as a worthwhile and capable person, and learns the skills necessary to manage her life.

Establishing the Relationship

Case managers and clients begin by getting to know each other and establishing the trust that will enable them to work closely together for three years. This bonding process sometimes takes months for clients whose lifelong experiences of abuse and abandonment taught them not to trust anyone. They find that time spent in the car with a client is valuable because they can talk together at length with relatively little distraction; they do not have to make eye contact if a woman is uncomfortable with that, and silences are not uneasy.

At the first home visit, the case manager identifies and addresses immediate problems such as obtaining clothes and diapers for the newborn or locating temporary housing; activities that demonstrate from the beginning that the case manager cares and can be trusted to follow through. Within the first few weeks, the case manager sets the ground rules, or defines the nature of the relationship. She may explain:

- "We'll have a three-year working relationship, not a three-year friendship."
- "You can trust that I will be with you through ups and downs: there will be times you don't like me. It's okay if you disagree with me, but we have to keep communication open."
- "I'll always be truthful with you. I won't lie to you, or for you."
- "My role is not to continually respond to your crises, but to help you move beyond crisis and toward achieving your goals."
- "If you take one step, I'll take two."

Case managers work within the context of the client's family, and establish rapport with the other children, the husband or significant other, and members of the extended family. As mothers, our clients are at the center of this network of relationships, in which everyone is involved in some way with her substance abuse and related problems. Family members may have powerful influence over the woman, and they will all be affected by critical changes the woman makes as she attempts to break long established behavioral patterns. Gaining the family's trust is a preliminary step that then allows the case manager access and the opportunity to communicate with this important group throughout the intervention.

Clients sometimes disappear for weeks or months at a time, leaving the children with family members. Having a close relationship with the family allows the case manager to continue to provide services on behalf of the children, as well as to learn the whereabouts of the missing client. Most missing clients inevitably reconnect with their case manager when they experience a crisis event. A client may experience several cycles like this before she begins to recognize that she herself will have to change her behavior, that it's tremendously beneficial to have the advocate's help, and that the clock is ticking on her time left in the program.

Identifying Client Goals: Assessment and Planning

In treatment planning, the more individualized and accurate the client assessment, the more useful it will be. PCAP developed the "Difference Game" card sort assessment to enable clients and case managers to work together to identify client needs (Grant, Ernst, McAuliff, and Streissguth, 1997). The Game is easy to administer and interpret, is engaging and meaningful, and can be a powerful strategy for intervention when used as a stimulus for identifying client goals. Clients often know what needs to be changed, but because of low outcome expectancy and a poor sense of self-efficacy, they feel helpless and incompetent to begin to solve problems on their own.

The Difference Game is a concrete, hands-on activity. Adapted from a scale developed by Dunst et al. (1988), it consists of a set of 31 laminated cards, on each of which is written an item that is a possible client need (e.g. "housing," "drug or alcohol treatment," "more education") and including a "wild card" representing any additional need the client may choose. The case manager asks the client to sort the cards into two piles, those items that would "make a difference" in her life, and those that "no, would not make a difference." The client is then asked to select from the "yes" cards the 5 items that represent her most important needs. Finally, she ranks these 5 cards in order of her priorities.

The case manager and client use these top 5 cards as the basis for discussion and for planning a course of action that will "make a difference." The client identifies specific, meaningful goals that she would like to work on during the next 4 months, and together they come to an agreement about realistic steps they can take toward meeting those goals. They record each goal, the small steps required to reach the goal, and who will be responsible for accomplishing different tasks. It is critical that some of the steps, no matter how small, are attainable by the client in a 4-month period, because it is as she observes herself accomplishing desired behavior that her sense of self-efficacy develops.

Goals are evaluated and reestablished every 4 months because this length of time allows clients 1) to accomplish short-term, concrete tasks (e.g. complete paperwork for housing waiting lists, or enroll in a neighborhood parenting class), and 2) to make progress on long-term goals (e.g., enter long-term residential treatment). It is not unusual for a client to specify a single, major issue (e.g., stay in recovery, or not see a former abusive partner), as a continuous goal every 4 months throughout her PCAP participation.

The effectiveness of the Difference Game is that it requites the *client* to think about and choose her most meaningful priorities, instead of someone in a professional capacity determining those for her. The focus is on possibilities and desired outcomes as opposed to problems, weaknesses, or negative conditions. The Difference Game, used in conjunction with the development of meaningful goals, is a logical method that illustrates to clients within the context of their own lives the continuum from making a decision, to taking definite steps, to ultimately reaching a goal that makes a difference.

Case Study: Using the Difference Game With a Client

The following event occurred in a family preservation project. A client completed the Difference Game with her therapist, selecting the Wild Card as her top card and designating it as a "need for make-up." The therapist was less than optimistic about letting this client set the direction for case planning, but she nevertheless returned to the client and asked her to explain the "story" behind each card selected (and particularly the "make up" card, knowing there were more pressing issues in the family). The client's story revealed a problem she had previously been unwilling to talk about. For years her spouse had physically and emotionally abused her, and refused to let her wear cosmetics. The client believed if she could be courageous enough to wear make up, it would be the first step toward leaving the relationship and beginning a new life. The make-up was her symbol for change. The therapist supported the client's reasoning. The woman made a plan and successfully set it in motion over the following months.

Finding a Voice in the Service Provider Network

PCAP case managers do not provide direct services, such as substance abuse treatment or health care, but instead connect clients with appropriate providers and experts in the community. They provide practical assistance and emotional support to clients in a manner that cannot be duplicated by service providers who have high caseloads, specific agendas, and time constraints. Professional and agency effectiveness can increase when the case manager tackles barriers (e.g., lack of housing, transportation, and/or child care) that could otherwise hinder or defeat a provider's aims for a client. A physician, for example, can more fully focus on a family's health care needs when a case manager addresses the family's environmental issues.

In the initial stages of the intervention, PCAP clients typically have poor negotiating skills. The case manager role models telephone etiquette and interpersonal behavior that is likely to elicit support and help, and practices with the client. She helps the client organize her thoughts and articulate concerns and goals. After releases of information are signed, she arranges meetings or conference calls to bring members of a client's provider network together, with the client present whenever possible. The case manager functions as a liaison for communication within this network, and works to facilitate development of a service plan that gives voice to the client's needs, creates realistic expectations, and addresses providers' concerns. The case manager then helps the client follow through with the plan.

In practical terms, this strategy means that a mother in recovery will not be faced with trying to comply with a court's stipulation that she attend outpatient treatment five mornings a week in one part of town, while the housing authority assigns her to a unit in a neighborhood requiring her to make two bus transfers to get to treatment, and Child Protective Services grants her reunification with her two children with no contingencies for childcare (a true scenario). When a woman learns to speak up in a way that demonstrates respect for herself and others—and with her case manager as guide and advocate—providers will listen, recognize the realities of her circumstances, and design a plan that will help her succeed in her recovery, rather than set her up for another failure.

In some situations, a "strong arm" in the form of a written contract is beneficial, and clients are more likely to adhere to goals when they participate in establishing the concrete, logical steps of such a document. Case managers may work with clients and providers to draw up agreements that define explicit responsibilities and timelines. The case manager refers to the contract both in supporting her client and in upholding the position of an agency. Personalized agreements heighten service providers' awareness of the possibilities of working successfully with this high-risk population.

Role Modeling, Teaching Basic Skills

Role-modeling and teaching basic life skills are critical case manager strategies. It is clear that the clients' bleak backgrounds have done little to prepare them for adult life or parenting. For example, problems with landlords and bill collectors are common. Few of these women have lived in a household that was "managed," nor have they had adequate training to prepare them for basic functioning within an economic system. In addition, they may have cognitive impairment as a result of prenatal exposure to alcohol/drugs and their own years of substance abuse. Case managers find that the most effective teaching techniques with clients are those that are explicit, hands-on, and experiential.

"My case manager handled a lot of situations, and I learned through her how to deal with and talk to people." — PCAP Client

"My case manager had a big influence on me and how I deal with things in my life." — PCAP Client

The Mother/Infant Dyad

On the most basic level, case managers first help mothers attend to the quality of the home environment, to make it safe and comfortable for children. They help the mother learn to turn away former acquaintances who drop by to party with her, or who need a place to sleep. They help her learn how to reduce the level of stimulation from loud music and other noise, clean the house, and keep potentially harmful items out of the baby's reach. Because our clients typically live in low-income or substandard housing, case managers are frequently involved in extended negotiations with a landlord to make repairs in electrical wiring or broken windows.

As basic environmental needs are addressed, the case manager begins to give a mother information about her child's particular developmental stage, and teach her to have appropriate expectations. For example, a baby who is learning to pick up and eat Cheerios from a tray in front of her is likely to scatter the cereal. The case manager helps the mother learn to show the baby and demonstrate delight in her progress, rather than shout or slap because the baby "made a mess."

An important home visit activity is to simply help the mother observe the baby playing and responding to various stimuli. Case managers teach a mother to pay attention, to observe, and to understand that her baby has a personality and communicates with every facial expression and gesture. They may record with the mother what the baby can do as they observe and interact for 20 minutes, to illustrate to her the diversity and complexity of her baby's behavior. The case manager may then ask the mother to repeat this again before the next home visit,.

Interface with the Child Welfare System

PCAP staff are mandated to report child abuse and neglect. As regular home visitors, they are in a unique position to identify problems that may place children at grave risk in families who would otherwise have disappeared from notice by health and social service providers. They instigate removal of children from the home when necessary.

The issue of child custody is a recurrent theme in clients' lives because a majority of the women have had children removed from their care by the state. Regaining custody is a common goal stated by clients in their first year in the program, although case managers do not necessarily concur that reunification is in the best interests of the child/ren. The turning point for successful resolution of child custody issues occurs when the mother realistically comes to terms with her ability to parent, and is willing to consider the best interests of the child. For some mothers this means deciding to relinquish custody to a foster family who has bonded with the child and would like to adopt. For others it means staying in recovery and doing whatever is necessary to resume or maintain custody of her child/ren. Regardless of who has custody, case managers work on behalf of the child to secure a safe home environment and regular health care.

The following case study illustrates how case managers are able to continue to work with clients after reporting to Child Protective Services (CPS).

> C. delivered a medically fragile infant, and had custody of the baby after she was released from the hospital. It soon became obvious to the case manager that C. was using drugs, was not eating for days at a time, and was not capable of keeping the baby on a feeding and medication schedule. Her case manager was open and honest with C. and explained that she was recommending removal of the child by CPS until the mother could provide competent care. The baby was removed, and CPS wrote a contract with the mother stipulating drug treatment and parenting classes specific to medically fragile infants. Although C. was initially angry and distant with her, the case manager offered to help her comply with the CPS recommendations. The case manager attended parenting classes with C., maintained her trust, kept in close contact with the CPS social worker, and kept the client informed. C. completed 90 days of inpatient treatment, followed by six months of outpatient treatment. The CPS worker drafted a permanency plan stipulating that the baby be adopted by the foster mother, but the case manager intervened because C. was complying successfully with the written contract. The baby was ultimately returned to C. Her former boyfriend, a crack user, disappeared now that C. was mothering a special-needs child. C. began to believe in her worth as a person and in her abilities as a mother, fully and gratefully accepting responsibility for her child.

PCAP case managers teach clients about behaviors that are normal and appropriate for children of different ages; they role model alternative ways of responding to a child's behavior; they enroll clients in parenting classes and accompany them if necessary. Clients are sometimes impatient and harsh with their children, but case managers rarely observe signs of deliberate injury. If a case manager suspects that someone else in the household (for example, a boyfriend) is abusing a child, they involve the mother and Children's Protective Services with the immediate aim of stopping harm to the child. The next step is to teach the mother to pay attention and recognize problems, resist pressure from "friends" who pose a risk to her family, and protect her children (or lose them).

In general, PCAP and child welfare services work closely together. However, child welfare recommendations can be inconsistent depending on the social worker if decisions are based on biased attitudes and beliefs, or lack of information and experience. It is not uncommon for a woman to comply with her contract stipulations in order to regain custody of her child, only to learn that her social worker will recommend child removal at a court hearing. As advocates, PCAP case managers help clients comply with their individual contracts and act as liaisons between the agency and the client. They keep careful documentation and maintain releases of information so they can communicate with all parties, verify compliance or non-compliance, and advocate accordingly to uphold agreements made in the contract.

It is not uncommon for PCAP case managers to voice objections to child welfare workers over decisions to not investigate, or to close cases early without adequate follow-up oversight. This is particularly true in cases where the client is an alcoholic mother. Service providers do not necessarily understand that although alcohol is a legal substance not detectable on urine screening, it can be a dangerous drug. We know that a mother who has a chronic, untreated alcohol problem poses a serious risk to children in her care because of the potential for neglect, including malnutrition and accidents. In cases like these, PCAP case managers and/or supervisors make referrals to child welfare and continue to do home visits and maintain a watchful eye while the woman remains in the program. Clearly, our work is made more difficult if we do not have the strong arm of the civil agency charged with child protection. In extreme cases PCAP asks the police to go to a home and intervene on behalf of the children.

Accepting Setbacks

Any undertaking that requires a person to make fundamental changes in long established behavior patterns (for example, losing weight or quitting smoking) may entail setbacks. Relapse should not be a surprise in the recovery process, particularly among clients with a long history of drug or alcohol abuse. PCAP clients are not asked to leave the program because of noncompliance, setbacks, or relapse. Instead, they are taught to learn from their mistakes. This policy has resulted in clients' increased likelihood of overcoming shame after relapse, contacting the case manager quickly, resuming recovery (or treatment), and repairing the damage done. Case managers use relapse experiences to help clients examine events that triggered the setback, and to develop resiliency strategies. When a client is able to successfully rebound from a relapse event, she develops self-efficacy as she observes herself coping, overcoming a crisis, and moving on. Two PCAP Case Studies: Jane and Laurie

Jane

Jane was a Native American woman who enrolled in PCAP when she was 18 years old. Her birth mother had been an alcoholic and it was suspected that she drank heavily during her pregnancy with Jane. Jane was now pregnant with her first child and had been a heavy drinker during the first few months of the pregnancy.

As a baby Jane had been adopted by a middle class white family, and was subsequently raised only by her adopted father. Her youth was not that of a typical middle class child. She had difficulties in school. She frequently ran away and got into fights. By the time she was 14 she was in a group home for juveniles. One day she severely beat another girl, almost killing her. Jane was sent to a juvenile detention center until she was 17. When she was transitioned from there into another group home, Jane began using alcohol and marijuana again. Soon after her release at the age of 18, she moved in with a man nearly twice her age, became pregnant, and was referred to PCAP.

Not surprising, Jane was slow to trust her PCAP case manager and rarely asked for help. The case manager continued to call and show up at her home, offering help. Eventually, Jane began initiating the calls to ask for help. As a first time mother (and her partner a first time father), they needed assistance with the basics of parenting. The case manager spent a lot of time with both parents, on parenting skills, budgeting, and helping them communicate with each other. It was obvious that Jane had a hard time managing the demands of daily life.

The unexpected happened when Jane had a psychotic break, becoming extremely paranoid, hearing voices, expressing suicidal ideation and having thoughts of hurting her child. Her case manager facilitated Jane's admission to a psychiatric hospital where she was diagnosed with bipolar disorder. By now the case manager had a strong and trusting relationship with Jane, and had established herself as someone whose advice Jane could trust. This positive and close relationship helped Jane accept the diagnosis more readily, and she began outpatient psychiatric treatment and medication. Even though a Child Protective Services case was opened, she and her partner were able to retain custody of their child. After a year, Jane's mental illness symptoms stabilized. She left the father of her baby and entered art school. PCAP helped her obtain subsidized housing and connected her with a long-term case management program that would work with her after she left our program. At the time she left PCAP, she was sometimes struggling with her mental health condition, but she had a strong support network in place.

Laurie

Laurie was a typical PCAP client. She came from a family where drug use was the norm. She had been molested as a child. She was in family placements and foster care, and she never knew her father. She had been involved in gangs and her older brother had been murdered. Her mother and aunt were in prison for drug-related crimes. She herself had served time for a drug-related crime, and she was facing sentencing for another.

At age 29 she had just given birth to her second child. She had abused cocaine and alcohol throughout the pregnancy. Her 7 year old daughter had been removed from her care the year before, due to neglect. She had had a hard life and didn't trust anyone, but was willing to be in PCAP because she was told it would "look good" to Child Protective Services. But she didn't really want anyone in her business.

Her PCAP case manager had a hard time getting involved in Laurie's life. The case manager was only "allowed in" to help with things like clothes and transportation. There were many missed appointments. Still the case manager persisted. She left phone messages and notes, and sometimes visited the home unannounced.

After about a year in PCAP, the client's life fell apart. She was facing jail time and she became pregnant again. This time she turned to PCAP. With the case manager's help, Laurie completed inpatient substance abuse treatment for pregnant women. Upon discharge she continued with her outpatient treatment. The judge allowed home detention sentencing, provided she did not re-offend. Her housing situation stablized, she began mental health treatment, and she gave birth to a healthy son. She now recognized when she needed help and called her case manager *before* a crisis developed. She entered a welding program at the local community college and graduated. She invited her PCAP case manager to the graduation.

As she leaves PCAP, Laurie is in permanent stable housing, has obtained full-time employment, and is no longer on welfare. She has been clean from drugs and alcohol for over a year. She has regained custody of her older daughter. In addition she now has custody of her two younger sisters, who were being neglected in a family placement, so she is parenting a total of five children.

Had Laurie been enrolled in a typical social services program, she would have been discharged for non-compliance, or program services would have ended long before Laurie had learned the lessons that took time to learn. She would have lost custody of all of her children and she'd be back in prison. Lauries PCAP case manager was a persistent presence in her life, and was there when the client decided she wanted to change and needed help.

Strategies for Helping Mothers Enter and Complete Treatment

While it is desirable for a woman to acknowledge her own substance abuse problem and ask for help, it may not happen soon enough. Often the criminal or civil dependency court system will require the client to obtain treatment. Once in a treatment setting, clients have no choice but to hear the stories of other women like themselves, including those who acknowledge their addiction. In this setting they are able to detoxify, begin to listen, and examine their own lives. With the client's knowledge, PCAP case managers sometimes ask the court to mandate treatment, and find that these formerly resistant clients become some of our most successful.

Unwillingness to be separated from their children is the most common barrier to getting women to enter and stay in treatment. Long-term, gender-specific residential treatment programs are almost always the first choice of PCAP case managers for their clients, and we are fortunate to have these available in Washington State. These residential programs are designed for children to accompany their mothers, and for mothers to learn and practice their parenting skills for a period of up to 6 months. They give families an opportunity to live in a safe place, free of the chaotic environment to which they are accustomed. The extended length of stay gives mothers and their case managers time to set up the support systems they will need when they leave, particularly clean and sober housing.

PCAP case managers are familiar with the treatment programs in their area and establish good relationships with the administrators and counselors. They can facilitate admitting their client to the program they believe may be best suited to the client's needs. They are instrumental in walking women through the many steps required to become eligible for funding for treatment and medical care. Case managers find that it is important to gain the cooperation of the client's family and support system because they can be a source of motivation and practical help while the woman is in treatment. Women who are able to build connections with healthy, drug-free family members are most likely to succeed.

While women are in treatment, the PCAP case manager visits regularly to provide emotional support and problem-solve issues that may jeopardize her staying in treatment (for example, by supervising child visitation). They may support the client by helping her obtain clothes and toiletries; they may write letters of encouragement. They will participate in case staffing and discharge planning and help make plans for the woman's life after treatment, particularly by exploring options for safe, stable housing.

After leaving treatment, the PCAP case manager works with her client on immediate needs and long-term goals. While engaged in activities together they talk about stressors, relapse triggers, and relapse prevention strategies. Clients are most likely to succeed if they are active in after-care programs, so the case manager will introduce her to groups and will perhaps attend 12-step meetings with her until the client is comfortable attending alone.

Through all of this, the message is that the client can succeed. If a relapse occurs, it's a temporary setback and an opportunity to ask for help in getting back on track.

Strategies for Helping Mothers Choose a Family Planning Method

The family planning objectives of the Parent-Child Assistance Program are to reduce the incidence of future alcohol and drug-exposed births, and to reduce the incidence of unintended pregnancies. While we know that one way to achieve this is to motivate clients to use an appropriate family planning method, the choice to do so is entirely the client's. PCAP is not a pregnancy prevention program. Many clients who achieve a stable and sober lifestyle choose to become pregnant because for the first time they'll experience a healthy pregnancy and have the opportunity to raise their own child. Case managers help clients understand that sex is a natural and enjoyable part of life, and that "family planning" means planning pregnancy to occur at an optimal time.

It is essential that case managers connect clients with family planning clinics or health care providers who provide physical examinations, identify potential contraindications for specific birth control methods, and determine the safest and most appropriate method for the woman. Case managers who accompany their client to these visits can then review the material periodically to make sure the client understands. The necessary knowledge base includes:

- the basics of female and male anatomy;
- how family planning methods work and how they may be contraindicated because of a preexisting health condition;
- the range of family planning options available and what the options require from the client (some options may not be wise choices because of a client's life style);
- the side effects of various methods;
- the long-term health risks of unsafe sex: e.g., risks of contracting sexually transmitted diseases, hepatitis C.

Introducing the concept of family planning, educating, motivating, and helping a client obtain a method is not necessarily a straightforward process for reasons ranging from the intensely personal and familial, to those imposed by lawmakers or the insurance industry. The process takes time, and may involve setbacks, missed appointments, birth control side effects or failure, or subsequent unintended pregnancy. Understanding this can reduce case manager frustration. The important points are to be sensitive to the client's perspective, including cultural and religious factors, to follow-up and take the next step, and to be persistent in meeting client and program goals.

The conversation with a client about family planning will be an ongoing one. Case managers use motivational interviewing strategies to help clients examine the reality of their situation and the consequences of another pregnancy. The process is gradual and thoughtful so that decisions are long lasting, grounded in the client's own belief system, and based on her individual choices. PCAP case managers don't argue with clients about family planning because developing resistance and conflict will be counterproductive.

When a case manager introduces the topic of family planning, she often discovers that a client has already been thinking about it, or has tried a method previously. We may hear reservations like the following:

- "I am not sexually active now, so I don't think I need to use birth control."
- "I haven't gotten pregnant for the last 2 years and I haven't been using birth control, so why would I need it now?"
- "I tried it, but it made me gain weight."
- "I don't like to put chemicals in my body."

Case managers encourage clients to discuss previous experiences, fears, and expectations. It is especially helpful to acknowledge ambivalence and elicit ideas about the pros and cons of another pregnancy in very concrete terms. Case managers write down the client's ideas in her own words so the client can recognize her own thought processes when they revisit the topic. By not imposing concepts or suggestions that have no bearing on a client's beliefs and feelings, she demonstrates respect and avoids creating frustration on both parts.

Role modeling can be an important part of family planning intervention with clients, and particularly with women who have FASD. Case managers may choose to talk with their clients about methods they've used in the past, decision-making processes they've gone through, and what has worked well for them. In this way clients observe a person they respect taking care of themselves and making conscious choices.

As the case manager continues goal-setting exercises with the client every four months, they explore how having another child might affect the client's ability to achieve her objectives.

PCAP Intervention with Women Who Themselves Have FASD

While neuropsychological deficits and other adverse outcomes associated with prenatal alcohol exposure have been well documented for over 30 years, interventions for individuals with FASD have not been systematically developed and evaluated. In 1999 PCAP expanded its eligibility criteria to enroll a sample of women with FASD. In 2001 we conducted a 12-month pilot study to examine more specifically how these women could be helped within the existing framework of PCAP (Grant et al., 2004). A total of 19 clients with FASD (n = 11) or suspected FASD (n = 8) were enrolled in the pilot study. Their average age was 22 years, most were unmarried (84%) and poorly educated (47% had a 9th grade education or less), and almost all had been physically or sexually abused as children (94%). Among the 15 who were mothers, the mean number of children was 2.3 (range 1-6); on average, only half of the children were living with their biologic mother. All reported many unmet basic service needs.

In considering the special cognitive deficits associated with FASD, we realized that to meet the needs of these women we would have to develop specific strategies to increase connection to community services and improve quality of services delivered. The pilot community intervention consisted of delivery of the standard PCAP model enhanced in two ways: 1) by modifying PCAP in order to accommodate clients with FASD; and 2) by educating community service providers to accommodate clients with FASD.

Modifying PCAP to Work with Clients with FASD

This adaptation required staff training and development, a process that also served to alert case managers to the possibility that some of the high-risk mothers they were already working with might be fetal alcohol affected. University of Washington researchers and clinicians educated PCAP case managers and supervisors on topics including biologic mechanisms of fetal alcohol exposure, teratogenic effects across gestation, diagnostic characteristics, and central nervous system and behavioral problems across the lifespan. An FAS expert and author trained staff on the day to day management of individuals with FASD, and facilitated a staffing session on management issues case managers had encountered in working with clients with FASD who were among their PCAP clients. PCAP staff observed the diagnostic process at the university FAS diagnostic clinic. Case managers helped clients assemble documentation required by the diagnostic clinic, including copies of birth or other records verifying extent of prenatal alcohol exposure, early childhood photos, growth charts, and school records. PCAP located a neuropsychologist in the community who facilitated the diagnostic process by evaluating clients, and negotiated with state agencies to pay for these exams. As FASD enrollment got underway, PCAP case managers met in weekly case consultations with supervisors to review assessment data, develop and monitor tailored interventions, address service barriers, and, as necessary, solicit additional consultation from an experienced staff clinical psychologist.

Educating the Community to Work with Clients with FASD

Clinical practice recommendations for FASD patients call for coordinated, multi-systemic management. However, as we began our work we found that most providers knew very little about FAS and its implication for practice, and had little direct experience with this patient population. With that in mind, we identified key providers who could deliver quality service to our clients with FASD, who were interested in the problem, and who were willing to work with a client with FASD as a case study in close collaboration with her PCAP case manager. We conducted FASD training with providers at 15 major clinics and agencies, and offered consultation as questions arose in treating these young women.

Recommendations to Providers

The community providers and PCAP case managers brought different but complementary skills to the intervention. Experienced case managers helped providers understand the relationship between the clients' organic brain damage and their sometimes socially inappropriate and otherwise puzzling behaviors, and how to respond in helpful ways. For example, clients with FASD typically experienced difficulties in the following areas as a result of diminished executive function skills: translating information from one sense or modality into appropriate behavior (e.g., hearing into doing); generalizing information from one situation to another; and comparing, contrasting, sequencing, predicting, and judging events and experiences in their lives. Clients' poor short-term memory often resulted in information or instructions being quickly forgotten. Although their long-term memory could be fine, their information storage was often disorganized, so information was difficult to retrieve. Their expressive language or articulation was often better than their receptive language or comprehension.

Case managers recommended to community providers the following strategies to communicate more effectively with FASD clients:

- Talk in concrete terms, avoid using words with double meanings or idioms, and say exactly what you mean.
- Give simple step-by-step instructions, and then have the patient demonstrate understanding by showing a skill, rather than relying on a verbal affirmation that she understands.
- Give simple (5th grade level) written instructions, with illustrations if possible.
- Re-teach and repeat important points at each visit, and remember that instructions are unlikely to generalize to a similar situation.
- Provide consistency both in the environment and in the people providing care. If the primary provider must change, create a transition period for the current provider to introduce the new provider.
- The aim of treatment should be to stabilize presenting problems rather than to pursue a cure for permanent disabilities in reasoning, judgment and memory.

Skilled PCAP case managers found that working with FASD clients was far more difficult than working with the typical PCAP clients for whom the intervention was designed, i.e., substance-abusing women with complex problems. The impact of the neuropsychological deficits on their FASD clients was obvious, and required that case managers modify their traditional intervention approaches. Case managers found it helpful to remind these clients that the reason they had difficulty with memory and daily living functions is because of brain damage caused by their mother's alcohol drinking during pregnancy. This strategy helped clients understand the importance of not repeating the pattern, and provided motivation for them to abstain from drugs and alcohol and/or use a family planning method.

While typical PCAP clients can be taught how to improve access to services by defining and articulating needs and problems, locating an appropriate provider, making appointments, and using transportation systems, the FASD clients were either unable to learn these skills or they learned them very slowly. Case managers had to assume a far more directive role as they introduced clients to community services and helped them comply with appointments and recommendations. As one case manager said, "She just doesn't get it," referring to the client's lack of comprehension, poor memory, and difficulty executing a plan even with assistance. Therefore, while this pilot project did not necessarily result in FASD clients developing the ability to access services independently, PCAP assistance did result in clients' increased use of services. By combining education with follow-up hands-on experience, we demystified the FASD disability for the providers, who were then able to deliver services appropriately tailored to the specific needs of FASD patients. In addition, the pilot resulted in relatively stable contacts for clients with providers, a critical step in improving retention and adherence to provider recommendations over time.

FASD Case Study

Michelle came into PCAP the same way most women do. During pregnancy her drug of choice was methamphetamine, and she also drank occasionally. Although she had permanently lost custody of four other children, she was allowed to keep custody of her newborn son because she had made significant progress since relinquishing her parental rights. It was clear from the beginning that Michelle had multiple problems; her case manager was frustrated at her inability to "get it." The PCAP clinical supervisor suspected FASD at intake and met with Michelle's mother to interview her about her drinking during pregnancy. Her mother initially denied alcohol use, but readily admitted to using heroin. When the supervisor asked if it were possible that she drank before she knew she was pregnant the mother said yes, she had "partied just like everybody else, and had loved Black Russians." After alcohol exposure was verified, Michelle had a neuropsychological evaluation. Her IQ was 73 and she had significant problems with memory and processing information.

Within a year and a half of her son's birth, Michelle gave birth to a second child, a girl, and moved with her two children into a clean and sober home for women with substance abuse issues. It became clear that Michelle could not keep track of both children at the same time; her son had disappeared on several occasions. Only with the assistance of the group home staff and the other residents was she able to parent as well as she did. A child welfare report was made and she lost custody of the children, not because she was a bad mother, but because she couldn't manage the two children simultaneously. Michelle's case manager arranged to have her evaluated at a brain injury clinic at a local hospital, where they formulated a treatment plan including occupational therapy and memory tools. Michelle was able to recognize her own improvement, stating, "Hey! I can multitask now!"

Michelle's children were eventually allowed to have longer visits at her home, and she appeared to be able to track and process the children's activities. Unfortunately, Michelle did not get custody of her two youngest children because of her past history. However, the family they were placed with allowed liberal visitation, and Michelle was able to be an active part of their lives. Michelle chose to have a tubal ligation because she knew she would be able to stay in contact with her children, and she could not stand the grief of relinquishing a future child.

Our small pilot study convinced us that an experienced and clinically supported case manager, working in collaboration with her client and a network of educated providers, might reasonably expect to accomplish a number of important steps over a 12-month intervention. These steps, not necessarily sequential, include the following:

- Securing stable housing, and safe, secure placements for the children; this may include connecting clients with parenting classes, support groups and respite care; helping clients make decisions about their ability to adequately care for all of their children; mediating with child welfare services and the courts.
- Assisting clients in obtaining inpatient or outpatient treatment and supportive aftercare, for those actively abusing alcohol or drugs.
- Assisting clients in evaluating family planning needs and choosing a contraceptive method, keeping in mind that a long-term, more reliable method may be the best option because of memory and judgment impairment.
- Establishing an educated network of service providers who will continue to work with clients after the case manager's services are no longer available.

- Obtaining DDD (Division of Developmental Disabilities) status for clients as appropriate in order to secure a measure of financial stability for the future.
- Identifying committed, experienced and/or trained mentors for clients, as most individuals with FASD will require long-term support and assistance.

These interventions may not only improve the client's current quality of life, but may also establish an enduring foundation for preventing crises long after a program's services are no longer available, thereby mitigating the social and familial burden associated with the long term care of these individuals. Caregivers who have become exhausted or alienated may be willing to resume a supportive mentoring role after a case manager has helped a client stabilize.

We cannot alter the permanent organic brain damage associated with a diagnosis of FASD or the difficult life circumstances these patients have experienced. The formidable challenge remains that these young women, and most individuals with FASD, will continue to need some kind of coordinated assistance across the lifespan.

Gatekeepers of health and social services must recognize when their systems are ineffective, and examine different approaches to working with challenging clientele. Our experience has demonstrated that with the expertise of a knowledgeable and dedicated staff, and with the commitment of strong community partnerships, we have the potential to serve mothers and children affected by alcohol and drug abuse, improve their quality of life, and ultimately prevent the births of future alcohol-damaged children.

REFERENCES

Aos, S., Lieb, R., Mayfield, J., Miller, M., & Pennucci, A. (2004, July 6). *Benefits and Costs of Prevention and Early Intervention Programs for Youth* (p. 1-20). Olympia, WA: Washington State Institute for Public Policy.

Bandura, A. (1977). Self-efficacy: Toward a unifying theory of behavioral change. *Psychological Review, 84*, 191-215.

Bobo, J. K., McIlvain, H. E., & Leed-Kelly, A. (1998). Depression screening scores during residential drug treatment and risk of drug use after discharge. *Psychiatric Services, 49*, 693-695.

Burns, K., Melamed, J., Burns, W., Chasnoff, I., & Hatcher, R. (1985). Chemical dependency and clinical depression in pregnancy. *Journal of Clinical Psychology, 41*, 851–4.

Centers for Disease Control and Prevention (CDC). (2004). Alcohol Consumption Among Women Who Are Pregnant or Who Might Become Pregnant — United States, 2002. *Morbidity and Mortality Weekly Report, 53*, 1178–1181.

Coles, C. D., Platzman, K. A., Smith, I., James, M. E., & Falek, A. (1992). Effects of cocaine and alcohol use in pregnancy on neonatal growth and neurobehavioral status. *Neurotoxicology and Teratology, 14* (1), 22–33.

Driessen, M., Meier, S., Hill, A., Wetterling, T., Lange, W., & Junghanns, K. (2001). The course of anxiety, depression, and drinking behaviours after completed detoxification in alcoholics with and without cormorbid anxiety and depressive disorders. *Alcohol and Alcoholism, 36*, 249-255.

Dunst, C. J., Trivette, C. M., and Deal, A. G. (1988). *Enabling and empowering families: Principles and guidelines for practice.* Cambridge: Brookline Books.

Ernst, C. C., Grant, T. M, Streissguth, A. P., & Sampson, P. D. (1999) Intervention with high-risk alcohol and drug-abusing mothers: II. 3-year findings from the Seattle Model of Paraprofessional Advocacy. *Journal of Community Psychology, 27*(1), 19–38.

Famy, C., Streissguth, A. P., & Unis, A. S. (1998). Mental illness in adults with fetal alcohol syndrome or fetal alcohol effects. *American Journal of Psychiatry, 155,* 552–554.

Finkelstein, N. (1993). Treatment programming for alcohol and drug-dependent pregnant women. *International Journal of the Addictions, 28*(13), 1275–1309.

Grant T. M., Ernst C. C., McAuliff, S., & Streissguth A. P. (1997). The Difference Game: Facilitating change in high-risk clients. *Families in Society: The Journal of Contemporary Human Services, 78*(4), 429–432.

Grant, T., Ernst, C. C., Pagalilauan G., & Streissguth, A. P. (2003). Post-program follow-up effects of paraprofessional intervention with high-risk women who abused alcohol and drugs during pregnancy. *Journal of Community Psychology, 31*(3): 211–222.

Grant, T. M., Ernst, C. C., & Streissguth, A. P. (1999). Intervention with high-risk alcohol and drug-abusing mothers: I. Administrative Strategies of the Seattle Model of Paraprofessional Advocacy. *Journal of Community Psychology, 27*(1), 1-18.

Grant, T., Ernst, C., Streissguth, A., & Porter, J. (1997). An advocacy program for mothers with FAS/FAE. In: Streissguth, A.P. and Kanter, J. (Eds.) *The Challenge of Fetal Alcohol Syndrome: Overcoming Secondary Disabilities* (pp. 102-112). Seattle: University of Washington Press.

Grant, T., Ernst, C., Streissguth, A., & Stark, K. (2005). Preventing alcohol and drug exposed births in Washington State: Intervention findings from three Parent-Child Assistance Program sites. *American Journal of Drug and Alcohol Abuse, 31*(3), 471-490.

Grant, T., Huggins, J., Connor, P., Pedersen, J., Whitney, N., & Streissguth, A. (2004). A pilot community intervention for young women with fetal alcohol spectrum disorders. *Community Mental Health Journal, 40*(6), 499–511.

Grant, T., Huggins, J., Connor, P., & Streissguth, A. (2005). Quality of life and psychosocial profile among young women with fetal alcohol spectrum disorders. *Mental Health Aspects of Developmental Disabilities, 8*(2), 33–39.

Greenfield, S. F., Weiss, R.D., Muenz, L. R., Vagge, L. M., Kelly, J. F., Bello, L. R., et al. (1998). The effect of depression on return to drinking: A prospective study. *Archives of General Psychiatry, 55,* 259-265.

Greenhouse, L. (2000, October 5). Justices consider limits of the legal response to risky behavior by pregnant women. *The New York Times,* p. A26.

Harwood, H., Fountain, D., & Livermore, G. (1998). *The Economic Costs of Alcohol and Drug Abuse in the United States, 1992.* Washington, D.C.: National Institute on Drug Abuse and National Institute on Alcohol Abuse and Alcoholism.

Institute of Medicine [IOM]. (1996). *Fetal Alcohol Syndrome: Diagnosis, Epidemiology, Prevention, and Treatment* (p. 21). Stratton, K. R., Howe, C. J., Battaglia, F. C. (Eds.). Washington D.C.: National Academy Press.

Jacobson, J. L., Jacobson, S. W., & Sokol, R. J. (1994). Effects of prenatal exposure to alcohol, smoking and illicit drugs on postpartum somatic growth. *Alcoholism Clinical and Experimental Research, 18*(2), 317–323.

Jacobson, S. W., Jacobson, J. L., & Sokol, R .J. (1994). Effects of fetal alcohol exposure on infant reaction time. *Alcoholism Clinical and Experimental Research, 18* (5), 1125–1132.

Kessler, R. C., Crum, R. M., Warner, L. A., Nelson, C. B., Schulenberg, J., & Anthony, J. C. (1997). Lifetime co-occurrence of DSM-III-R alcohol abuse and dependence with other psychiatric disorders in the national comorbidity survey. *Archives of General Psychiatry, 54,* 313–321.

Marcenko, M. O., & Spence, M. (1995). Social and psychological correlates of substance abuse among pregnant women. *Social Work Research, 19,* 103–110.

Marlatt G. A., Somers J. M., & Tapert S. F. (1993). Harm reduction: Application to alcohol abuse problems. *NIDA Research Monograph, 137,* 147-166. Review.

Marlatt, G. A., & Tapert, S. F. (1993). Harm reduction: Reducing the risks of addictive behaviors. In J.S. Baer, G.A. Marlatt, and R. McMahon (Eds.), *Addictive behaviors across the lifespan* (pp. 243-273). Newbury Park, CA: Sage Publications.

Miles, D. R., Svikis, D. S., Kulstad, J. L, & Haug, N. A. (2001). Psychopathology in pregnant drug-dependent women with and without comorbid alcohol dependence. *Alcoholism: Clinical and Experimental Research, 25,*1012–1017.

Miller, J. B. (1991). The development of women's sense of self. In J. D. Jordan, A. G. Kaplan, J. B. Miller, I. P. Stiver, & J. L. Surrey (Eds.), *Women's growth in connection* (pp. 11-26). New York: Guilford.

Miller, W. R. & Rollnick, S. (1991). *Motivational interviewing: Preparing people to change addictive behavior.* New York: Guilford Press.

Nelson, J., & Marshall, M. F. (1998). *Ethical and legal analyses of three coercive policies aimed at substance abuse by pregnant women.* Charleston, SC: The Robert Wood Johnson Foundation.

Olds, D., Kitzman, H., Cole, R., & Robinson, J. (1997). Theoretical foundations of a program of home visitation for pregnant women and parents of young children. *Journal of Community Psychology, 25*(1), 9-25.

Paltrow L. M., Cohen, D., & Carey, C. A. (2000). *Year 2000 overview: Governmental responses to pregnant women who use alcohol or other drugs.* Philadelphia: National Advocates for Pregnant Women of the Women's Law Project.

Pharis, M. E., & Levin, V. S. (1991). "A person to talk to who really cared": High-risk mothers' evaluations of services in an intensive intervention research program. *Child Welfare, 70*(3), 307-320.

Rice, D. P. (1993). The economic costs of alcohol abuse and dependence: 1990. *Alcohol Health and Research World, 17*(1), 10–11.

Sherman, B. R., Sanders, L. M., & Yearde, J. (1998). Role-modeling healthy behavior: Peer counseling for pregnant and postpartum women in recovery. *Women's Health Issues, 8(4),* 230-238.

Streissguth, A. P., Bookstein, F. L., Barr, H. M., Sampson, P. D., O'Malley, K., & Young, J. K. (2004). Risk factors for adverse life outcomes in fetal alcohol syndrome and fetal alcohol effects. *Developmental and Behavioral Pediatrics, 25,* 228-238.

Streissguth, A., Porter, J., & Barr, H. (2001) *A study of patients with fetal alcohol syndrome spectrum disorders (FASD) who became parents.* 24th Annual RSA Scientific Meeting, Le Centre Sheraton, Montreal, Quebec, June 23-28.

Substance Abuse and Mental Health Services Administration (SAMHSA). (2002). *Results from the 2001 national household survey on drug abuse: Volume 1: Summary of national findings*. Rockville, MD: U.S. Department of Health and Human Services, Substance Abuse and Mental Health Services Administration, Office of Applied Studies.

Substance Abuse and Mental Health Services Administration (SAMHSA). (2004). *The NSDUH Report: Women with Co-Occurring Serious Mental Illness and a Substance Use Disorder*. Rockville, MD: U.S. Department of Health and Human Services, Substance Abuse and Mental Health Services Administration, Office of Applied Studies. Retrieved September 2, 2004 from: http://oas.samhsa.gov/2k4/femDual/femDual.htm.

Will, G. F. (1999, November 1). Paying addicts not to have kids is a good thing. *Baltimore Sun*, p. 15A.

In: ADHD and Fetal Alcohol Spectrum Disorders (FASD)　　　ISBN: 1-59454-573-1
Editor: Kieran D. O'Malley, pp. 95-102　　　© 2008 Nova Science Publishers, Inc.

Chapter 6

NEUROPSYCHOLOGICAL PROFILES OF CHILDREN AND ADOLESCENTS WITH FETAL ALCOHOL SPECTRUM DISORDERS AND ADHD

Donald S. Massey[*] and Valerie J. Massey[*]

Research over the past 25 years on Fetal Alcohol Syndrome (FAS) has established the teratogenic effects of alcohol on the developing fetus, both in animals and humans. Results of this research have clearly described the presence of a syndrome of neurodevelopmental, neurocognitive and neurobehavioural deficits that persist through the lifespan, regardless of race or ethnic origin (Jones, et al 1973). FAS is now commonly seen as a pattern of physical malformations, growth deficiency and growth retardation, coupled with intellectual and developmental disabilities that are a direct result of prenatal exposure to alcohol in utero. Although the effects of alcohol use in pregnancy had been described in ancient literature Jones and Smith in 1973 presented the topic again to the medical community in the 20th Century, resulting in an explosion of research in virtually every field connected to health and education.

The initial focus of this current research on FAS was not only to establish alcohol as the specific teratogen causing the malformation in the structure and function of the brain and body of the developing human fetus (Jones, et al 1973), but also to develop a set of specific characteristics that define the syndrome well enough to be accepted by the American Academy of Pediatrics in 2000, and the International Classification of Diseases with respect to the syndrome's full or partial presentation. Early definitions describing FAS in children pointed to growth deficiency or retardation of prenatal onset, which typically continued postnatally (Rosett 1980). Characteristic physical malformations included a list of abnormal facial features with short palpebral fissures, flattening of the midface, thin upper vermillion border, hypoplastic or underdeveloped philtrum, shortening and upward canting of the nose, flattening of the nasal bridge and/or epicanthal folds as the major indicators. Other less prominent physical malformations included skeletal anomalies, heart defects, urinary and/or kidney deficits, neural tube deficits, and in some cases, malformation of the sexual organs.

---

[*] Doanald S. Massey and Valerie J. Massey, Neuropsychologists in Private Practice and Adjunct Professors. Department of Education Psychology, University of Alberta, Canada

Evidence of central nervous system abnormality and/or dysfunction was also required, and this included microcephaly, mental retardation, motor impairment, tremors, and attentional deficits with or without hyperactivity.

Current research is more focused on describing the effects of the syndrome through the age span including the cognitive, developmental, behavioural and psychosocial problems known to cause lifelong primary and secondary disabilities. The modal deficits across the lifespan have been isolated and described by pioneer researchers such as Streissguth and colleagues in North America (1993, 1994), as well as Spohr, et al in 1993 and Aronson , et al in Europe in 1985. These studies have provided a clearer picture of the persistent abnormal cognitive and behavioural deficits of alcohol-affected individuals and their lack of age-appropriate social, emotional, and day-to-day functioning. Specific research is also underway from the developmental perspective of children and adolescents since this is the first noticeable manifestation of the effects of the syndrome. The pattern of cognitive deficits encompass the broad range of weaknesses or delays in language, comprehension, memory, learning, intelligence, abstract reasoning and judgment, and cause-and-effect learning. Behavioural deficits include attentional problems, oppositional behaviour and conduct, poor social and adaptive functioning, impulsivity, lying, stealing, delinquencies, legal problems, chemical dependency, moodiness, inappropriate sexual behaviour, and other mental health problems (Streissguth 1986).

Among these various concerns, it has been established that neurobehavioural and social problems are perhaps the most prominent set of symptoms, particularly from the pediatric neuropsychological perspective (Steinhausen, et al 1993, 1994, Mattson, et al 1998, Roebuck, et al 1999 Mattson and Riley 2000, Mattson, et al 2001, O'Malley and Nanson 2002). These variables are often the most common presentation of the partial syndrome, also known as Alcohol Related Neurodevelopmental Disorder (ARND), particularly when the physical manifestations of the syndrome are not observable. Specific research is being conducted in the most common symptom areas, which include Attention Deficit Hyperactivity Disorder (ADHD) and other neurodevelopmental deficits closely associated with FAS. While ADHD has been separately classified as a specific disorder of childhood in the DSM-IV, FAS does not enjoy its own classification in the same manual even though it is the most prevalent cause of preventable mental handicap in North America (Abel and Sokol 1987). The close association of FAS with ADHD deserves closer attention since it appears to be a co-morbid condition, particularly in children and adolescents with FAS. This chapter will examine the association between children and adolescents with FAS from a clinical and practical neuropsychologial perspective. The aim of the review is to familiarize the clinician with typical and frequently occurring neuropsychological deficits seen in FAS and ARND children and adolescents in order to provide a common ground for future discussion and research in the field of pediatric neuropsychological practice.

INFANCY TO PRESCHOOL PERIOD

Manifestation of the full or partial syndrome in infancy depends on a number of factors including the amount, duration and timing of alcohol consumption during pregnancy of the mother, the mother's age and general health condition, as well as socio-economic factors.

Initially, only the full syndrome may be diagnosable at birth based on physical malformations and growth deficits, and the history of the mother. The partial syndrome may be suspected and the child scheduled for follow-up although neuropsychological assessment is not possible at this early stage. Developmental assessments can, however, provide a general index of delays in basic sensory, motor, language and behavioural functioning.

Jones and Smith in 1973 reported that, with heavy prenatal alcohol exposure, one would expect to find the characteristic craniofacial features (microcephaly, short palpebral fissures, epicanthal folds, maxillary hypoplasia, cleft palate, micrognathia), growth deficiency (pre-and postnatal), physical deformities and anomalies such as limited range of motion at the elbow, interphalangeal and metacarpal-phalangeal joints, hip dislocation, altered palmar crease pattern, other physical anomalies (cardiac, external genitalia capillary haemangiomata) fine motor dysfunction (tremulousness, weak grasp, poor eye-hand coordination), developmental delay and disorders of the central nervous system due to changes in brain structure and function (Jones and Smith 1973, Clarren, et al 1978, Peiffer, et al 1979, Wisniewski, et al 1983, Coulter , et al 1993, Riley, et al 1995, Johnson , et al 1996, Sowell, et al 1996, Roebuck, et al 2002,Mattson , et al 1996, Roebuck, et al 2004).

Smith and Jones also described the first necropsy performed on a FAS stillborn infant which clearly demonstrated the dysmorphogenesis of the brain which they felt was responsible for some of the functional abnormalities noted in the syndrome (Jones and Smith 1973). This included the displacement or disorientation of the neuronal and glial elements of the brain in the stillborn as well as the incomplete development of specific components of the brain including the corpus callosum. They concluded that some of the more functional deficits noted in this syndrome were, in fact, related to the dysmorphogenesis observed in their stillborn specimen. They also indicated that some of the secondary features of FAS including microcephaly, delays in general development, fine motor skills, and joint abnormalities related to neurological impairment of the fetus (Jones and Smith 1973).

In their study of three newborns (one stillborn), Smith and Jones described the similarity of two of the infants with FAS in some detail, indicating that both children had serious problems with respiratory adaptation and one had difficulty with biochemical adaptation including hypoglycemia, hypocalcemia and hyperbilirubinaemia, all of which have serious implications for later brain functions as noted among other medically at-risk children such as prematures or low birthweight infants who also demonstrate a number of neurodevelopmental deficits throughout childhood and adolescence (Massey ?). They observed microphthalmia in both infants and suggested that the small palpebral fissures observed in FAS was secondary to reduced ocular growth (Jones and Smith 1973). They observed that the prenatal-onset growth deficiency noted in one of their subjects persisted though the postnatal period despite high caloric feedings and that length was more adversely affected than weight gain, without any obvious indication of nutritional deficiency for the pregnant mother, aside from iron deficiency. Smith and Jones suggested that the results of this small study were significant as they believed that the risk of FAS in the offspring of pregnant mothers was very high unless maternal alcoholism is controlled. Smith went on to describe the syndrome and reported that, in 1979, there were approximately 6550 cases of alcohol-affected children born annually and approximately 1800 born annually with the full syndrome reported in the literature (Smith 1979).

Other studies, including Peiffer, et al examining fetuses, newborns, infants and young children in 1979 reported that chronic maternal alcohol abuse during pregnancy resulted in a number of serious malformations of the brain including arhinencephaly, porencephaly, agenesis of the corpus callosum, hydranencephaly, microdysplasias such as a reduced gyration of the dentate nucleus and inferior olives, malformation of the cerebellar hemispheres, agenesis of the cerebellar vermis, demyelinated white matter, abnormal development and smaller size of the medulla oblongata, abnormalities of the spinal cord and brain stem, spongiform loosening of the hypothalamic and thalamic areas, in addition to congenital heart defects and craniofacial anomalies (Peiffer, et al 1979). They also established additional criteria for the diagnosis of FAS including the main symptoms of delayed intrauterine and postnatal growth, microcephaly, psychomotor retardation, enlargement of the ventricles, hypotonia of the muscles, craniofacial anomalies (short nose, epicanthus, ptosis, small lips, micrognathia, and congenital heart deficts. They too found deficits in the migration of glial and neuronal cells, heterotopias in the leptomeninges, and brain stem malformations leading to hydrocephalus internus. These 6 cases enlarged the spectrum of morphological anomalies, indicating that the embryo is susceptible to teratogenic influence by alcohol. They also concluded that, while the clinical phenotype of children with alcohol embryo and feto pathology was indeed very similar, the spectrum of neuropathological findings was much broader and one could not conclude a specific type of malformation caused by alcohol (Peiffer, et al 1979).

Clarren and his colleagues studying brain malformations in FAS children suggested that microcephaly and mental retardation were the principal features of FAS (Clarren, et al 1978). They proposed that the mental deficiency was caused by diminished brain growth due, in part, to ethanol exposure in utero. Their necropsy studies on four perinatal subjects exposed to high levels of alcohol during gestation demonstrated very similar types of brain morphogenesis with leptomeningeal and neuroglial heterotropia the most prominent features. They described this as a sheet of aberrant neural and glial tissue that covered some of the brain surface and partially incorporated the pia mater. They also postulated that, in comparison with what is known about normal neuronal migration and timing, the observed dysmorphogenesis likely occured prior to 45 days gestation for cerebellar and brainstem develpment, and by 85 days gestation for cerebral abnormalities. These malformations were also correlated with heavy maternal alcohol consumption with chronic and intermittent high consumption producing similar results. They estimated that, while intermittent high peak doses of alcohol could damage to the fetus, the specific mechanism of brain morphogenesis was unknown at that time (Clarren, et al 1978). This is not surprising as the severity of effects may relate to a number of variables including dosage, gestational timing, and fetal resistance, or the response of the individual fetus to the ethanol. Clarren and his colleagues noted that only two of the four subjects determined to have ethanol-induced brain malformations were considered to meet the criteria for full FAS, suggesting that, in some infants, brain structure and function may be the only major abnormality resulting from alcohol exposure in utero while in other infants, more pervasive problems are noted.

These brain malformations would have a substantial negative impact on the structure and function of the developing brain throughout childhood. Early researchers observed that 44% of the offspring of heavy drinking mothers demonstrated borderline mental deficiency at age 7 even though only 32% had multiple clinical features of FAS (Jones and Smith 1973). Aronson , et al reported in a Swedish study (Aronson, et al 1985) that the children born of alcoholic mothers compared to matched controls, demonstrated IQ scores 15 to 19 points below controls (p<0.01) with their group mean -1.6 SD below the control mean. Significant differences between the groups were also noted on other variables central to the early development of children including impaired visual perception, impaired human figure drawings, impairments in emotional stability, hyperactivity, distractibility, short attention span, and perseveration , among the FAS sample with none of these disturbances noted for the controls reared either in foster homes or biological homes. Despite very few systematic studies linking the relationship of physical characteristics to psychological variables such as cognition, perception and development, this relationship has been well established in the literature with more studies now evaluating other aspects of psychological development in children with or without complete FAS features.

Early studies in Sweden using the WISC noted significantly lower scores for FAS children on measures of eye-hand coordination, hearing and speech functions, practical reasoning, visual form perception, concept formation, and attention span. The profiles of these children were also more uneven compared to controls although no difference between the Verbal or Performance scales of the WISC was noted (Aronson, et al 1985). Lower scores were also obtained on human figure drawings for FAS children in these early studies, suggesting global cognitive and developmental delays, and there were increased indicators of emotional instability on these drawings. These same studies noted additional behavioural characteristics such as hyperactivity, distractibility and short attention span in most of the children with FAS but in none of the control subjects. Other problems included difficulties with understanding verbal instruction with a corresponding need for smaller class sizes. In the area of perceptual difficulties, the FAS children were noted to have considerable difficulty, with many of the subjects demonstrating severe impairment in interpreting sensory input related to auditory and visual stimuli. This led to additional insecurity and lower self-confidence. Hyperactivity, attentional deficits, and perseveration were again noted in at least half of the study subjects, further complicating the learning environment.

The researchers pointed out that a number of studies reported mental retardation in FAS children with average IQ at around 68 and discrepancies in scores (Jones, et al 1974). Aronson, and colleagues indicated in their Swedish study in 1985 that the physical characteristics of FAS were significantly associated with decreased intellectual performance, consistent with in other studies reported in the literature at that time. They also observed, however, that children in their study group without the physical traits of FAS were also significantly lower in IQ than controls. They concluded that neurological and psychological disturbances existed without somatic FAS traits, as reported by other researchers (Jones, et al 1974, Clarren, et al 1978). They further observed that their study group differed significantly from controls on the subscales of the WISC as well with their subjects' variations being much greater on the measures.

This prospective Swedish study was the best example of the range of variables examined in young children although one of its drawbacks was that the consumption of alcohol in pregnancy of the 30 mothers was generally unknown. This study is still important to the field as matched controls, with children in foster and biological homes, were used. Study subjects also demonstrated full and partial features of FAS. The researchers emphasized that cognitive, perceptual, attentional and behavioural deficits existed with these children and combined to form more global problems with learning, particularly at the classroom level. Many of their subjects had been placed in foster homes early on suggesting that these learning difficulties were of prenatal origin and that good foster care was not able to fully compensate for prenatal handicaps.

Examples of more recent research on young children in the 1990s can be found in a 10-year European study by Spohr and colleagues evaluating long-term outcome and developmental consequences of 60 children diagnosed with FAS in infancy and childhood (Spohr, et al 1993). The researchers noted that from a morphological perspective, the characteristic craniofacial features of FAS tended to diminish with time but that microcephaly, short stature, and, to a lesser extent, lower body weight (in boys only) persisted. Even severely dysmorphic children showed some "catch up" in growth, height and weight but not in head circumference as microcepahaly persisted in 65% of the sample at follow up. They noted that improvements were also seen in internal organ malformations, skeletal abnormalities, and specific neurological symptoms on follow up. Severely affected children, however, continued to demonstrate the typical characteristics of FAS well into adolescence. They concluded that intrauterine alcohol exposure was more noticeable in boys than in girls. The researchers noted that, with respect to intelligence, results were stable over time with only a few children demonstrating better post-test performance. A small percentage of the sample of FAS children demonstrated lower post-test performance 10 years later (normal intelligence previously) with several of these children diagnosed as learning disabled and at least one had mental retardation. In addition, a substantial deterioration in school status was observed with approximately half of the children registered in special education centers in adolescence whereas 10 years prior they attended regular schools or preschools. The examiners concluded there was a tendency for impaired intelligence to increase with severity of dysmorphological observations at initial assessment even though there was no statistical association. In other words, not all children with mild dysmorphology showed normal intelligence and not all severely FAS children showed mental retardation. They also concluded there was no significant statistical association between IQ and the standard predictors of morphological damage including head circumference (Spohr, et al 1993). They did, however, note substantial changes in the residential situation of these children since initial assessment as many of them were no longer living in their biological homes and most had been placed with surrogate parents, foster homes, or adoptive parents in early childhood.

These results suggest that one can expect lower scores on intellectual ability tests but not always in the expected direction. Some studies have reported average to high average IQs, suggesting that IQ variations are frequently noted and these measures may be of limited diagnostic relevance unless of course significantly deficient overall performance is observed. It is also important to note that standardized IQ tests such as the WISC-III or WAIS-III were never designed to evaluate brain damage and norming studies excluded such subjects. It is no surprise therefore that their diagnostic utility is limited to educational prediction and additional variables related to language and non-language processing. There is no obvious "profile" on these tests demonstrating the diverse impairment present in children and adolescents with FAS or the partial syndrome. Clinically, however, alcohol-affected children have the greatest difficulty with language and comprehension tasks. They also struggle with output ability and some aspects of nonverbal reasoning. Overall scores on the Wechlser scales also vary a great deal, particularly when children with partial presentation of FAS are assessed.

Current Perspectives on ADHD and FASD . . .

REFERENCES

Abel EL, Sokol RJ (1987) Incidence of fetal alcohol syndrome and economic impact of FAS-related anomalies. *Drug Alcohol Depend* 19: 51-70

Aronson M, Kyllerman M, Sabel KG, Sandin B, Olegard R (1985) Children of alcoholic mothers. *Acta Paediatr Scand* 74: 27-3519.

Clarren SK, Alvord EC, Sumi SM, Streissguth AP, Smith, DW (1978) Brain malformations related to prenatal exposure of ethanol. *Journal of Pediatrics* 92: 64-6721.

Coulter CL, Leech, RW, Schaefer GB, Scheithauer BW, Brumback RA(1993) Midline cerebral dysgenesis, dysfunction of the hypothalamic-pituitary axis, and fetal alcohol effects. *Archives of Neurology* 50: 771-775

Committee on Substance Abuse and Committee on Children with Disabilities, American Academy of Pediatrics (2000) Fetal alcohol syndrome and alcohol-related neurodevelopmental disorders. *Pediatrics* 106: 358-361

Johnson VP, Swayze VW, Sato Y, Andreasen N (1996) Fetal alcohol syndrome: Craniofacial and central nervous system manifestations. *American Journal of Medical Genetics* 61: 323-339

Jones KL, Smith DW, Ulleland CN (1973) Pattern of malformation in offspring of chronic alcoholic mothers. *Lancet* 1:1267-1271.

Jones KL, Smith DW (1973) Recognition of the fetal alcohol syndrome in early infancy. *Lancet* 2: 999-1001

Jones KL, Smith DW, Streissguth AP, Myrianthopoulos NC (1974) Outcome in offspring of chronic alcoholic women. *Lancet* 1: 1076-1078

Massey DS: *Premature birth and learning disabilities*

Mattson SN, Riley EP, Sowell ER, Jernigan TL, Sobel DF, Jones KL (1996) A decrease in the size of the basal ganglia in children with fetal alcohol syndrome. *Alcoholism: Clinical and Experimental Research* 20: 1088-1093

Mattson SN, Edward PR (1998) A review of the neurobehavioral deficits in children with fetal alcohol syndrome or prenatal exposure to alcohol. *Alcoholism: Clinical and Experimental Research* , 22: 279-294

Mattson SN, Riley EP (2000) Parent ratings of behavior in children with heavy prenatal alcohol exposure and IQ-matched controls. *Alcoholism : Clinical and Experimental Research* 24: 226-231

Mattson SN, Schoenfeld AM, Riley EP (2001) Teratogenic effects of alcohol on brain and behavior. *Alcohol Research and Health* 25: 185-191

O'Malley KD, Nanson J (2002) Clinical implications of a link between fetal alcohol spectrum disorder and attention-deficit hyperactivity disorder. *Canadian Journal of Psychiatry* 47: 349-354

Peiffer J, Majewski F, Fischbach H, Bierich R, Volk B (1979) Alcohol embryo and fetopathy. *Journal of the Neurological Sciences* 41: 125-137

Riley EP, Mattson SN, Sowell ER, Jernigan TL, Sobel DF, Jones KL (1995) Abnormalities of the corpus callosum in children prenatally exposed to alcohol. *Alcoholism: Clinical and Experimental Research* 19: 1198-1202

Roebuck TM, Mattson SN, Riley EP (1999) Behavioral and Psychosocial Profiles of alcohol-exposed children. *Alcoholism: Clinical and Experimental Research* 23: 1070-1076

Roebuck TM, Mattson SN, Riley EP (2002) Interhemispheric transfer in children with heavy prenatal alcohol exposure. *Alcoholism: Clinical and Experimental Research* 26: 1863-1871

Roebuck-Spencer TM, Mattson SN, Marion SD, Brown WS, Riley EP (2004) Bimanual coordination in alcohol-exposed children: Role of the corpus callosum. *Journal of the International Neuropsychological Society* 10: 536-548

Rosett HL (1980) A clinical perspective of the fetal alcohol syndrome. *Alcoholism: Clinical and Experimental Research* 4: 119-122

Smith DW (1979) The fetal alcohol syndrome. *Hospital Practice* 14: 12-26

Sowell ER, Jernigan TL, Mattson SN, Riley EP, Sobel DF, Jones KL (1996) Abnormal development of the cerebellar vermis in children prenatally exposed to alcohol: Size reduction in Lobules I-V. *Alcoholism: Clinical and Experimental Research* 20: 31-34

Spohr HL, Willms J, Steinhausen HC (1993) Prenatal alcohol exposure and long-term developmental consequences. *Lancet* 341: 907-910

Steinhausen HC, Wilms J, Spohr HL (1993) Long-term psychopathological and cognitive outcome of children with fetal alcohol syndrome. *Journal of the Academy of Child and Adolescent Psychiatry* 32: 990-994

Steinhausen HC, Willms, J, Spohr HL (1994) Correlates of psychopathology and intelligence in children with Fetal Alcohol Syndrome. *Journal of Child Psychology and Psychiatry* 35: 323-331

Streissguth AP (1986) The behavioral teratology of alcohol: Performance, behavioral, and intellectual deficits in prenatally exposed children, in West JR (ed): *Alcohol and Brain Development.* , 3-44 , New York, Oxford

Streissguth AP (1993) Fetal alcohol syndrome in older patients. *Alcohol and Alcoholism 2*: 209-212

Streissguth AP (1994) A long-term perspective of FAS. *Alcohol Health and Research World* 18: 74-81

Wisniewski K, Dambaska M, Sher JH, Qazi Q (1983) A clinical neuropathological study of the fetal alcohol syndrome. *Neuropediatrics* 14: 197-201

In: ADHD and Fetal Alcohol Spectrum Disorders (FASD)   ISBN: 1-59454-573-1
Editor: Kieran D. O'Malley, pp. 103-124   © 2008 Nova Science Publishers, Inc.

Chapter 7

ADULT NEUROPSYCHOLOGY OF FETAL ALCOHOL SPECTRUM DISORDERS

Kathy Page[*]

INTRODUCTION

Recognizing FASD is difficult, perhaps more so than for any other disability. After many years of teaching others to recognize and work with FASD, it still creeps up on me, wearing its disguise of simple sociopathy. For example, as I was backing out of a parking space at WalMart here in Susanville, California, my way was blocked by an obese woman, smoking, in an old, dusty car. She glowered at me, as she saw me blocking *her* way in to the space.

I glared back at her impatiently and signaled that unless she backed up I could not move. She backed up, I pulled out, she pulled in... many smugly grumbling moments later I was humbled by the realization that what we had here was probably some combination of the following:

- Poor motor planning
- Impaired spatial perception
- Sequencing difficulties
- Difficulty reading social cues
- Slow processing speed
- Poor cause-and-effect reasoning

...and, I further realized, we had every indication of a good smattering of the "secondary disabilities" that accrue to those whose cognitive impairments haven't been recognized or addressed. Signs of poverty and tobacco and food addiction were there, and some of the others, like unemployment, school failure, depression and trouble with the law lurked just below the surface in my imagination, possibly unwarranted but certainly not unreasonable. In

[*] Kathryn W. Page, Ph.D., Clinical Director, FASD Project, Pathways to Child and Family Excellence, 1345 Paul Bunyan Road, Suite B,. Susanville, CA 96130, (530) 257-0243

short, especially in light of the very heavy alcohol use in my rural town (half again as much as the state average [Vega, et al, 1993]), I may well have engaged in a parking-lot tussle with someone with the malfunctioning brain of fetal alcohol spectrum disorder (FASD).

And maybe not, of course. Current substance use, mental illness and traumatic brain injury are only a few of the other possible causes of her behavior and her demeanor. But prenatal alcohol exposure is a likely culprit, and the perspective of this chapter is that it would be helpful to this woman and to the community at large to figure out if that is indeed her case.

Recognizing, sorting out and working with FASD in adults is complicated well beyond the same task with children. Understanding the workings of the adult with FASD is equally if not more important to attempt, however, for many reasons including those below.

Along with unraveling the extra complexities that adults with FASD present (and trigger in others) and attempting to convince the reader of the worthiness of that endeavor, this article will provide a map of the component parts of fetal alcohol damage as they appear in adulthood, and share a glimpse into the lived experience of people with FASD. We also look at misleading signposts and shifting landmarks in the territory as it has been mapped by others, and mark the effect of that mismapping. And not to leave the reader in the slough of despond that so often accompanies a deeper understanding of FASD, the article then comes back home to the more hopeful territory of what we can do to help.

WHY IT IS HARDER TO RECOGNIZE AND WORK WITH FASD IN ADULTS THAN IT IS IN CHILDREN

Children

Seeing through "bad" behavior to the nervous system dysfunction that drives or exacerbates it is hard enough with children. Disobedience, disruption, lying, not following directions, stealing lunches, lying about stealing lunches (with evidence in hand, visible to all), not playing well with others, running with scissors, —this pattern is easily recognizable as the bane of grade-school teachers. It is also a common pattern with children who have FASD. These behaviors tend to trigger, at a minimum, an immediate reaction of impatience. Nevertheless, children have been graced with the near-universal appeal that keeps their caretakers coming back, and with the mutability that often rewards on-target intervention with gratifying change. Children are supposed, by definition, to still be growing and changing, and the adult world is inclined to give them a pass (at least in theory) when they lag behind their peers in development of academic, linguistic or social skills. "He'll catch up" is a phrase commonly heard with reference to such children.

Even so, without special insight or coaching, it is common for teachers or other adults to see children with CNS dysfunction of the particularly irritating FASD variety as "doing it on purpose", as manipulative: "He has selective memory—he only remembers what he wants to." "I know she can do this; she did it yesterday. She just isn't trying." "That child really has YOUR number." "He pitches a fit every time he doesn't get his way." "He's really smart—he can read above grade level—so he's just being lazy when he doesn't get his homework done." "She is so rebellious she insists on coloring outside the lines." "I don't know why that boy can't learn to take turns."

However, in many cases, with a little help and coaching, many teachers and caregivers have made the 180 degree paradigm shift that enables them to recognize CNS dysfunction and put in supports and accommodations that succeed in helping children achieve a calmer, more successful state. Improvement in learning, growth, self-regulation and healthy relationships can be relatively quick, ratifying the diagnostic impression of fetal alcohol damage that prompted those supports in the first place. As FASD awareness spreads, more and more teachers are seeking to identify and support the children in their classes with this condition. (Kleinfeld and Wescott, 1993)

Adults

"He'll catch up" is never heard, on the other hand, with reference to the adult who doesn't follow the rules, constantly interrupts others, does not tell the truth or respect others' property. Add poor hygiene to that, and the small measure of understanding and patience that might exist for this guy disappears altogether in the average person. He becomes another irresponsible character who just doesn't care how he affects others. Feelings are hurt, offense is taken, relationships fall apart, jobs are lost and mind-altering substances are one appealing refuge.

The question that usually arises in conversations about FASD, especially with people in positions of societal authority, has to do with distinguishing voluntary, purposeful behavior from behavior that is largely spurred by central nervous system (brain) dysfunction. In this country with its very strong belief in individual freedoms, rights and responsibilities, the idea of "excusing bad behavior" is always suspect.

Separating out fetal alcohol damage from manipulative or sociopathic behavior in adults is complicated by several factors: unrealistic expectations; the moralistic, punitive, angry or misguidedly "helpful" reactions when these expectations are unmet; off-putting defensive traits; the snowballing detritus of secondary disabilities including mental illness; and a cruel quirk of fetal alcohol damage that leaves people with an illusory competence in expressive language. .

Unrealistic Expectations

There is a natural expectation that adults who do not appear to be developmentally disabled have mastered the basics of communication, responsibility, integrity, impulse control, reasoning, self-care and so on. Most of us hold both ourselves and others to this expectation. People with prenatal alcohol damage, whose disabilities so often "fly under the radar" in ways that other disabilities do not, are particularly prone to unrealistic expectations from others—and often from themselves as well. A person with the standard unrecognized disabilities of FASD is likely to be given tasks that require competence with all the above domains, and to readily--even eagerly--take them on, including those that are well beyond his or her actual capacity. When memory fails, stimulus overload occurs, auditory comprehension is blocked or logic goes missing—for starters—the task at hand will fall apart, disappointment will result, and the deal is broken. The general assumption is that these failures are a result of the person's unwillingness to "get with the program".

Of course, for people with FASD, it is a matter of inadequate connections in the brain. The thinner corpus callosum, smaller cerebellum, nucleus accumbens and caudate nucleus, the neurotransmitter imbalances, and the lower frontal lobe glucose-uptake (along with the rest of the neurophysiology we have yet to discover about FASD) all conspire to keep even the person with a normal or high IQ from being able to reach the expected level of functioning in any practical sense.

Compounding the problem of expectations regarding compliance with societal norms is the belief that all people learn from their mistakes, learn from consequences, grow inevitably into "responsibility"—and that if they don't it is because they just don't want to. That expectation of normal maturation overall or the more specific ability to learn from a particular consequence is, to varying degrees, unrealistic with fetal alcohol damage.

Another unrealistic expectation is based on consistency: if a person can do something one day, not doing it the next day is usually seen as an issue of motivation. With the dyscontrol that pervades FASD comes an unevenness of mood, performance, focus, even motor control. It is a little like a fluctuating but never entirely recovered hangover.

There are moral expectations: we expect people to tell us the truth, to "own up to" their misdeeds, to keep their promises, and to respect private property (that is, not to steal). These too are foiled by the peculiar difficulties of the prenatal alcohol-damaged brain.

And there are expectations of hygiene and grooming. A person who consistently smells bad gives off a powerful "stay away" message; messy, wrinkled or dirty clothing has the same effect, and with the perceptual difficulties of FASD such shortcomings may not even be registered by the person inside this off-putting package.

It is impossible to parse out all the expectations we hold for normal behavior as they are limitless and often unconscious, revealed to us only in our reactions when they are broken. The ones mentioned above are merely the most commonly problematic. Making the shift in interpretation--from the other person's deliberate non-cooperation to one's own unrealistic expectations--can make all the difference in effective intervention.

Reactions from Others

Most of the layers of our society depend to some degree on the fulfillment of the above expectations, and when those expectations go unmet beyond the standard margin of error we allot each other, the response can range anywhere from well-intentioned but badly-aimed "help" to the cold fury of incarceration. But whatever the reaction, absent a good and workable understanding of the neuropsychological impairments that get in the way of normalcy, it is bound to be worse than ineffective.

We should note, however, that it is equally unrealistic to expect uninformed others-- authorities, caregivers, friends and family or society in general—to recognize fetal alcohol damage when they see it, or to easily amend expectations and reactions even if they do. Those of us in this field must exercise the same patience, understanding and respect with these others as we want them to exercise with the victims of prenatal alcohol exposure. We are asking them to step outside everything their instincts tell them, coming from traditions as old as humanity itself.

The normal reactions to adults with moderate to severe FASD--who blow up on the job, don't show up on time, make promises they do not keep, take things that don't belong to them and then lie about it, or who chronically ignore basic standards of hygiene—center around anger and distancing. We humans are wired, evolutionarily, to move toward others who send off signals of trustworthiness and to move away from those who send the opposite: signals that they might cause our tribe to be betrayed to the enemy, and the cave overtaken. It is very difficult to unhook from the instinct to reject (angrily, sometimes violently) people who behave in ways that do not conform to our most basic norms. We have moral frameworks that justify this instinct: some people are just plain "bad", in the most primitive frame. As we move up the twin ladders of sophistication and good intentions, the frames get fancier, but the basic message is the same: the person's character is defective, not to be trusted. We have humanistic explanations of poor parenting and ineffective teaching, psychological explanations of unresolved inner conflict or "fear of success", religious explanations involving the devil, sociological explanations of the disenfranchising effect of poverty...and the list could certainly go on.

All these might be true for any given person. (And who actually knows about the devil.) But the reason that our fetal alcohol-affected neighbor cannot "get over it" as he or she is so often exhorted to do is that the very basic ability to connect cause and effect, to learn from consequences, is not there, or is there in very short supply. Any approach that assumes this person can change if only they try hard enough--or if WE try hard enough--will run aground, and only add a layer of despair to an already raw and mangled sense of self in the affected person. But expecting people in relationship with a fetal alcohol-affected person to "get over it" themselves, and move toward encouragement and support, is also unrealistic unless we interject some vivid and accurate understanding, as well as a fair measure of support and encouragement, for them as well.

Taking FASD-related behavior personally is one of the most difficult habits to break, and one of the most destructive. Chronic promise-breaking, for example, so common in relationships with alcohol-affected people, is often a trigger for anger and retribution. Relationships of all kinds break apart, leaving another stain of bewilderment, shame and humiliation behind.

Some Individuals' Reactions to Their Own Unidentified but Probable FASD

Example 1. A 45-year-old woman (V.) struggling through a junior college class came in one day after 3 hours' sleep; she had tried her best to complete a long assignment, only got halfway through, and felt terrible about not finishing. Her face sagging with weariness and defeat, she dismissed the prospect of support from the Learning Disabilities department: "I should do this on my own". V. is beginning to realize that she probably has fetal alcohol damage. A recovering addict/alcoholic who has been in prison; V's children were removed by Child Protective Service. She always felt like "some kind of Martian" growing up, separated from other children's play by an incomprehensible but powerful force. To this day her interactions are awkward and somewhat stilted, with occasional startling bursts of affection. V.'s attitude toward her difficulties has long been that there is just something wrong with her, a "bad seed".

Until recently V. found a semblance of comfort in substances. She has a long history of isolating, hiding from anyone who came along looking for her. Describing (without knowing it) all the features of depression, she attributes her failures to some basic inadequacy as a person. Every time she forgets to do something she gives herself another whack. It has never occurred to her to ask anyone for help, or even for their patience.

Adults with conditions along this spectrum of fetal alcohol disorder experience a variety of difficulties and varying severities. V. is one of the luckier ones, in a sense, as she has come up from a swamp of self-loathing and behaviors born of desperation to a place where she is getting support from some who understand. She has the wherewithal to succeed with schoolwork and help others in recovery. After much persuading, V. is now willing to use the accommodations that are her right, including reduced assignment length and oral presentation of material. Her relief is palpable

Example 2. A 37-year-old man in prison, listening to a talk about FASD, sat shaking his head slowly, looking down at the table. Asked if he wanted to share his thoughts, he just looked up and said quietly "It's been a nightmare. Everybody always blamed me for everything, and I always thought they were right. They WERE right. I always screw things up, no matter how hard I try to get it right. Nightmare…" Later on in the morning he raised his hand and tentatively asked where, on the outside, he might find some kind of support group for people like himself. Of course the answer was that there is nothing yet, but that we're working on it, and that he might be instrumental in forming such a group. He did not look encouraged.

Adult Children of Alcoholics

A group whose purported issues are largely unexplored in this chapter deserves at least a brief mention. Adult Children of Alcoholics (ACAs) have been the subject of a a great deal of popular literature, research and clinical intervention in recent decades. (Brown, 1999). Self-help, therapy groups, 12-step groups and individual therapy have all aimed at undoing the detritus of alcoholic parenting, without a moment's attention to any connection between prenatal alcohol exposure and the problems in work, school, relationship and material aspects of life that so famously plague ACAs. AD/HD, learning disabilities, hypersensitivity to environmental stimuli, difficulty with planning and judgment, even increased health problems are widely noted in ACA literature, attributed to poor parenting. Psychotherapy offices are brimming over with ACAs earnestly working on their "issues", in hopes of unraveling the unconscious conflicts that must be the culprit behind the "passive aggressive" pattern of forgetting, or the "fear of success" manifested as difficulty keeping jobs or managing money.

Example 3. M, whose mother misunderstood her daughter's sloppy coloring in grade school as rebelliousness, and her chronic losing of precious items as personally meaningful, spent years in therapy trying to improve her character. A good and obedient psychology patient, Mary believed that she must be acting out intractable unconscious conflict, intractable only because she must not really want to get better. Upon hearing the hypothesis that her mother's heavy drinking may have contributed to these difficulties, M. was able to cast off debilitating depression, put practical supports in place and let her true gifts blossom.

One research study (Page, 2001) suggests that signs of prenatal alcohol damage are common among ACAs, and that once this possibility is broached, supports for brain dysfunction can replace the endless digging through family history…and life can become simpler and more successful.

Defenses

Another reason that serious disability is rarely recognized or addressed in adults with FASD has to do with the layer of defenses that accrete , pearl-like, over the profound irritants of a janky nervous system and malfunctioning brain.

A not uncommon stance, especially among the young or the mistreated, is "There's nothing wrong with me. My only problem is you people trying to tell me what to do." It is the rare (and independently funded) helping professional who will persist in efforts to find out and address the underlying causes for the swarm of maladaptive behaviors if this help is actively rejected by a person who has chronologically reached the age of consent. Even if some astute agency staff member does hypothesize FASD as the underlying reason for someone's chronic failure, the person may well reject such a hypothesis as yet another insult. The person with undiagnosed FASD has found himself on the receiving end of scorn, rejection and grievous misunderstanding for too many years and by too many people to immediately open to "help", even of the most accurate and kindly variety. For many, a defensive posture that favors the fiction of purposeful, premeditated, self-controlled "bad" has become the one slim tether to self respect, and it is often a convincing one at that.

Talking the Talk: Deceptively Competent Language

Adding to the "stealth" quality of this condition is a language feature common to FASD that clinicians refer to as "superficial fluency": the ability to sound as if one is carrying on a meaningful conversation when in fact very little is being exchanged. There is difficulty articulating one's own real feelings and thoughts and difficulty grasping the meaning behind others' utterances, but sometimes an astonishing ability to produce a reasonable facsimile of conversation. If you don't listen carefully and double-check what you hear, you will think the person's cognitive processes are in fine working order. This is a cruel and common trick of FASD, a sleight of tongue that leaves expressive language intact but dampens many of the faculties that language normally conveys.

Secondary Disabilities

Another pair of complications comes with the veils of secondary disability that may mask—at the same time as they should highlight—the brain damage. Secondary disabilities (Streissguth, 1996) are the legal troubles, joblessness, chemical dependency, educational failures and other detritus of misunderstood brain damage. First, there is often such a welter of needs, crises, brushfires to put out that little time or energy is left for the intensive and subtle sleuthing it takes to lift the cover off and look underneath. Second, the effects of the constant stress and substance use may mimic or exacerbate, and will certainly confuse, the role of FASD in the troubles in the first place.

Mental illness, another of the secondary disabilities of unaddressed FASD, can further muddy the waters of underlying brain dysfunction among adults with FASD. Even when the process of neuropsychological or other testing has at last been accepted and funded and is underway, mental health issues so prevalent with fetal alcohol damage can interfere with getting a clear read on qualities and abilities: "state" trumps "trait" if it is strong enough. Depression can cause impairment in processing speed, retrieval of information and flexibility of thinking, lowering scores artificially; anxiety can exacerbate poor impulse control, causing quick, incorrect leaps; of course the psychologist is expected to factor in issues of mental health, but at times these more subtle shadings are lost in the chaotic patchwork characteristic of FASD.

Further, since much psychological testing relies on self-report, it is unlikely that an accurate history can be gleaned without corroborative sources. Asking the client a question like "How long have you felt this way?", tapping, as it does, a requirement for estimation of time, could yield guesses of "five minutes", "twenty years" or the honest "I don't know". Asked to describe elements of performance, family, medical, employment or academic history, the person with FASD will rarely be able to give anything like a realistic report. Yet with the typical ability to sound like an accurate historian, most clinicians do not think to double-check information given.

Information-Gathering

Finally, while a child is still in school, records and descriptions of behavior are easy to gather; maternal drinking history may be difficult. Once in adulthood, however, these records, descriptions and history become much harder to find. Self report, as noted above, is even less reliable if the person does suffer from FASD.

WHY WE SHOULD BOTHER ANYWAY

There are good reasons not to go to the expense and trouble of recognizing and addressing the particular neuropsychology of adults with fetal alcohol damage. It is too late for early diagnosis; there are no services for adults with FASD; the person may not be interested in exploring the diagnosis—and may in fact be actively opposed to the idea. And unlike children, who have a readymade "external brain" in school, if not in their parents, adults generally cherish the right to live independently and make their own decisions; "there is nothing wrong with me" is the conceptual ticket to never having to ask for or receive help.

BECAUSE…

Until We Do, The Cycle Continues and Expands

People with FASD are filling up and repeatedly failing in our public systems, and without adequate recognition and support they are more likely to stay in the cycle of substance abuse, homelessness, failure in general—and in the process create another generation of alcohol-affected, brain-damaged children in foster care.

People with fetal alcohol damage may cherish--fiercely--the right to independence, but in fact they rarely attain it (only 20%, according to Streissguth, 1996). As noted above, our current lack of identification and support for this condition is a setup for unrealistic expectations and the resulting chronic, often disastrous, failure to meet those expectations across the board— in relationships, jobs, rehabilitation, housing, money or time management. It is thought by most in the field that moderate to serious fetal alcohol damage afflicts a high percentage of the clients filtering through various systems of public assistance and it is likely that there is an even heavier concentration of FASD among the users of those systems who keep coming through. (There is no research on this yet, partly because of the paucity of diagnostic resources.)

An element of rehabilitation is expected in most of these systems, criminal justice being a do-it-yourself version. Welfare-to-Work, Child Protective Services, Vocational Rehab, chemical dependency treatment, criminal justice and mental health all operate on the assumption that lessons will be learned and change will occur. It is commonly expected that there will always be a subset of clients who do not change, and who may cycle through the system (or several parts of it) over and over. Some women have multiple children removed; some addicts never escape the cycle of relapse; some people cannot keep a job; some criminal offenders are incarcerated repeatedly and some mentally ill clients appear unwilling to engage in the self care that could improve their circumstances. For these people, change does not occur, and in fact the problematic behavior threads down through several generations. Failure to change is usually attributed to unwillingness, and the client's supports removed. With policies informed by fetal alcohol awareness, it is likely that many of these chronic failures could be eliminated.

With Understanding, Change is Possible and Can Make a Huge Difference to the Individual and Society

During a recent training with Native American home visitors for women with at-risk pregnancies, the supervisor realized to her chagrin that she had been forcing her workers to drop those women from their caseloads who chronically failed to show up for rides to the doctor, for example, or who seemed in some way "resistant" to ostensibly helpful advice. She suddenly recognized the likely connection between these clients' own histories of prenatal exposure and the behavior that reflected significant impairments in memory, planning and judgment. With tears in her eyes, she declared that she would never again drop these clients from the program, but would instead concentrate on identifying and addressing the gaps in functioning that kept them from successful connection.

Shifting the perceived inadequacy from client to program is all too rare, so far. Examples abound of well-intentioned, conventionally-trained staff members carrying out policies that completely miss the boat, FASD-wise. In Welfare-to-Work classes, clients with brain dysfunction are given homework which they agree to do, with every sign of having understood the instructions, then they show up the next week with "the dog ate my homework"-type excuses for not having done the task. They are either ignored, berated or eventually dropped from the program. In chemical dependency treatment, clients are confronted for "talking the talk but not walking the walk", having sincerely meant to walk the talk they uttered in the meeting but forgot all about as soon as they walked out the door. And getting to an unfamiliar office for a drug test may cause such overwhelm that the destination is never reached. Child Protective Service might ask a client to attend a parenting class, much of which focuses on organizing a child's schedule and systematizing discipline. The pro forma sticky charts and requisite "consistency" are entirely beyond the reach of someone whose own scattered brain barely gets her out of the house with all her clothes on right side out. Yet she will sincerely and convincingly promise to use this technique, about as possible as a trip to Mars.

People with FASD are so often at the center of staff anger at being "manipulated", "conned" and "used" that their departure from programs is sometimes celebrated rather than mourned. What goes unrecognized is the toll this trail of broken promises and failures takes on the person him- or herself.

Our fetal alcohol damaged ones, the "frequent flyers" through multiple systems, need a different approach to rehabilitation. This approach is spelled out further below, but the key components include realistic expectations, simplicity, a close connection with one FASD-savvy person, and plenty of logistical support. And most will need some degree of this support for the rest of their lives.

Diagnosing adults with fetal alcohol damage is necessary but not clearly not sufficient to creating adequate supports. Certainly it is crucial: without understanding the neuropsychology of our alcohol-affected brothers and sisters, we will continue to labor under the delusion of their willful noncompliance, and we will continue to set them up for, and then blame them for, their inevitable failures. But without changing the professional and community response to meet the particular needs of people with FASD, though we may understand the reason for the failures we will continue to be helpless to stop them from happening.

MAP OF NEUROPSYCHOLOGICAL FEATURES OF FASD IN ADULTHOOD

It has been said (Kapp and O'Malley, 2001, O'Malley and Storoz 2003) that fetal alcohol spectrum disorders cause dyscontrol across all systems: attention and focus, activity level, mood, behavioral self-regulation, speech, coordination and balance, sensory-motor input and outgo, cognition, reality-testing, estimation, planning and so on through the infinite number of ways to slice human functioning. There is controversy over the existence of a "behavioral phenotype" of fetal alcohol spectrum disorders and scientific research on this subject is notably lacking. Nevertheless, there is agreement among professional and family caregivers as well as individuals with FASD that the following aspects—in no particular pattern but quite often at least smattering of each—are among the most troublesome and consistent.

Attention Deficit/Hyperactivity Disorder (AD/HD)

The hallmark of AD/HD is disorganization—of thoughts, work, material possessions, relationships, impulses and on through self image. Impulsivity is the predominant thread with hyperactivity and inattention in varying severity.

AD/HD of the inherited "garden variety" can be found in high proportion among air traffic controllers and brain surgeons, for example, professions well-suited to the need for high stimulation, laserlike focus and multitasking. (Hallowell and Ratey, 1994). But AD/HD symptoms of the fetal alcohol variety, complicated as they are by difficulties in self-regulation, memory, sensory integration and cause-and-effect thinking, are part of a different and much more problematic beast. In this volume the reader will encounter further information about specific differences between AD/HD with and without prenatal alcohol exposure: differential treatment, specific attentional features and the implications of both.

It should be noted that in the abundant research on AD/HD, prenatal alcohol exposure is almost never factored out, resulting in an entire body of literature that is very likely contaminated: what has been studied as AD/HD is almost certainly in some part actually fetal alcohol damage. The exceptions are Clare Coles (2001) who has studied AD/HD with and without prenatal alcohol exposure, and Kieran O'Malley (Kapp and O'Malley 2002, O'Malley and Storoz 2003) who writes aboutAD/HD symptomatology in FASD. Many of us who are involved in large-scale diagnosis of FASD have noted informally that nearly all of the people qualifying for a diagnosis somewhere on the fetal alcohol spectrum either have or could qualify for a diagnosis of AD/HD as well.

Neuromotor Difficulties

Neuromotor effects associated with FASD include problems with balance, coordination, fine motor control, visual-motor skills, motor planning, perception and sensory integration. (From personal clinical observation over the years, it appears that large muscle movement is not notably impaired in fetal alcohol damage.) Sensory integration (Kranowitz, 1996), refers to the system of processing incoming stimuli through the senses. For most of us, the five senses are calibrated to a level of sensitivity that allows us to enjoy this incoming information and alerts us to danger or need through discomfort. For some people, the level of sensitivity is either too high, too low or both in any or all of these areas. Prenatal alcohol exposure often causes such imbalance: the tags on the back of shirts are irritating, only certain foods taste right, one has to keep changing body position, the bell at school sets off a flight reaction—or, in the opposite direction, wounds are not noticed, food is rejected even when needed, sleep is the last thing on a child's agenda when tired. A person with sensory integration difficulties will seem to overreact frequently, often entirely unaware of the trigger. Children with impaired ability to filter out sensory information will easily lose control in a crowded market, for example, regressing to much younger behavior than normal. Witnesses (including the well intentioned parents) to the resulting meltdowns are prone to attribute such behavior to failures on the part of the parents, which inevitably adds a layer of stress and intensity to the experience. Adults with this same impairment are physically and psychologically uncomfortable much of the time, At the higher range of functioning, an adult with sensory integration difficulties might find herelf beginning to panic in holiday shopping (beyond the expectable level), or have to leave busy conference meetings and take time out to decompress. At the lower end, adults with sensory issues may feel constantly barraged by incoming stimuli, overwhelmed to the point that nothing but complete isolation brings relief.

The fragile central nervous system of FASD has been compared to the "Princess and the Pea"—where the princess was so bothered by a tiny pea under a whole pile of mattresses that the kingdom was mobilized to create a soft enough bed for her to get to sleep on. Self regulation is one of the expected tasks of maturation, but if the messages arriving to the brain are of the Red Alert variety, to ask the person to "lighten up", "just get OVER it", or otherwise ignore the perceived physical imperative is to ask the impossible. Especially in the absence of the abilities to reason, remember previous (survivable) similar conditions, or come up with flexible, creative solutions to the problem at hand—all qualities that are affected by impairments in executing function.

Executive Functioning

Executive functioning refers to the ability to integrate separate pieces of information into a process of reasoning which is necessary for judgment, deliberate decision-making and generally getting along in the community. Recognizing patterns over time and situation, generalizing from one situation to another, putting oneself in another's shoes, relating cause and effect and being able to predict future events are all components of executive functioning. People with alcohol-related brain damage (and many people with brain damage in general) are often well able to grasp isolated pieces of information, but the ability to put them together to make accurate sense of the whole is affected. Without such connections, the "big picture" is lost--one's view of reality is not only limited to the immediate and most proximal moment, but it is also bent by the prism of the emotion of that moment. If a person is afraid, for example, other people's neutral or even positive actions can seem frightening. (This is a natural human reaction, but with effective executive functioning we can reason ourselves through it and avoid acting out.) Such limited and fragmented perception leads to great difficulty managing basic issues of time, estimation, truth and relationships—to "doing life".

To further illustrate the idea of executive functioning, imagine, literally, a big picture. A sailboat bobs on the ocean; birds fly above and fish doubtless swim below. An enormous steamship is heading directly for the sailboat. If your field of vision is somehow limited to the scene directly facing you, your interpretation of the picture will be in separate pieces "It's a sailboat"…"It's some birds"…"It's a steamship". There will be no sense of relationship between the elements even if you can keep the other elements in memory as you move from one side of the picture to another. There will be no ability to predict the crash or to theorize how it could be avoided, and certainly no extrapolating the presence of fish.

Executive functioning can be impaired independently of IQ, upbringing, other talents or intention. Gaps in this area of functioning are particularly frustrating when the person with FASD has a normal or above average IQ, as discussed above in "Expections." If our executive functioning is impaired, if we can only see the little piece of reality directly in front of us, it is unlikely that we will be able to do the following, so necessary for successful, independent living:

- Make plans
- Talk ourselves out of doing things that appeal in the moment but may be destructive in some way
- Act thoughtfully toward other people or understand their reactions when offended
- Keep promises
- Remember what we came into the room for
- Respect traffic signals if we're in a hurry
- Explain our actions
- Understand that our actions have consequences

- Resist taking other people's things that appeal to us
- Recognize and remedy our mistakes
- Predict what will happen
- Try another solution when our approach fails
- Benefit from any kind of program that relies on reward or punishment
- Take either credit or blame for our contribution

It is the experience-based belief of this writer that poor executive functioning is behind most of what we normally call "irresponsibility", and behind a great deal of what we attribute to deliberate bad choices and weak moral character. It is an inability to make use of abstract concepts like responsibilities, good choices and strong morals. People with FASD may be able to parrot these principles by rote; they cannot apply them meaningfully to their own lives.

Memory

Several types of memory are commonly impaired by prenatal alcohol exposure. Observation suggests that memory is most problematic when related to action: remembering what happened, or what one was going to do, or putting into action what one is supposed to do, for example, appear to be harder than remembering a piece of pure information. Part of executive functioning, as mentioned above, entails keeping more than one piece of information in mind.

Example 4. G, a Ph.D. with probable fetal alcohol brain damage, describes his difficulty remembering all the tasks involved in taking a shower: he brushes his teeth, washes his body, shampoos his hair, and shaves. He says if he doesn't keep repeating these items to himself he is apt to leave one out. As with the rest of the faculties necessary for a logistically successful life, memory takes a further nosedive in the presence of stress. During the period surrounding his orals, G had to make lists for himself down to the items of clothing he put on.

"Moral Retardation"

This phrase has been used by parent groups for some years now (McKinney, 1997) to connote the oddly disjunctive misbehavior of the moral variety that we see in homes where children with FASD are raised with solid moral values and typically good parenting. It has long been a puzzle how a person of supposedly normal intelligence, raised to be an upstanding citizen, rewarded for honesty and punished for dishonesty, can wind up with entrenched habits of lying, cheating and stealing.

These terms of course are the pejorative version, and the ones most likely to be used by society at large if not the family itself. (And sometimes the person with FASD him- or herself as well, although that requires a level of self awareness rare in this condition.) Breaking down the components necessary for truth-telling or respecting rules and personal property, we can see the broken strands of executive functioning gumming up the works.

Telling the truth requires

1. accurate recollection of events,
2. the ability to override the fear-driven if myopic impulse to get out of trouble at any cost,
3. recognition of the chances that a lie will probably be discovered,
4. understanding the very abstract concept of integrity.

Resisting the impulse to take a shortcut by ignoring rules requires a similar set of capacities. The person who fills out a time card with more than the hours worked, for example, is not thinking of the consequences of getting discovered, operating with an understanding of integrity, putting himself in the boss' shoes or remembering what happened the last time he did that. And stealing adds the particularly FASD-typical inability to recognize boundaries: the emotion of the moment, "I really want that", overrides any sense of respecting the other person's reality, let alone awareness of the possible consequences.

These "moral" failings are perhaps the most destructive outgrowths of the neurological impairment of FASD. Poor reasoning and judgment can be understood and forgiven, as can lapses of memory. Even the meltdowns and panics and fidgets connected to sensory issues are manageable. But as mentioned toward the beginning of this chapter, we humans are wired up to reflexively distance ourselves from others who seem to be capable of hurting us, and lying, stealing and cheating—no matter how understanding the other might be—will inevitably take a serious toll on relationships of all kinds.

Emotions

Remember the Bozo Clown, the inflatable toy with sand in the bottom? We could knock it down and it would always bounce back up again. No matter how hard we hit it, we could always count on its resilience. There is a bell curve to resilience, as there is to practically everything—on one end, there are people who can bounce back from catastrophically painful events, and on the other end there are those who are laid low by the smallest things, and there they stay. As with the sensory integration patterns mentioned above, people with FASD are on the fragile end of the resilience scale in terms of emotional reactivity. There isn't much sand in the bottom of this nervous system which is easily knocked down and slow to re-establish balance.

Parallels have been drawn between FASD and Borderline Personality Disorder—there are many shared features, including intensity—and totality--of emotions without the ability to call on "big picture thinking" to help ride out the storm. For the person with FASD, an emotion that most of us would recognize as passing or limited is likely to color the perception of the entire world at that moment, translating immediately to forever, in the person's mind. Suggestions for alternative interpretations often go astray, prompting accusations that the helpful other "just doesn't get it!". Good advice regarding problem-solving is met with air-tight "yes but". Flexibility and patience are not on the map; MUST DO SOMETHING takes up the whole space.

As feelings congeal into moods, the ability to climb out of anxiety or the blues decreases, never having been strong in the person with FASD to begin with. Mood disorders are common with FASD, and acting out is the common response. Given the slim likelihood of independently gaining perspective, or reasoning one's way out, or the flexibility of trying various solutions, it will be important to address the mood imbalance in the most effective way possible; otherwise, intervening in any other aspect of the person's life will meet with insurmountable obstacles situated right in the heart of that person herself.

Fluctuation

A complicating feature of FASD is the fluctuating pattern of central nervous system functioning. One day the powers of reasoning and memory can be relatively high, with little disturbance from sensory input; the next day functioning can plummet. Fatigue, overwhelm, poor nutrition or stress of any kind can be the cause, and it takes a lot less to send the CNS of a person with FASD into a tailspin than it does with a "normie", and sometimes there is no discernible cause whatsoever.

This fluctuation is another aspect of FASD that leads to unrealistic expectations and the concomitant misplaced disappointment or anger; "I know you can do it. You did it yesterday. Obviously you just don't care."

Immaturity

The combination of impulsivity, easy overwhelm and "princess and the pea" complaints, poor ability to reason, impaired memory, totality and intensity of emotions, and inconsistency from day to day—plus perhaps some other mystery ingredients—add up to a global, generalized immaturity in the person with FASD. Parent lore has it that there is often a maturational spurt in the mid-20's but on the whole and again independent of IQ, the person with fetal alcohol damage is likely to behave and perceive—but not speak, remember—like a much younger person. The Vineland Adaptive Behavior Scale has been promoted (Streissguth,1996) as a better indicator of functional capacity than the often-deceptive IQ; this window of developmental age provides a framework for understanding FASD that is far more helpful than psychological reports or psychoeducational testing, in many parents' experience. When a fetal alcohol affected child moves into young adulthood, a parent can be swayed by the normal developmental wishes for separation, increasing freedom and responsibility to manage money, time, obligations and relationships. It is difficult to impose restrictions appropriate to a 12-year-old on someone ten years older, but without such restrictions the yearned-for freedom very often leads to trouble.

A judge (McGee, 1999) related his court's success with adolescents with FASD: one component was a cadre of volunteer grandparents. Asked whether his often gang-related youngsters didn't feel "uncool" being shadowed by old people, Judge McGee said "Don't forget—these 16-year-olds are really about eight or nine. You'd be amazed at how glad they are to have a surrogate grandparent." The tender youngness lying beneath a tough exterior took the mother of a 23-year-old gang wanna-be by surprise as she discovered (at the bottom of the bag of clothes that he had carried around from house to house) an old ragged bunny from his childhood and a bright yellow fluffy chick from his ex-girlfriend.

INTERVENTIONS AND SUPPORTS THAT WORK

R. and the Group Home

Example 5. R., an 18 -year-old with a long history of foster care, group homes, juvenile hall—and an alcoholic mother, came to us at the diagnostic clinic with his grandmother. R.'s grandmother was now his staunch supporter, his only real anchor to family. R. was diagnosed with Fetal Alcohol Syndrome: his IQ in the 80's, he had particular difficulty connecting cause and effect, and developmentally he fell within the range of 9-12 years old. The diagnosis was helpful in re-routing him from the rough prison-like center he was headed for—the judge sent R. to a group home where it was hoped that he would be guided into a productive adulthood, now that they knew the cause of his misbehavior. At first the house seemed to be a success, but R. was a smoker and the house prohibited smoking. R. was caught, sanctioned, and kept on smoking. Finally the house staff decided they would use the biggest guns they had, and threatened him with loss of visits with his grandmother if he smoked again. He ran…to his grandmother's house.

Obviously diagnosis wasn't enough. The house staff didn't include FASD information to shape policies in any useful way, and R. was inadvertently set up to fail again.

A key principle in intervention with FASD is to stop what isn't working, find out what's the hard part, and see what you can do to help. (Evensen, 2004). Threatening R. to get him to stop smoking was not working, nor was removing privileges. Cajoling, reasoning and demanding were not working. Finding out what the hard part is might involve questions like the following, with practical responses:

1. Is he physiologically addicted? If so, he may benefit from medical treatment for his nicotine addiction.
2. Is he self-medicating? (Tobacco has been called in some circles "poor man's Ritalin") If so, he may need a medication evaluation.
3. Where is he getting the cigarettes—staff member? Need to stop the window of supply.
4. Is there any staff role-modeling of smoking? Need to stop the staff indulgence in substances forbidden to residents.

Taking into account R.'s developmental level, his crucial attachment to his grandmother, and his history of impulsivity, it should have been predicted that he would run, faced with the prospect of losing touch with his grandmother. R.'s difficulty grasping cause and effect should have pointed to the futility of using behavior modification techniques. In R's case, as with so many people with fetal alcohol problems, it is not so much R we need to direct our change effort toward, but the environment and the system, internal as well as external. Only then will R.'s internal world settle enough to accept the helpful scaffolding we put up around him, so he can begin to heal the terrible wounds of his lifelong exclusion from anything approaching normalcy.

Settle, Scaffold, and Heal

The steps to a happy, productive life for a person with a fetal alcohol-affected brain begin with accurate identification of that condition. The areas of deficit and strength are mapped out and the chaotic nervous system is settled. Then a supportive scaffold is constructed around mood, life habits and relationships, and the emotional healing can begin. This cycle of settling, scaffolding and healing goes around repeatedly, revised and refined to the point that in the end, the person reaches a point of self advocacy and valued contribution.

Of course this is ideal, and assumes the absence of intractible issues like serious attachment problems, severe mental illness, or entrenched sociopathy. But the experience of many successful families tells us that it is attainable.

Identification

Identification is commonly thought to be the most effective intervention for people with FASD. (Streissguth et al 2004). Once the maladaptive behavior is unmasked as biologically based rather than deliberate, expectations can become more realistic. Other people's natural reactions of distancing or anger can be tempered, and root causes of difficulties can be addressed realistically

Diagnosis by an inter-disciplinary team that understands this disorder would ideally include evaluation of cognition, memory, executive functioning, ability to distinguish between truth and fiction, developmental level, communication, neuromotor (including sensory integration) functioning and mental health. In the best of circumstances, brain imaging would accompany this evaluation.

Sometimes, of course, the person doesn't want to be seen as defective, go through any more tests, sign up for any more "services"—long experience has taught that offers of help inevitably lead to further complication and blame. In that case some pre-diagnostic alliance must happen: link arms with the person, together look at (and as soon as possible laugh about) signs of malfunctioning brain parts—sympathize with experiences of failure, as specifically as possible, and get the person interested in exploring the possibility of CNS damage.

In the meantime, until the formal diagnostic process can take place, more informal information-gathering can be quite useful in forming a picture. The following are just a few examples of simple observational windows into some aspects of the neuropsychology of a person affected by fetal alcohol exposure:

Table 1.

Cohesion and sequencing: During a narrative of an event, listen for coherent beginning, middle and end
Memory: Watch for missed appointments, lost papers, forgotten tasks
Neuromotor: Look at handwriting, ask about sports activities
Sensory integration: Ask about tags on clothes, food, experience in big stores like Costco
Perception: Notice bad grooming or hygiene, copying shapes
Reasoning: Listen for cause-and-effect connections
Rigidity of problem-solving: Play 20 Questions

A formal and comprehensive diagnosis is frankly almost impossible for the average person to obtain at this point. Some compromise version can be extremely useful, as we put together a hypothesis about a) the existence of alcohol-related brain damage, and b) areas of strength and weakness. The number of clinicians who are willing and able to identify fetal alcohol damage is small, their methods vary widely, and the diagnosis is still controversial. Nevertheless, this hardy band is growing in number, skill and consistency, and the growing demand will continue to spur them on.

Settling

Example 6. Listen to this 55-year-old teacher's description of her internal reality:

"... an inner world in which all the parts swell and shrink from day to day, like a bunch of sea cucumbers. Identity, mood, physical well-being, perceptions, memory, impulse control, sensitivity, ability to make sense of heard information, cognitive clarity in general...all so much more changeable than for the normal person. I get a sense of these swirling, competing priorities that that can energize me or paralyze me, and I have times of huge and sudden fatigue. It is almost impossible for me to generate an orderly system to my life, and so a lot of the time I'm just chasing after all the loose ends of things I haven't done, or stuff I've forgotten, or promises I made that I can't even remember what they were. What I wish I had is something like the old camp coffee technique, where you add eggshells to the boiling mess of coffee grounds and water, and they bind to the grounds and sink to the bottom so the rest of the coffee is clear."

Settling the swirling loose ends and competing priorities, the fragments of remembered tasks, the sense of self that won't stay consistent, the jangling sensory assault, or the energetic bursts and shutdowns—settling this roiling inner world would be so welcome to her. It would release her true gifts and joys into being, uncluttered with the frantic and largely fruitless attempts to maintain order.

The prerequisite for any lasting settling is an understanding of the cause of all this inconsistency in the first place—identification, in this case, of the underlying fetal alcohol damage.

Providing an explanatory context has helped many who suffer from this condition. It lifts the constant search for what might be wrong, the blame that casts about looking for a place to land. It allows for forgiveness, both by the person and of the person. And it sets the stage for the scaffolding to follow, shoring up the areas that do not work right.

Settling an out-of-control central nervous system requires more than just theory, of course. The physical fact is that equilibrium is hard to come by, and must be actively protected. The mechanism must be attended to like an old cranky Porsche: tuned up frequently, given the best oil and gas, kept in the garage at night and so on. Translated to the human mechanism, the fragility of the fetal alcohol-affected nervous system means that issues like blood sugar, nutrition, sleep, exercise, and recreational substances have a much larger impact than they do for unaffected people.

When choices and habits like the above are not enough to settle the tempestuous inner landscape, medication may be necessary to provide enough calm to begin the larger changes necessary to move ahead.

Scaffolding

Once settled, we begin to scaffold: we help put up supports to help the person build a life that allows his or her true nature to bloom, and to become an integral member of the community.

Careful to walk a line that respects both the person's difficulty in generating appropriate structure and the need for as much autonomy and dignity as possible, the helping professional here must elicit the client's own wishes and values but also serve as a reality check. Improved relationships, a decent job, safe housing, getting children back and parenting well, education, better money management are common goals. These are attainable. Getting a Lexus and a mansion in Beverly Hills are also common goals among our clients—these are not attainable, at least not if the employment obtained is legal. Since no amount of scaffolding will bring those about, it is our job to grasp the underlying wishes and translate them into the achievable: respect from the community, esthetic pleasure, material comfort.

We put practical, relevant supports in place. It is often necessary to keep them in place through another person—suggestion is not enough, usually, and head-nodding and verbal agreement does not necessarily portend success. Some of these supports will be simple, logistical and not too loaded. Supports for a poor memory, for example, might include a watch with a beeper and text to tell you why it's beeping, or phone calls before important events, or calendars and clocks in every room, and the use of lists.

Supports for sensory issues might include help choosing clothing that will not irritate, repeated reminders of the particular triggers for that person, or practice with finding refuge in overwhelming situations.

Other supports will be more difficult.

One of the hardest involves getting the person to ask for help, and extends to budget assistance, perhaps a third-party payee. Establishing routines may necessitate the presence of a helper, or at least visual or audible reminders of this structure. Recreational opportunities, social or therapeutic groups, gradual introduction into the community through volunteer work or limited, specific activities all serve to help keep the person on track.

One of the most important elements of the suggested scaffolding is the education of the people in the lives of our client. Harder than it sounds, this involves helping spouses, children, co-workers, psychotherapists—everyone—to understand that the very maddening or disappointing behavior they experience must not be taken personally, and that gentle reminders must be substituted for accusations or emotional trauma. It involves some healing of those others as well, as they have often suffered deep wounds in the context of this relationship.

Healing

Healing the heart and spirit is an area that often takes a back seat—or more often has to run alongside the car—in agencies that support people with troubles of the kind that accompany fetal alcohol. It is already very difficult to maintain the logistical network necessary for safe and acceptable life practices; healing is, if addressed at all, referred to "Mental Health", usually a county agency whose staff has no experience in FASD. (Not that privates ones do either.)

Traditional client-centered psychotherapy has not typically been helpful in addressing the organically-based issues that keep people from relating to themselves and others in a positive way. More helpful is an approach that recognizes and helps the person address the central nervous system malfunctions, and provides a safe place for experience to be unpacked and normalized.

For example, a client comes in and says "I feel like there's something wrong with me. I have always felt different, like I just don't get it." The traditional cognitive-behavioral therapist will see this as an irrational belief, the psychodynamic therapist will see it as a product of inadequate parenting, the interpersonal counselor will see it as a spiritual void. These clinicians will roll up their sleeves and get to work on dismantling what is obviously a distorted self image. A clinician will training in fetal alcohol, on the other hand, will elicit information about the specific ways the client doesn't get it, the ways he or she feels different, and what exactly does he or she think is wrong. If this material maps onto the pattern of fetal alcohol implications, the next question will be regarding maternal drinking.

And there the stage is set to flesh out the possibility of FASD (never disregarding the other interpretations as well!), and then begin to address the nervous system's glitches. From there the healing of emotional trauma and self image can proceed.

Support groups have been successful in providing a safe place for adults to share their experiences, feelings, problems and solutions. Few of these exist currently, but reports are coming in from the ones that do, with news of growth, belonging and community.

The reader might well ask who is the agent of all this support. While there are some systems in place for people with officially recognized developmental difficulties, or with diagnosed mental illness, a really workable system does not yet exist for our clientele, who may actually qualify for not just double but triple or even quadruple diagnoses in addition to the specific peculiarities of fetal alcohol damage. We in this field are proposing that such a system needs to be created. The principles described here are by no means universally agreed-upon, but are the product of ongoing conversation among people dedicated to understanding and helping those with FASD.

Principles of Intervention

In contrast to the principles of most programs, it appears that people with FASD will not be served by a system of rewards and punishments; they will not benefit from the usual aim of total independence; they cannot manage a fragmented array of services from different people spread out all over town; and they may continue to have trouble with truth-telling, hygiene or recognizing the boundaries of personal property.

What they will benefit from is, first, accurate diagnosis of the cause of their misbehavior; second, interventions that serve to settle the wildly fluctuating and chaotic nervous system; third, ongoing protective structure to shore up malfunctioning areas; fourth, attention to healing the heart and spirit. An understanding other appears to be essential to this structure, as are careful environmental adjustments, including the deep education of the people closest to them. Ultimately, they will benefit most from widespread recognition of the pattern of behavior that comes from brain damage, not from malicious intent.

CONCLUSION

In a story by a well-known foster dad and group-home leader ("I've helped over 900 kids!"), a young man wants a job. Dad has already categorized him as lazy and told him he will not recommend him at the auto body shop. He nevertheless tries out for the job at the shop. The boss tells him to shelve the new parts and toss the old ones. Left alone for several hours, he works diligently but throws away the new parts and shelves the old ones. The boss is furious, and tells our boy that he obviously doesn't really want the job. The dad, confirmed in his contempt for the boy, tells him he'll never get anywhere, that he is the poster child for the irresponsible ones who will wind up one the street. Dad is half right: unless this boy gets some help from someone who understands, either through training or intuition, the processes and principles that help people with fetal alcohol damage, he is in fact very likely to wind up on the street.

When I told the story of the woman in the car behind me in Susanville during a training someone asked me if—big proponent of self awareness that I am—I would ever consider telling someone like her that I thought she had brain damage. Although the thought did occur to me in an unkind, slightly explosive and totally useless form at the moment...of course not. But my own belated shift in awareness lifted a burden from my soul in a most unexpected way.

I believe it hurts us at a deep level, society as a whole, to continue to condemn people to lives of incarceration, isolation, ridicule and shame, at the same time as the knowledge exists that could support these same people to live with dignity and the profound happiness that comes with being a positive contributor to the community

The best prevention of future generations with fetal alcohol damage comes from a whole community that recognizes it for what it is, wraps those who already have it in a 24/7, seamless safety net, and certainly provides treatment for women with substance abuse problems.

REFERENCES

Brown, Stephanie. (1999). *The Alcoholic Family in Recovery: A Developmental Model*. New York: Guilford Press.

Coles, Claire (2001). Fetal alcohol exposure and attention: moving beyond ADHD. *Alcohol Research and Health, 25*,199-203.

Evensen, Deb (2004, personal communication)

Hallowell, Edward M., MD, and John J. Ratey, MD (1994). *Driven to Distraction: Recognizing and Coping with Attention Deficit Disorder from Childhood through Adulthood*. New York: Simon and Schuster (Touchstone).

Kapp , FME and O'Malley KD (2002) Watch for the Rainbows. True stories for educators and other Caregivers of children with Fetal Alcohol Spectrum Disorders. Revised 1st edition, September , Publisher Frances Kapp Education, Calgary, Canada

Kleinfeld, Judith and Wescott, Siobhan. (1993). Fantastic Antone Succeeds. University of Alaska Press.

Kranowitz, Carol. (1998). The Out-of-Sync Child. New York: Penguin Putnam (Perigee).

McGee, Charles (1999, personal communication)

McKinney, Vicky (1997, personal communication)

O'Malley, K. D. and Storoz, L. (2003) Fetal alcohol spectrum disorder and ADHD: diagnostic implications and therapeutic consequences. Expert Rev. Neurotherapeutics 3 (4), 477- 489

Page, K. (2001). Dissertation: Signs of Prenatal Alcohol Damage Among Adult Children of Alcoholics, Center for Psychological Studies, Albany, CA.

Streissguth, A.P., Barr, H.M., Kogan, J., and Bookstein, F.L. (1996). Understanding the occurrence of secondary disabilities in clients with fetal alcohol syndrome and fetal alcohol effects. Final report to the Centers for Disease Control and Prevention (CDC), August, 1996 (Tech. Rep. No. 96-06). Seattle, WA: University of Washington.

Streissguth , AP, Bookstein, FL, Barr, HM, Sampson, PD, O'Malley K, Kogan Young J (2004) Risk factors for adverse life outcomes in fetal alcohol syndrome and fetal alcohol effects. Developmental and Behavioral Pediatrics, Vol. 25, No. 4, 228-238

Vega, William (1992). *Profile of Alcohol and Drug UseDuring Pregnancy in California* , submitted to California Dept. of Alcohol and Drug Programs by University of California, Berkeley , School. of Public. Health, Sept. 1993.

In: ADHD and Fetal Alcohol Spectrum Disorders (FASD) ISBN: 1-59454-573-1
Editor: Kieran D. O'Malley, pp. 125-160 © 2008 Nova Science Publishers, Inc.

Chapter 8

SEXUALLY INAPPROPRIATE BEHAVIOR IN PATIENTS WITH FETAL ALCOHOL SPECTRUM DISORDERS

Natalie Novick-Brown[*]

INTRODUCTION

It was late afternoon when she heard the phone ring with the call that would change her son's life and her own forever. She moved slowly across the room and quietly lifted the receiver. She heard the deep voice on the other end ask her if he had reached the Smith residence. "Yes," she replied. "This is the Sheriff's Department, Mrs. Smith. I am afraid I have some bad news." She had become somewhat accustomed to calls from school personnel and neighbors over the years reporting minor problems involving her son Jim and his behavior with other children or adults. Early in Jim's life, these reports were frequent and varied and typically involved minor rule breaking behavior, temper tantrums, or social problems with children his age. But Jim was now 20 years of age and seemed to have grown out of many of his problems. He was even working part-time at a local grocery store and appeared to be doing well.

Diagnosed as "different" since infancy, no one really seemed able to pin down the real cause of his problems. First, his doctor, and later elementary school staff, suspected Jim might be slow or even mildly retarded. They later decided he was learning disabled and had him placed in a special education program. By the time he entered adolescence, the professionals had decided he probably suffered from Attention Deficit and Hyperactivity Disorder (ADHD) with severe deficits in concentration and impulse control that affected his ability to learn and relate to others. Most recently, when the school suggested that Jim would benefit from a vocational training program, the professionals hinted that he might be suffering from Fetal Alcohol Syndrome. Jim's mother didn't know exactly what that meant, but she did know she was tired of all the labels and how much hard work she had done to get Jim through his youth. She admitted to herself that she had gone through a "wild period" around the time of Jim's birth and probably had more alcohol at times than she should have had. But no more

---

[*] University of Washington's Fetal Alcohol and Drug Unit in Seattle. FASD expert in private practice.

than other young women her age, she thought. It had sent shivers through her when they first suggested that Jim's problems might have been the result of her own short period of experimentation with alcohol and marijuana. However, she rejected any such explanation given how many times the professionals had been wrong and given Jim's good progress over the past two years.

She could hardly decipher the words as she heard them: Child Rape? Sexual Exploitation of a Minor? "You must be mistaken! It can't be Jim," she heard herself stammer. Her mind drifted away as she barely heard the officer's assurance that the perpetrator was indeed her son Jim. How could this be?, she thought. Jim hardly seemed aware of sexuality. He seemed to have no interest in sex, only a passing interest in females, and never asked any questions about his sexual development. In fact, he almost appeared to be asexual, she thought to herself. During all the years of his struggles in school and in the community, she had never recalled anyone, including professionals, saying anything about Jim's sexual behavior or sexual development. It suddenly occurred to her that she did not have the faintest idea about her son's sexuality. She seemed paralyzed and unable to comprehend anything she was hearing until the officer's words pierced her inner world: "Felony rape with the possibility of 10-15 years in prison." How could she have been so blind? How could she have let her son down like this?

Sadly, stories such as this are hardly unknown to parents of special needs children and have becoming alarmingly common in recent years. While parents, teachers, mental health professionals, and caregivers have focused on the many perplexing and demanding symptoms, behaviors and deficits of special needs populations, little attention or research has been directed at understanding such persons as sexual beings. Predictably, little in the way of education, assistance, or therapy has been available to these youth, who almost certainly face the very complex world of sexuality and sexual relationships with a combination of trepidation, confusion, misunderstanding, guilt, impulsivity, and intense attraction. As a psychologist who has specialized for many years in the evaluation and treatment of violent sexual offenders, this author has witnessed and studied the remarkably complex and often contorted development of severe sexual pathology on the part of so-called 'normal' individuals without cognitive and neurological impairments. One might imagine that from the standpoint of an adolescent or young adult suffering from ADHD or Fetal Alcohol Spectrum Disorder (FASD), the developmental journey through understanding one's sexuality and sexual development and finding appropriate methods for sexual expression might simply be overwhelming. It would be gratifying to report that having recognized the paucity of knowledge and limited practical assistance available to such clients and their caregivers, we have undertaken research that will soon alleviate such ignorance. Unfortunately, nothing could be further from the truth. The shroud of secrecy, discomfort, isolation, and mythology that surrounded the study of "normal sexuality" at the time of the seminal studies of Kinsey and Masters and Johnson appears still to attach to the understanding and study of sexuality in special needs populations. It appears to be generally unsettling for many of us to think of "those people" as sexual beings with powerful (and normal) sexual drives.

The purpose of this chapter is to provide an initial review and understanding of what little we do know about the sexuality of special needs populations, with emphasis on those suffering from the cognitive and neurological deficits inherent in ADHD and FASD. This author first provides a review of the limited empirical research on the subject, which is restricted at this point to incidence data. Next, there is an analysis of how to conceptualize sexually inappropriate behavior: deficits in sexual socialization or sexual deviancy, with additional emphasis on the effect of childhood sexual abuse on sexual development. Following a basic review of the functional deficits in ADHD and FASD and historical overview of diagnostic symptomatology, the next section presents an intriguing area of research that has received little empirical attention: comorbidity of the two conditions. The chapter then turns to how primary functional deficits in ADHD and FASD might lead to the emergence of sexual behavior problems, with an assessment of the possible scope of the problem as identified in FASD research. Individual and environment factors that play a role in sexual expression are identified, with emphasis on the problem of hidden disabilities that make identification and assessment very difficult. Next, the chapter focuses on normal sexual development, followed by abnormal sexual development, and then highlights how special needs youth are significantly disadvantaged in this complex developmental process. Protective factors that may mitigate against the expression of sexually inappropriate behaviors are identified as well as aggravating risk factors that are likely to potentiate sexual misconduct. The chapter culminates in a discussion of the legal challenges faced by special needs clients who act out sexually, with a review of the critical elements that should be included in risk assessment, treatment, and community management. Suggestions for future research are offered at the close of the chapter.

Literature Review

There are two widespread myths about the sexuality and sexual behavior of individuals with cognitive disorders and developmental delays: either they are childlike and sexually innocent, or they are hypersexual and out of control. With respect to both perspectives, there is no definitive research on sexual offenders that shows individuals with cognitive and neurological disorders are either more or less prone to commit sexual offenses than normal populations. The few studies that address this issue suggest slightly higher rates of sexually offending for people with cognitive disorders (e.g., Day, 1997), but this may reflect the relative ease with which their sexual misconduct is detected or other factors rather than sexual deviancy. Nonetheless, because sex offense is dealt with so harshly in our society today and so little is known about the sexuality of individuals with cognitive and neurological impairments, it is important to begin addressing this issue in order to better protect the interests of the mentally disabled as well as the interests of the community. While it matters little to victims why someone has sexually assaulted them, accurate identification of cognitive and neurological deficits in sex offenders is imperative not only to assess level of culpability but to determine the specialized services they will need in order to prevent recurrence.

What little research has been done in the area of cognitive deficits and sexual behavior has looked generally at the proportion of cognitively impaired sex offenders compared to the proportion of non-impaired sex offenders. A comprehensive but early review of sex offenders found that 10% to 15% of all sexual offenses are committed by people with mental retardation, which is only slightly higher than the incidence rate in the general population of around 9% (Murphy et al., 1983). Another study conducted two years later (Gross, 1985) found that almost 50% of incarcerated offenders with developmental disabilities and 34% of those living in the community had been convicted of sex offenses. However, Gilby and colleagues (1989) found that the frequency of sexual behavior problems in juveniles with mental retardation did not differ significantly from the frequency of similar problems in non-impaired juveniles. In a more recent study (Day, 1997), sex offenses were found to be the second most common crime among people with developmental disabilities, and sex offenses were the crimes for which most offenders with developmental disabilities were incarcerated. A nationwide study that surveyed 243 community agencies found the most common sexual offenses among individuals with cognitive deficits were inappropriate sexual behavior in public (62.2%), sexual activity involving minors (42.6%), and assaultive/nonconsensual sexual activity with adults (34.5%) (Ward et al. 2001). In comparison, the most common sexual offenses in the general population are offenses against children, genital exposure, and rape (Murphy et al., 1983). While these statistics may appear similar, other studies have found that cognitively impaired sex offenders tend to commit more "nuisance" sex offenses as opposed to serious sex crimes involving emotional and/or physical injury to the victim (Gilby et al., 1989; Day, 1997). As there is no body of research on the nature and scope of sexual offending by individuals with cognitive and neurological impairments, no conclusions on incidence rates can be drawn. However, as this chapter will note, there is reason to suspect that Central Nervous System (CNS) deficits play an important role in the behavior of some sex offenders.

SEXUAL DEVIANCY VS. INADEQUATE SEXUAL SOCIALIZATION

Accurate understanding of the reason why someone has committed a sexual offense is important because of the harsh manner in which sex offenders, with their presumed sexual deviancy, are dealt with in our society today. However, as Hingsburger and his colleagues (Hingsburger, Griffiths, and Quinsey, 1991) point out, it is often quite difficult to distinguish between sexually inappropriate behavior and sexual deviancy, even in the rare situations where the attempt is made. According to these authors, behaviors that may seem sexually deviant – such as exhibitionism, inappropriate touching, and even more intrusive sexual assaults against children and adults – may not be motivated by sexual deviancy at all but rather by other factors. *Counterfeit deviance* is a term they have used to describe sexual behaviors that appear to have criminal and deviant sexual intent but which are, upon analysis, the result of other factors, such as lack of sexual socialization.

Because we live in a system that generally does not support appropriate and timely sex education, dating, and social experimentation (i.e., learning experiences) for people with cognitive disorders, lack of sexual socialization may be a primary factor underlying sexual offenses committed by these individuals. Instead of recognizing that individuals with CNS impairments have the same sexual urges and desires as non-impaired persons and teaching them the range of behaviors involved in appropriate sexual expression, caregivers generally ignore their sexuality until problems develop. Then, instead of providing treatment that essentially addresses what these individuals could have learned in childhood and adolescence had their caregivers been better informed, these individuals are instead incarcerated, civilly committed, or medicated and sent to supervised residential facilities. In all of these settings, they are expected to understand the reasons for their legal sanctions and to simply stop their inappropriate sexual behaviors. In the small percentage of cases where treatment is offered, it often is not provided by mental health professionals trained to work with this special population.

As Hingsburger et al. (1991) note, there are many possible explanations other than sexual deviancy why persons with cognitive and neurological deficits might sexually offend, including:

- living in environments that prohibit appropriate sexual expression;
- lack of opportunities to meet and develop relationships with appropriate sexual partners;
- lack of knowledge about basic social skills such as sexual versus nonsexual touch and public versus private behavior;
- lack of understanding and skills to deal with sexual urges and impulses;
- inappropriate modeling by others who have sexually abused them; and
- no training on boundaries between self and others.

All of these factors having to do with lack of sexual socialization stem from a single underlying problem: failure to recognize the importance of teaching responsible, normative socio-sexual expression to youngsters with cognitive impairments and developmental delays.

SEXUAL ABUSE

Although many sex offenders were sexually abused in their childhood, there is no empirical support for the conclusion that childhood sexual abuse "causes" someone to become a sexual offender. However, childhood sexual abuse may cause children – cognitively impaired or not -- to engage in inappropriate sexual behaviors. In general, children who have been sexually abused often display more sexual behaviors in childhood and adolescence than children who have not been abused (Friedrich et al., 1987, Friedrich and Luecke, 1988). Learning theory postulates that children learn about sexual expression from observing significant adults in their lives (Groth, 1979; Longo, 1986) and that sexual abuse causes sexuality to become a central developmental focus of the child, around which other developmental tasks continue but often at a delayed pace in comparison to non-abused children (Gil and Johnson, 1993). Others suggest that some children mimic their sexual abuse as a form of repetition compulsion in response to being overwhelmed by feelings of helplessness, terror, anxiety, and vulnerability (Breer, 1987). Based on this theory, the child who acts out sexually takes on the perpetrator role as opposed to the victim role and thereby gains temporary relief. Other children may become eroticized by their caregiving environments (Yates, 1987), such as children who are regularly exposed to adult sexual activity or masturbation. If they also experience separation anxiety, random physical abuse, or abrupt rejections, this only intensifies the relief they might possibly gain from sexual expression. Yates (1982) also notes that many preschoolers do not differentiate between affectionate non-sexual and sexual relationships and consequently become sexually aroused by routine physical or psychological closeness with others. Whatever the explanation, because of their deficient coping skills, children with FASD and ADHD may be more prone than their unimpaired counterparts to engage in inappropriate sexual behaviors following their own sexual victimization.

PRIMARY FUNCTIONAL DEFICITS

Two broad and interrelated functional deficits contribute to the problem of counterfeit deviance: *attention deficits* (particularly, social attention) and *deficient impulse control*. Proficiency in attention involves a complex cognitive process that encompasses many sub-skills beyond the ability to sustain focus on a target stimulus without being distracted by extraneous stimuli. These sub-skills include the ability to distinguish between important versus irrelevant social information, accurately perceive and understand subtle social cues and social context, understand verbal information and communicate effectively, perceive boundaries between the self and others, and retain and retrieve information in working memory (Barkley, 1990). Proficiency in impulse control involves sub-skills such as an ability to delay gratification, consider consequences and social taboos, inhibit inappropriate thoughts and intentions, generalize past mistakes to current situations, and temper an egocentric view of the world (Barkley, 1990). Although researchers who study adolescent and adult sex offenders find strong evidence for impulse control deficits in individuals who commit sexual offenses (e.g., Knight and Prentky, 1990; Prentky et al., 1995; Knight, 1989) and in sex offenders who recidivate (see 2004 meta-analysis by Hanson and Morton-Bourgon), there is almost no research on impulse control or attention deficits in offenders with cognitive and neurological impairments. There also is very little research on whether either deficit category distinguishes sex offenders from their non-impaired counterparts. The sole exception appears to be a recent article by Baumbach (2002) that suggests deficits in response inhibition may be a key factor in the lack of self-control exhibited by sex offenders with Fetal Alcohol Spectrum Disorder (FASD).

FETAL ALCOHOL SPECTRUM DISORDERS (FASD)

The term Fetal Alcohol Syndrome (FAS) was first introduced in 1973 by researchers who described a pattern of facial dysmorphology, growth deficiency, and Central Nervous System (CNS) dysfunction (e.g., learning difficulties, poor impulse control, problems in social perception, deficits in receptive and expressive language, poor capacity for abstraction or metacognition, deficits in mathematical skills, memory problems, brief attention span, and poor judgment) in a small sample of women who chronically abused alcohol during their pregnancies (see Jones and Smith, 1973). Partial Fetal Alcohol Syndrome (PFAS) and Alcohol Related Neurodevelopmental Disorder (ARND) were terms that were later added by the American Institute of Medicine (IOM, 1996) to classify variations of the disorder. The IOM also created the term Alcohol-Related Birth Defects (ARBD) to address physical disabilities such as deformities in skeleton and internal/sensory organs. PFAS, also called Fetal Alcohol Effects (FAE), involves CNS impairment and associated neurodevelopmental problems without the facial dysmorphology associated with FAS. ARND, on the other hand, involves CNS defects and developmental abnormalities without facial dysmorphology and growth defects.

Today, while there is still variation in terminology, Fetal Alcohol Spectrum Disorders (FASD) is becoming widely used as an umbrella term encompassing all diagnostic categories associated with damage from prenatal alcohol exposure.

While it is not precisely known how many individuals with FASD are committed to juvenile facilities or incarcerated in adult prisons for sexual misconduct, recent research suggests disproportionate representation, which may be due to factors unrelated to sexual deviance as noted earlier in this chapter. The scope of the problem appears to be quite large, as discovered in post-hoc research by Streissguth et al. (1997). In that study, it was found that approximately 50% of adolescents and adults had experienced trouble with Sexually Inappropriate Behaviors. More generally, this study found that 60% of adolescents and adults had experienced trouble with the law, and 50% had been confined involuntarily under civil or criminal law. It was not addressed in this study how many of these legal problems were due to sexual misconduct.

ATTENTION-DEFICIT/HYPERACTIVITY DISORDER (ADHD)

ADHD has a much longer empirical history than FASD and is one of the most frequently studied childhood disorders. First identified in Heinrich Hoffman's 19th century descriptions of "Fidgety Phil" (Arnold and Jensen, 1995), one of the earliest papers on the subject was a three-part article by Still (1902) which described children with ADHD as suffering from defects in "moral control" and "volitional inhibition." Researchers in the late 1940s were impressed by the similarity between the behavioral problems of ADHD children and those with brain injury. As a result, overactivity, distractibility, inattention, and poor impulse control were believed to be characteristic of brain injury despite the absence of definitive neurological evidence (Strauss and Lehtinen, 1947). In the 1960s, the emphasis on hyperactivity as the hallmark symptom of the disorder took precedence in the absence of scientific methods to detect brain injury (Chess, 1960; Clements, 1966). However, as more measures were developed to assess additional constructs associated with the disorder, it became apparent that attentional deficits and impulse control problems also were primary symptoms as well as hyperactivity (Douglas, 1972). Although abundant evidence accumulated in the 1970s and 1980s to support this tri-dimensional construct of ADHD (Douglas 1980, 1983), more recent research has shown that the Predominantly Inattentive Type of the disorder may be qualitatively different from the Predominantly Hyperactive-Impulsive Type (Barkley et al., 1990; Barkley, DuPaul and McMurray, 1990). The Diagnostic and Statistical Manual, Fourth Edition (DSM-IV), now describes three subtypes of the disorder: the predominantly hyperactive-impulsive category, the predominantly inattentive category, and a combined subtype.

Categorized under the broad category of Inattention are deficits in primary skills, such as ability to sustain attention and mental effort on tasks or activities, follow through on rules and instructions, give close attention to details, listen when spoken to directly, organize tasks and activities, maintain focus in the context of extraneous stimuli, and remember things necessary for tasks or activities (Barkley, DuPaul and McMurray, 1990). Primary disabilities included under the subtype Hyperactive-Impulsive include: fidgetiness; staying seated when required; moving, running, and climbing more than most children; playing noisily; talking excessively; interrupting others' activities; and being less able than others to wait in line or take turns in games (American Psychiatric Association, 2000). The problems associated with disinhibition typically arise in the preschool years; problems associated with inattention often arise later in childhood between ages 5 to 7 (Hart et al., 1996; Loeber et al., 1992). Although children with ADHD often display problems in the two major symptom dimensions noted above, they also display a number of other symptoms that affect social cognition and behavioral inhibition including motor coordination and sequencing (Barkley, DuPaul, and McMurray, 1990; Mariani and Barkley, 1997), working memory and mental computation (Barkley, 1997, Mariani and Barkley, 1997; Zentall and Smith, 1993), planning and anticipation (Barkley, Grodzinsky, and DuPaul, 1992; Douglas, 1983), verbal fluency and confrontational communication (Grodzinsky and Diamond, 1992; Zentall, 1988), effort allocation (Douglas, 1983; Voelker et al., 1989), application of organizational strategies (Hamlet, Pellegrini and Conners, 1987; Voelker et al., 1989; Zentall, 1988), internalization of self-directed speech (Berk and Potts, 1991; Copeland, 1979), adherence to restrictive instructions (Barkley, 1985; Roberts, 1990), self-regulation of emotional arousal (Barkley, 1997; Douglas, 1983), and diminished moral reasoning (Nucci and Herman, 1982; Simmel and Hinshaw, 1993).

Similar to children diagnosed with FASD, children with ADHD appear more likely than normal children to have deficits in general intelligence (Barkley, 1997a), problems with academic achievement (Barkley, 1990; Cantwell and Satterfield, 1978), poor peer acceptance (Johnston, Pelham and Murphy, 1985; Pelham and Bender, 1982), and deficits in adaptive functioning (Barkley, DuPaul and McMurray, 1990). Children with "pure" ADHD (i.e., ADHD not associated with comorbid disorders) are likely to have problems primarily in school performance (Paternite and Loney, 1980) and are often described as "underachieving." Those with associated aggression and conduct problems appear to have far worse outcomes such as predelinquent or delinquent behavior in the community (Barkley et al., 1990) and have symptoms of the disorder that persist into later adolescence (Biederman et al., 1996). As young adults, between 30 and 60% of individuals with ADHD continue to have problems with restlessness, inattention, impulsivity, low self-esteem, and depression (Manuzza et al., 1993). Many of the above characteristics associated with ADHD have also been found in sexual offenders (e.g., see Hanson and Bussiere, 1998, and Hanson and Morton-Bourgon, 2004).

As in the FASD population, longitudinal research suggests that children with ADHD are at greater risk than normal children for arrest and incarceration as adults (Manuzza et al., 1989). Several studies of adult male prisoners also have found unusually high rates of ADHD in male prisoners (Curran and Fitzgerald, 1999; Rasmussen et al., 2001; Eyestone and Howell, 1994). However, as with FASD, almost no literature exists on the possible role of ADHD in sexual misconduct, although anecdotal clinical data suggests the possible role of the disorder in childhood sexual aggression and in adult hypersexuality and inappropriate sexual behavior (Hallowell and Ratey, 1994). In addition, research with the Child Sexual Behavior Inventory finds that parents of ADHD children more often report interpersonal boundary problems and excessive masturbation than parents of children without this disorder (Friedrich, 1994).

COMORBIDITY

The comorbidity of FASD with ADHD also has received little empirical attention, although research is now beginning to focus on this issue. ADHD symptoms of inattention, impulsivity, and hyperactivity seem to be almost universal in individuals suffering from FASD (Snyder et al., 1997). When Nanson (1990) compared the behavior of FAS children against those with pure ADHD and normal children, children with FAS had similar behavioral ratings compared to children with ADHD, although the children with FAS were more cognitively impaired than the children in the other two groups. Thus, the distinction between the two diagnoses may be one of degree rather than quality in some individuals.

Early research showed an association between maternal alcohol consumption and smoking during pregnancy and symptoms of ADHD in children born of such pregnancies (Bennett, Wolin, and Reiss, 1988; Nichols and Chen, 1981; Streissguth et al., 1984). According to Nanson and Hiscock (1990), maternal alcohol consumption during pregnancy, even in small amounts, is associated with inattention and restless behavior in preschool children, and preschool children of social drinkers appear to display behavior similar to preschoolers who are later diagnosed with Attention Deficit Disorder (ADD). In this early comparison of children with FASD and ADD, it was found that FASD and ADD children, regardless of their intellectual abilities, were considered by their parents to be hyperactive and inattentive compared to normal children. Thus, this preliminary evidence suggests that children diagnosed with ADD may include a number of individuals whose symptoms were caused by prenatal exposure to "social" amounts of alcohol.

Also interesting in terms of a link between the two conditions and their association with sexual behaviors are studies in the mid-1990s (Niccols, 1994; Stratton et al., 1996) that found hyperactivity in 85% of children with FAS. Another study in the mid-1990s (Friedrich, 1994) found that parents reported an unusually high incidence of interpersonal boundary problems and increased masturbation in children diagnosed with ADHD. Concurrently, Streissguth (1997) noted that some children with FASD were out of control even as preschoolers, displaying behaviors seen in children diagnosed with ADHD (i.e., physical aggression, fire setting, marked hyperactivity, incorrigibility, and *unusual sexual behavior.*)

A recent literature review by O'Malley and Nanson (2002) found emerging clinical, neuropsychological, and neurochemical evidence of a commonality in prenatal damage to the neurochemical and structural environments of the brain in individuals with ADHD and FASD. For example, research on FASD using Magnetic Resonance Imaging (MRI) has found anomalies in the corpus callosum and subcortical structures in the brains of individuals with FASD (Bookstein et al., 2002) and reduced brain size and density in the frontal lobes and striatum of individuals with ADHD (Castellanos et al., 1994; Hynd et al., 1993; Rapoport, 1996). This brain damage appears to manifest in very young infants as problems in mood and state regulation and self-soothing as well as hypersensitivity to external stimuli and is found in neonates diagnosed with ADHD (Thomas and Chess, 1977; Wittenberg, 2001) and in those diagnosed with FASD (Streissguth et al., 1984).

According to the literature review (O'Malley and Nanson, 2002), evidence of an etiological link between FASD and ADHD is also found in the neurochemical system. One body of research postulates that ADHD stems from dysregulation in the frontal-nigrostriatal dopamine system and the effect of this dysregulation on arousal states (Cyr and Brown,

1998). A second body of research theorizes that ADHD is caused by dysregulation in the noradrenergic system (Arnold and Jensen, 1995; Pliszka, McCracken, and Maas, 1996). In contrast, studies of the neurochemistry in FASD have been found in multiple systems, including the dopaminergic and noradrenergic systems (Gillespie et al., 1997). It may be that similar impairments in these two systems underlie ADHD symptoms seen in FASD subjects, such as hyperactivity, reactivity, attention deficits, inhibition deficits, and impaired habituation.

The DSM-IV notes that between 3-5% of children meet criteria for ADHD, and some studies suggest rates as high as 11% (Arnold and Jensen 1995). The incidence of FASD is lower, from 9.1 per 1000 live births (Sampson et al., 1997) to 10 per 100 in communities where alcohol abuse is common (Niccols, 1994). However, it should be kept in mind that these are merely the statistics for cases that have been identified and diagnosed. It is possible, and even likely, that these percentages significantly underestimate the actual numbers of children with these conditions. It also is possible that ADHD characteristics in some individuals may be the result of prenatal exposure to alcohol. According to Snyder and colleagues (1997), ADHD is one of the most frequent comorbid diagnoses in individuals with FASD at all developmental levels.

FROM FUNCTIONAL DEFICITS TO BEHAVIOR

What is it about attention and impulse control deficits that might lead to sexually inappropriate behavior in persons with cognitive and neurological impairments? In 1992, Carmichael Olson and colleagues (1992) studied the adaptive functioning of 61 adolescents and adults with FASD using the Vineland Adaptive Behavior Scales to measure daily living skills (e.g., social interaction, eating and meal preparation, toileting, personal self-care, domestic skills, scheduling and punctuality). Results showed that primary functional disabilities stemming from CNS dysfunction in turn led to more complex maladaptive behaviors that compromised not only adaptive functioning but sexual behavior as well. Some of these primary functional disabilities included emotional dependency, excessive need for attention, stubbornness, sullenness, social withdrawal or social intrusiveness, crying or laughing too easily, lack of consideration of others, failure to learn from mistakes, hygiene problems, behavioral disorganization, lack of initiative, and unresponsiveness to subtle social cues. A follow-up study that same year (LaDue et al., 1992) using the Symptom Checklist as well as the Vineland replicated the initial study but found more specifically that 31% of the 92 patients studied had histories of Sexually Inappropriate Behaviors, with males (38%) far more likely than females (18%) to have displayed these behaviors.

After these basic adaptive skills had been identified, researchers postulated that more complex maladaptive behaviors stemming from these primary deficits might have serious life-long consequences, including impaired sexual expression. A major four-year study in the mid-1990s undertaken to confirm this hypothesis discovered some rather surprising findings. Research on adverse life outcomes (termed "secondary disabilities") in 415 children, adolescents, and adults with FASD found that unexpectedly large percentages of this sample not only had histories of mental health problems, disrupted school experience, trouble with the law, involuntary confinement, and alcohol/drug problems, but almost half of those studied had a history of *repetitive Inappropriate Sexual Behaviors* (Streissguth et al., 1997). A number of specific sexual behaviors were identified under the broad category of Inappropriate Sexual Behaviors: inappropriate sexual advances, inappropriate sexual touching, promiscuous sexual behavior, exhibitionism, compulsive sexual behavior (e.g., compulsive masturbation), public masturbation, voyeurism (i.e., peeping), incest behavior, obscene phone calls, sexual activity with animals, other "unusual or worrisome" sexual behaviors, and contact with the law regarding sexual offending.

According to more recent research out of the same lab (Streissguth et al., 2004), the second most frequent adverse life outcome across the life span in FASD populations is repetitive Inappropriate Sexual Behaviors. (Mental health problems are the most common adverse life outcome.) Moreover, Inappropriate Sexual Behaviors appear to increase with each age category from 39% in children to 48% in adolescents and 52% in adults. In children, the most frequently noted Inappropriate Sexual Behaviors are exposing (20%) and inappropriate sexual touching (19%). In adolescents and adults, promiscuity (26%) is the most frequently mentioned Inappropriate Sexual Behavior, with twice the number of females (22%) engaging in this behavior as males (11%). Inappropriate sexual advances (18%) are the second most frequent Inappropriate Sexual Behavior for both adolescents and adults. Trouble with the law for inappropriate sexual behaviors occurred twice as much for males (19%) as females (8%).

Given these findings, it would not be surprising to find that both FASD and ADHD are over-represented in populations that sexually offend, although as previously noted, there is controversy in the literature regarding such a conclusion (Hingsburger and Tough, 1997). While individuals with these conditions may be more likely to be charged with a crime compared to those without such deficits because of their relative inability to hide their behavior, on the other hand, sexual offenses by people with cognitive deficits may go unreported since law enforcement officers and prosecutors tend to be unsure how to handle individuals with cognitive and neurological disabilities. Further complicating the issue is counterfeit deviance and the possibility that individuals with CNS deficits sexually offend because they do not realize their behavior is unhealthy, harmful, or illegal due to lack of sexual socialization (Hingsburger, Griffiths, and Quinsey, 1991).

INDIVIDUAL VS. ENVIRONMENTAL FACTORS

Two studies (Day, 1994; Griffiths et al., 1985) that have looked at *individual factors* in developmentally delayed sex offenders find traits also seen in clinical practice with sex offenders diagnosed with FASD and/or ADHD. In particular, these studies found that compared to adult non-delayed sex offenders, adult developmentally delayed sex offenders tend to:

- Be sexually naïve;
- Display significantly more social skill deficits;
- Lack interpersonal skills;
- Have difficulties interacting with the opposite sex;
- Commit fewer "serious" sex offenses but more minor "nuisance" offenses; and

- Show a low degree of specificity in terms of offense type, age, and sex of victim.

Adolescent male sex offenders who are developmentally delayed show similar qualities compared to their non-delayed counterparts, especially in that they are more likely to engage in inappropriate, non-assaultive, nuisance sexual behaviors such as exhibitionism and voyeurism (Gilby et al., 1989).

Individual characteristics found in general sex offender populations (Hare, 1991) also are found in FASD and ADHD populations (Streissguth, 1997; American Psychiatric Association, 2000), including:

- hyperactivity and restlessness, manifesting in general sex offender studies as attraction to high-stimulation and high-risk behaviors and irresponsibility;
- self-control problems, manifesting in sex offenders as impulsivity, failure to consider consequences and learn from past mistakes;
- social and interpersonal problems (, manifesting in sex offenders as egocentrism, intolerance, rigid thinking, interpersonal insensitivity, and manipulativeness;
- impatience, manifesting in sex offenders as a need for instant gratification and low frustration tolerance;
- emotional immaturity, manifesting in sex offenders as egocentrism and lack of empathy; and
- self-regulation deficits, manifesting in sex offenders as anger control problems and addictive behaviors.

Certainly not every person with FASD or ADHD develops a sexual behavior problem. However, in those who do, and particularly in those who go on to commit sexual offenses, comorbidity of FASD with ADHD may be a significant *individual factor* in terms of predisposition.

In addition to individual characteristics, there also appear to be a number of *environmental factors* that might lead a person with cognitive deficits to act out sexually (Hingsburger, Griffiths, and Quinsey, 1991), including:

- Inadequate social education;
- Lack of information about appropriate sexual behavior;
- Insufficient opportunity for sexual expression;
- History of sexual or physical abuse;
- Exposure to violence and/or pornography;
- Pervasive restrictions in daily life that reduce privacy; and
- Limited social access to prospective dating and sexual partners.

Individual characteristics due to CNS impairment are unchangeable; environmental factors that can either remediate or exacerbate the functional problems inherent in primary disabilities are subject to intervention, but only if the deficits are appropriately assessed and identified.

Hidden Disabilities

When brain damage is apparent because of intellectual deficits, learning delays, hyperactivity, and physical abnormalities, deficits in attention and impulse control are often assessed and identified as part of a comprehensive testing process, and interventions can be applied somewhat effectively in childhood (Novick, 1997). On the other hand, if the more obvious indications of CNS dysfunction are absent, these deficits and their socio-sexual implications may go undetected, with intervention occurring only after the individual has gotten into serious legal trouble in terms of his or her sexual behavior. According to LaDue and Dunne (1997), some people with fetal alcohol impairment may "sound" or "look" competent because of superficial verbal ability but nonetheless have underlying and pervasive cognitive deficits. This situation likely affects many undiagnosed persons with ADHD and FASD, many of whom may appear "normal" because of average IQs and no visible abnormalities but who nonetheless have significant CNS dysfunction that compromises executive skills, adaptive functioning, social cognition, and social behavior. Unfortunately, damage from fetal alcohol exposure is often very difficult to determine. As Streissguth notes (1997), mothers are rarely questioned about their alcohol use during pregnancy. Yet, recent animal research is showing that even a single exposure to high levels of ethanol in beer, wine, or hard liquor can kill nerve cells in the developing brain (e.g., Ikonomidou et al., 2000). Findings such as this may have far-reaching implications for individuals who are suffering from FASD and/or ADHD but have not been diagnosed as such.

Because ADHD and FASD become increasingly difficult to diagnose as an individual matures (Huebert and Raftis, 1996), the sociocognitive deficits often become hidden disabilities. In FASD, affected individuals tend to lose by adolescence the characteristic features that stereotypically Define the condition (i.e., distinct facial characteristics and growth deficiencies) and make early intervention more likely (Streissguth, 1997). In the case of ADHD, the hyperactivity in young children that frequently serves as a marker for the condition appears to diminish by adulthood (American Psychiatric Association, 2000). Without a diagnosis that signals CNS dysfunction, such individuals may be held fully accountable for their sexually inappropriate sexual behaviors as they mature. In fact, as Baumbach (2002) recently noted, the high incidence of FASD coupled with the frequency with which it may go undiagnosed make it "highly likely" that sexual offender treatment programs contain a good number of individuals with undiagnosed cognitive and neurological impairments caused by prenatal alcohol exposure.

Normal Sexual Development

There is a great deal of confusion in the general population about what is "normal" sexual expression. As Gil and Johnson (1993) note in their comprehensive treatise on the subject, sensuality and erotic behavior are part of normal human development from the earliest stage of infancy. These authors point out that infants even a few days old respond with sensual pleasure to being soothed, kissed, and caressed by caregivers. Infants soon learn that they can give themselves sensual pleasure by sucking on their fingers and toes or by stroking soft blankets and toys. Even before the age of 12 months, children sometimes discover the intense pleasure of orgasm that comes from self-stimulation. For some of these children, masturbation becomes a soothing sensual experience that provides tension reduction and distraction (Yates, 1990).

As they mature, children discover their genitalia and eventually may include others in their widening exploration of sensual experiences. As Gil and Johnson (1993) note, it is normal for school-age children who have not been sexually abused to become curious about others' bodies as well as their own. Normal sexual exploration often includes looking at or touching other children's genitals as well as their own, kissing and hugging, using profanity, and telling "dirty" jokes. Occasionally, non-abused children may even try to mimic coital positions and motions that they have briefly glimpsed on television, in movies, or in their homes and neighborhoods. During puberty, sensuality takes on an erotic and sexual connotation when most youngsters learn to associate pleasurable sensual feelings with their genitals. Self-stimulation and sexual play and exploration with peers in childhood frequently expands after puberty into kissing, hugging, fantasizing, genital fondling, sexual intercourse, and other sexual experiences between two people. According to researchers who have studied such childhood behaviors, approximately 40% of adults surveyed reported sexual activity before age 13 (Haugaard and Tilly, 1988) to 70% (Finkelhor, 1983; Goldman and Goldman, 1988). Similarly, when Finkelhor and Strapko (1992) surveyed mothers, 60% reported that their children engaged in sexual behaviors.

For the majority of children, the knowledge that sexual expression carries with it social "rules" comes naturally and easily. Sexual socialization, or the display of appropriate normative sexuality, is gradually learned directly and indirectly from parents, friends, and the social environment. Imbedded within these learning experiences are messages – often subtle – about private versus public behaviors, the physiology of sexuality, the meaning of "consent," male-female relationships, dating and courtship, marriage, and sexually transmitted diseases. The ability to learn and apply these rules of social-sexual conduct not only depends on the child's innate capacity to perceive, understand, assimilate, and respond appropriately to cues from the environment but also on the capacity of the environment to teach these rules in a manner consistent with the child's cognitive capabilities. When there are no social cognition deficits, the subtle cues are assimilated as well as the more direct lessons. However, in children with CNS deficits, even the direct lessons (if they are provided) often miss their target because the message is not delivered in terms that can be understood.

Evidence of sexual socialization failures can be seen in bizarre and unusual sexual behaviors in cognitively impaired populations, such as the preschooler who won't stop masturbating in the classroom or the elementary school child who persists in running up to female classmates and touching their chests. However, instead of recognizing these situations as the expected consequence of inadequate sexual socialization, more often than not the child is viewed as the entire problem. The child's cognitive and neurological deficits are either unknown or ignored, and the sexual behavior is seen as intentional and deliberately provocative.

INAPPROPRIATE SEXUAL BEHAVIORS IN CHILDHOOD

While caregivers, family friends, teachers, relatives, siblings, peers, television, print media, videos, and other sources of social communication all contribute to the sexual socialization of children, the home environment is by far the most important factor. However, according to Hingsburger and colleagues (1992), children and adolescents with cognitive disabilities tend to be inadequately socialized about emotional and physical boundaries, have not been given information on appropriate and safe sexual behavior, have not been taught social and relationship skills and given sufficient opportunities to practice those skills, and have not been given enough opportunities for sexual expression and intimacy. Other factors that appear to play a role are a history of sexual abuse, exposure to pornography, socioeconomic factors, pervasive use of restrictions in daily life that limit a wide range of social experiences, and denial that the individual has an interest in sex (Hingsburger, Griffiths, and Quinsey, 1991b). People react strongly and negatively to the idea of someone who is cognitively impaired learning about and expressing their sexuality. Caregivers in particular delay or avoid providing sexual education or sexual therapy to impaired youth. As a result, many individuals with cognitive and neurological deficits engage in inappropriate sexual behaviors as youth and, without effective intervention, often go on to commit sexual offenses.

This author's clinical experience with children, adolescents, and adults with the dual diagnoses of FASD and ADHD is consistent with the assessment of Hingsburger and his colleagues (1992b). Not only do many children with these disorders expose and engage in inappropriate sexual touching, many also engage in compulsive masturbation and/or public masturbation. Bizarre sexual behaviors are also seen in individuals diagnosed with FASD. For example, a young man diagnosed with FAS in childhood was referred to our clinic for sex offender treatment after his release at age 19 from a juvenile facility. His confinement stemmed from multiple charges involving sexual assault and lewd acts committed on five- and six-year-old males. Police reports described him walking into public restrooms, seeing unsupervised children using the urinal, and sexually abusing the children. His sexual acts involved rubbing an orange on his penis and drawing on his penis with a pen in front of the children. He also blew air through a straw onto one victim's penis. These behaviors were appropriately regarded as "sexual assault" and "lewd and lascivious" behavior by the authorities but, less appropriately, the behaviors were presumed to be sexually deviant in motivation. The young man was seen as willful and knowledgeable about the offensive nature of the behaviors. Evaluation eventually revealed that these assumptions were inaccurate. He was mimicking his own grooming and victimization earlier in his childhood by an adult uncle, perceiving that these behaviors were a "normal" preliminary step in friendship.

As research suggests (Gilby et al., 1989; Day, 1997), clinical practice reveals far more nuisance sex offenses in individuals with FASD, particularly those also dually diagnosed with ADHD, compared to their non-impaired counterparts. In FASD patients who display Sexually Inappropriate Behaviors during their youth, those who are the most disorganized and have the most difficulty with impulsivity and response inhibition, hyperactivity, and affect self-regulation in childhood (i.e., ADHD symptoms) may be the most prone to commit sexual offenses once they enter puberty. Anecdotal experience also indicates that these individuals may be inclined to develop compulsive sexual behaviors that bring them into frequent contact with the law (e.g., public masturbation, involving others in fetish behaviors).

Bonner and colleagues (1999) have developed a typology of sexually inappropriate behaviors in children that neatly classifies sexual behaviors into three broad categories in terms of victim invasiveness:

1. *Sexually Inappropriate Behaviors* that do not involve contact with another person (e.g., sexual remarks and gestures, touching or exposing one's genitals, self-injurious sexual behavior);

2. *Sexually Intrusive Behaviors* involving brief and inappropriate sexual contact with another person (e.g., running up to another child and momentarily touching his/her genitals before retreating, brushing up against another person in a sexually provocative way, briefly fondling someone's genitals until the other person objected); and

3. *Sexually Aggressive Behaviors* involving significant or prolonged sexual contact with another person resulting in completion of a sexual act such as oral sex, vaginal or anal penetration, and mutual masturbation.

Some Sexually Inappropriate Behaviors are illegal in adolescents and adults, such as exposing and voyeurism. All Sexually Intrusive and Sexually Aggressive Behaviors are illegal in adolescents and adults and generally result in charges of child molestation or lewd and lascivious behavior if the victim is a child and sexual assault, sexual battery, or rape charges if the victim is adult. Relating Streissguth and colleagues' (2004) research to Bonner et al.'s (1999) classification scheme, Inappropriate Sexual Behaviors in FASD youth tend to fall in all three of the above categories.

By age three, some children with CNS dysfunction begin to display inappropriate sexual behaviors in the first category noted above (i.e., Sexually Inappropriate Behaviors). By this age, children who have discovered the self-soothing properties of *masturbation* may begin to engage in this behavior compulsively and/or publicly. Although genital exploration in infancy is part of normal human development, the behavior may take on additional motivation for children with CNS impairments in terms of emotion modulation. The calming, pleasurable sensations from rhythmic rubbing of the genitals on something soft may be the child's only mechanism for self-soothing. This may be particularly true for young children diagnosed with ADHD as well as FASD as both groups have been found to have defects in emotion modulation. However, masturbation is an ineffective method of stress reduction because it precludes the individual from developing internal skills that can be used in any environment. Moreover, masturbation, if it becomes compulsive, can increase the negative emotional arousal that it was originally used to diminish. This counterproductive cycle is often seen in children who repeatedly self-stimulate in the presence of others as well as alone. Hyperactivity can fuel the compulsion, leading to frequent masturbation sometimes to the point of self-injury.

If sexual arousal during masturbation is paired in a child's mind with a particular object (e.g., his mother's silky nightgown), the child might develop *fetishism*. According to the DSM-IV, the sexual interest in fetishism involves the use of nonliving objects (the "fetish"), which may include women's underpants, bras, stockings, shoes, or other wearing apparel. Fetishism in combination with masturbation is frequently seen in individuals who engage in compulsive masturbation. The person with fetishism masturbates while holding, rubbing, or smelling the fetish object and may, when older, ask a sexual partner to wear the object during their sexual encounters. The condition tends to be chronic, and anecdotal clinical evidence suggests that compulsive fetish behaviors may be somewhat over-represented in cognitively impaired populations.

A case study illustrates how fetishism in combination with compulsive masturbation might manifest. A middle-aged client with FASD presented for sexual offender treatment with a history of sexual offense convictions in his late teens. His offenses involved having others dress in his fetish material (in this case, fuzzy one-piece pajamas). His victims were a young female child, a developmentally delayed adult male, and a developmentally delayed adult female. This client developed a sexual interest in pajamas during his childhood, several years after he began compulsively masturbating at home and at school. He cannot recall how the fetish material came to be paired in his mind with masturbation, but he does remember being raised in an abusive and chaotic household with caregivers who withheld affection and nurturing. Although his sexual offenses might suggest otherwise, his sexual fantasies through adolescence and into adulthood have consistently involved masturbating to the *sight* and *feel* of the fetish material rather than to thoughts of someone else wearing the material. He reports that wearing or seeing the fetish material soothes and comforts him, especially when he is masturbating.

Pantyhose and other items that are soft, silky, or furry may be preferred fetish material for individuals with impaired emotion modulation, as tactile experience of the soft material adds an extra element of soothing capacity to the masturbation activity. Sense of smell may add yet another sensory experience. While fetish sexual behavior itself is not a crime, individuals with CNS dysfunction tend to get into legal trouble by either involving someone else in their fetish behavior, as in the case study above, or by their method of acquiring the fetish. In the latter situation, cognitively impaired persons are often arrested for burglary after sneaking into neighborhood homes to steal fetish objects.

Another problem frequently encountered in clinical practice with cognitively impaired youth who display sexually inappropriate sexual behaviors is *promiscuity*. As noted previously in research by Streissguth and colleagues (2004), promiscuity is seen twice as often in females with FASD compared to males. Another case example may help to illustrate why cognitively impaired females have difficulty in this area. A 15-year-old teenage girl diagnosed with FASD and ADHD presented for therapy after her guardian (a paternal aunt) became frustrated with her oppositional behavior. Sexually abused by her biological father in early childhood, she'd been removed from her parents' home at age six and placed in a series of foster homes until her aunt agreed to become her caregiver. Although the aunt's home was highly structured, and the adolescent was closely supervised while at home, she had chronic social and behavioral difficulties at school. Shunned throughout her school years by peers her own age because she was immature and unpredictable, she'd tried socializing with younger children and other developmentally delayed youngsters in her special education classes, which was partially successful up through her junior high years. However, when she entered high school, she was rejected by her classmates because of her odd social behaviors (e.g., always needing to be the center of attention, talking non-stop about trivial things that had no interest to her peers, making up stories that were clearly outlandish in order to impress others, "tattling" to the teacher to get others in trouble). The only group that would accept her were other misfit youth involved in substance abuse, antisocial behaviors, and indiscriminate sexual activity. She learned quickly that in order to be accepted by this group, she needed to conform. She was an easy sexual target for the dozen or so boys in the group and, by the end of her junior year, she'd been sexual with all but one of them. Pregnant in her junior year, she was removed from high school and placed in a small group home where she could finish her education. Efforts by several well-meaning mental health providers to intervene in her promiscuous sexual behavior were ineffective as sexuality was the only "skill" this adolescent had learned in order to get her needs for acceptance and emotional intimacy met.

Adolescents with cognitive and neurological disorders also may have difficulties related to natural sexual curiosity if they lack sexual socialization skills. These difficulties may manifest in *exposing* behaviors or *voyeurism* that can result in arrest and incarceration. For example, a young adult male was referred for evaluation after being arrested and charged with his third voyeurism offense. Although he was diagnosed with one of the FASDs, he had an average IQ. He had been raised in a stable and nurturing home, but he was never provided social skills training or sexual education. He also was not given the opportunity to participate in organized social activities where he might have learned social skills on his own. He was arrested the first time at the age of 21 when he was observed crawling under the stall in a women's restroom on a college campus. In his psychosexual evaluation, he explained that he had never seen the female body prior to that incident and was curious about it. He also reported that he thought women would be pleased with his attention and want to start a relationship with him because "that's what happens in movies." Arrested and convicted the first time he engaged in this voyeuristic activity, he was placed on probation but immediately re-offended with exactly the same behavior. He evaded arrest and probation violation by absconding from the area where he'd committed the second offense. He traveled to another state and committed the same offense a third time on another college campus. Although his FASD diagnosis was known to the authorities, because of his average IQ and verbal proficiency, he did not appear disabled upon first impression (i.e., a hidden disability). Only after he was evaluated a second time by a mental health provider experienced in working with individuals with FASD was his cognitive disability identified.

While there is no linear progression with age from Sexually Inappropriate Behaviors to Sexually Intrusive and Assaultive Behaviors, there is a significant change in the nature of sexual acts once an individual reaches puberty. Sexual behaviors viewed in childhood as inappropriate take on a legal connotation once an individual reaches adolescence. Even if there has been no indication of sexual interest in childhood, hormonal changes during puberty create a heightened interest in sexuality and sexual expression. There is no empirical evidence that these hormonal changes affect cognitively impaired populations any differently than normal populations. Nor is there any evidence that cognitively impaired youth have any less of a drive for closeness and emotional intimacy than non-impaired youth. However, while the latter has been receiving and assimilating sex education in a variety of formats and from a variety of sources throughout their young lives, cognitively impaired youth have been largely left out of this process.

SEXUAL SOCIALIZATION

As a society, we tend to have a great deal of difficulty recognizing that people with disabilities are sexual beings and have the same needs for affection, intimacy, and sexual expression as those without disabilities. Unfortunately, misinformation and stereotypes also pervade the mental health community and legal system, both of which are ill-equipped to deal with inappropriate sexual behavior and sexual offending in individuals with cognitive and developmental deficits. In families, the sexual socialization of children with cognitive and neurological impairment is typically ignored until problems develop. Moreover, once inappropriate sexual behaviors occur, interventions are often ineffective because treatments typically do not address the special needs of this population. Swanson and Garwick (1990) neatly summarized the problem with the following observation: "...sexual offenses by individuals with mental retardation will be ignored as long as possible and then approached in a crisis-oriented, fragmentary and intrusive manner" (p. 155).

Significant deficits in social and interpersonal skills are hallmark symptoms of FASD and ADHD, even when affected individuals might seem normal because of an average IQ. While skill deficits are inherent in cognitive disabilities that affect normal social and emotional development, it is the response of the environment to these deficits that determines whether or not a youth will successfully navigate the difficult teenage and young adult years or will make mistakes that reveal lack of training far more than sexual deviancy. Typically, youth with cognitive impairments have had chronic difficulties making and keeping same-aged friends. However, once caregivers become aware of these difficulties, they typically respond by limiting their children's contact with peers in a well-meaning attempt to "protect" them from rejection. As a result, cognitively impaired youth are denied the natural social learning experiences, both positive and negative, that their non-impaired counterparts are exposed to on a daily basis. As their children enter their teen years, caregivers tend to become even more vigilant and protective. Flirting and dating are not permitted, and they typically limit their teenaged children from engaging in social activities with non-impaired teenagers. Unfortunately, if caregivers do not ensure that their cognitively impaired teenagers are exposed to adolescents who are appropriate in terms of age and developmental level, the natural learning process that occurs through social experimentation and feedback is denied to these youth. Instead, what often happens is that caregivers, believing that their teenagers are asexual, allow them to spend unsupervised time with children who are developmentally similar but chronologically much younger. It is often in these situations when normal sexual curiosity in the cognitively impaired teenager converges with opportunity to satisfy that curiosity. After the fact, when the legal system and mental health professionals are trying to determine appropriate interventions and/or sanctions, the disparity in age but similarity in development makes it very difficult to determine whether the sexual activity was a product of inadequate sexual socialization or sexual deviance. Typically, they err on the side of caution and choose deviance and punitive intervention.

Although affected youth are expected as they enter adulthood to become as independent and responsible as their disabilities permit, caregiver biases about their sexual innocence and need for protection and heightened levels of supervision by teachers and others in public settings impose strict rules on these youth and interfere with their legitimate entry into the adult world of relationships and sexuality. The following case study illustrates this point. A young man presented for sexual deviancy treatment after being released from prison and placed in a Community Protection Program. Raised by adoptive caregivers from a young age, he had been protected and nurtured throughout his childhood and adolescence. When he entered puberty at age 16, his parents decided not to tell him about sex, thinking that because he'd never showed any interest in the subject or in dating, he was asexual. They not only shielded him from sexually explicit print and visual media, they also decided not to involve him in social activities with other cognitively impaired youth as they wanted to protect him from possible victimization. By the time he was 22, he had been arrested twice for child sexual assault. He would run up behind young teenage girls in his neighborhood when their backs were turned to him and rub his body against their buttocks. During police interrogation, he agreed with the suggestion that he was "having sex" with the girls. Now on probation and in sexual offense treatment after spending almost ten years in prison, he is finally learning to tell the difference between appropriate and inappropriate sexual partners and learning basic information about meeting and establishing friendships with age-appropriate females who are developmentally similar. Very importantly, he also is involved in social skills training at a local mental heath clinic where he not only has the opportunity to practice his new social skills, he also can meet regularly with prospective dating partners in supervised social activities

PROTECTIVE FACTORS / RISK FACTORS

According to Streissguth and colleagues (1997), there are a number of factors that can decrease the likelihood that someone with FASD will display inappropriate sexual behaviors.

Table 1. Protective Factors

1)	living in a stable and nurturing home for over 72% of the individual's life;
2)	being diagnosed before age six;
3)	never having experienced violence against oneself;
4)	staying in each living situation for an average of 2.8 years or more;
5)	experiencing a good quality home between the ages of 8 to 12;
6)	being found eligible for developmental disabilities services;
7)	having a diagnosis of FAS rather than FAE (presumably FAS is more obvious than FAE, which may increase the probability of early detection and intervention); and
8)	having basic needs met for at least 13% of the individual's life.

As is clear in this table, the home environment appears to be a major determinant of whether a child will display inappropriate sexual behaviors. In particular, two major risk factors that affect prosocial functioning appear to be neglect and exposure to violence, physical or sexual. Compared to non-impaired children, vulnerability to neglect and violence appears particularly high for youth with cognitive and neurological disabilities. Statistics compiled by the National Clearinghouse on Child Abuse and Neglect Information found approximately 90,000 children were sexually abused in 2002 and that children with disabilities or mental retardation were four to ten times more vulnerable to sexual abuse than their non-disabled peers (National Resource Center on Child Abuse, 1992). Focusing more specifically on FASD populations, LaDue et al. (1992) found that youth with FASD were particularly vulnerable to abuse and neglect. Approximately 86% had been neglected, 52% had been physically abused, and 35% had been sexually abused. While a large meta-analysis found that being sexually victimized in childhood is not predictive of sexual offending as a teenager or adult (Hanson and Bussiere, 1998), this conclusion may not apply to populations with cognitive disabilities. For example, Streissguth and colleagues found in their 1997 FASD study that having been a victim of violence in childhood was a strong risk factor for inappropriate sexual behaviors later in life, increasing risk fourfold. This outcome may be because youth with FASD do not have the coping skills and resilience to deal effectively with victimization as these skills require sophisticated personal competencies such as the ability to recognize danger and adapt, distance oneself from intense feelings, and create relationships that are crucial for support (Mrazek and Mrazek, 1987).

LEGAL ISSUES

Once individuals enter their teen years, their sexual "mistakes" often bring them into contact with the law. People with cognitive and neurological disabilities tend to be disadvantaged by the legal and judicial processes due to several problems: 1) accurate assessment, 2) an informed support system, and 3) appropriate legal representation (e.g., Cockram et al., 1998; Hayes, 1997; Everington and Fulero, 1999). Even when a particular diagnosis is known, and there is adequate family support and legal representation, cognitively impaired sex offenders face a criminal justice system that is generally unaware of the impact of their disabilities on behavior. This lack of awareness causes a number of errors in the way these cases are handled – errors that not only affect the individual charged with a sexual offense but the community as well in terms of appropriate handling of the case. The problem is greatly magnified in cases where cognitive and neurological deficits are a hidden disability.

A major problem for populations with CNS deficits is the arrest and interrogation process. If they have never received appropriate sexual socialization, individuals with CNS impairment may engage in sexually inappropriate behavior without awareness that their behavior is illegal. More easily detected than individuals without cognitive impairment because they lack the "sophistication" to hide their behavior, they are more often arrested (Santamour, 1986). Once they are arrested, they typically undergo police interrogation. Police often use harsh tactics in interrogating a suspect, with the objective of exacting a quick confession and closing the case. The prosecutor may then use that confession upon which to build a case. On the opposite side of the courtroom, the defense attorney may represent the client without realizing there is a disability that might significantly affect the validity of the confession or, if the confession is valid, the degree of culpability. Plea negotiation is often the next step in the process, with both the prosecutor and the defense attorney (usually a public defender) trying to avoid the time and expense involved in a trial. It is during this phase that defendants may be told by prosecutors (and encouraged by their defense attorneys) to plead guilty in order to avoid the trial and the possibility of a long prison sentence. Even those without cognitive impairments find it difficult to withstand this kind of pressure. Once a conviction has been determined either by negotiation or trial, the judge may impose severe sanctions without taking the disability and its ramifications into account, even if the disability is identified. One of these ramifications is the defendant's vulnerability to sexual and physical victimization in prison. Considering the comparable disadvantages that affect every phase of the legal process, it perhaps is not surprising that people with cognitive deficits who engage in illegal behavior are more likely than non-impaired persons to be arrested, convicted, sentenced to prison, and victimized in prison (Santamour, 1986).

The criminal justice system's response in cases where the cognitive disabilities are known tends to be either dismissal of the behavior as unimportant or an overly punitive response (Mikkelsen and Stelk, 1997). The former does little to protect the community from recurrence of the behavior; the latter not only disregards the individual's legal rights and protections but also does a disservice to the community as well if the offender does not receive appropriate treatment. In the case of juveniles, youth are typically sent to juvenile residential programs involving strict supervision. When commitment includes treatment for sexual offending, youth with CNS deficits are often combined with non-impaired youth and quickly get lost in abstract treatment concepts and unattainable treatment expectations. Socialization skills are usually not even considered. Frequently, there is consensual and non-consensual sexual activity occurring in the facility outside the watchful eyes of staff. Youth with cognitive and neurological impairments tend to be sexually victimized by their non-impaired peers. As a result, these youth often emerge from their experience in a juvenile facility more sexualized than when they first entered and without the sexual training and social skills to manage successfully in the adult world. The situation is worse in adult prisons. While a few states have prison-based treatment programs for sex offenders (e.g., Kansas, Washington State), most don't. Those with such programs usually do not have specialized services or groups that target developmentally delayed prisoners. Sexual victimization is rampant in prison settings, and the developmentally delayed prisoner is often targeted.

Researchers have looked at the disadvantages faced in the legal system by those with cognitive deficits (e.g., Perske, 1991) compared to those without cognitive deficits. Some of their findings indicate that compared to their non-impaired counterparts, cognitively impaired individuals arrested for sex crimes tend to have the following additional problems (See table 2).

One of the most serious problems faced by cognitively impaired defendants in the legal system is *false confession.* Alarmed by processes and settings they do not understand and people who intimidate and pressure them, those who do not retreat into silence may admit behaviors that are partially or totally inaccurate and take responsibility for crimes they did not commit. The following case example is typical involves a young adult male defendant recently seen for a psychosexual evaluation following charges for burglary with sexual motivation. The charges stemmed from fetishism and involved his sneaking into people's homes to steal pantyhose that he could use during masturbation. He had burglarized four homes by the time he was arrested but had never encountered anyone at home during the commission of those crimes. Several months prior to the defendant's arrest on the burglary charges, he'd been arrested for setting a fire at a local high school. In that earlier case, he admitted under police interrogation that he set the fire, although he reported that he couldn't remember the details of how he had done it. He signed a confession, was convicted of the arson as a result of a plea agreement, and was sentenced to a year of house arrest. It was during this period of house arrest that the defendant was arrested for the burglary charges.

Table 2

Special problems faced by cognitively impaired persons in the legal system:
• They may display superficial verbal skills that often hide their underlying cognitive deficits and therefore present as fully competent;
• They may not accurately comprehend their legal rights but pretend that they do;
• They may not be able to understand and thereby respond appropriately to instructions from authorities;
• They may respond to questions with what they think officials want to hear rather than what actually happened;
• They may succumb to pressure during the interrogation process and confess to crimes they did not commit;
• They may become overwhelmed by police presence and shut down emotionally and verbally;
• They may become fearful and highly distressed by the detention process and attempt to escape;
• They may have significant difficulty in remembering and describing details of offense behavior;
• They may become easily confused about who is responsible for the crime and even whether a "crime" has been committed;
• They may acquiesce easily during plea negotiation, believing predictions by prosecutors (and perhaps their own attorneys) that they will face a very long prison sentence if their case goes to trial;
• They may serve longer sentences or a greater percentage of their sentences before being released on parole or probation; and
• They may get placed in maximum security facilities for segregation and "protection" needs.

Plea negotiations between the prosecutor and public defender on the defendant's burglary charges were intense. The prosecutor insisted on harsh penalties for someone charged with sex-related crimes who also had a history of arson behavior. According to the prosecutor, the arson conviction confirmed in her mind that the young man was a serious risk to the community in terms of his violence potential and, by extension, his potential for sexual violence. She was looking for a maximum sentence on the burglary charges, which included a lengthy prison term. However, shortly before the negotiations concluded, it was discovered that the defendant was innocent of his arson conviction. A teenager who actually committed the arson was arrested following a fire at a warehouse and confessed to the earlier high school fire during police interrogation. At the current time, several months after it was learned the defendant was not an arsonist, the prosecutor remains concerned that he is a dangerous sexual offender with violence potential.

ASSESSMENT

Counterfeit deviance and the assumption of dangerousness complicates the assessment of individuals with cognitive impairments who commit sexual crimes. However, if we do not identify the problem accurately, we cannot treat it effectively. The mental health system, as well as the criminal justice system, seems genuinely perplexed by how to assess and treat sex offenders with cognitive impairments.

In assessing sex offenders with cognitive disabilities to determine degree of culpability and risk of reoffense, a variety of factors should be considered. Of primary importance is accurately identifying the factors that undermine the individual's awareness of and control over his or her sexual behavior. The problem often begins during ***competency assessment***. Mental health professionals who do not have specific training and expertise in cognitive deficits often assume awareness and control based upon superficial responses to questioning. Competency evaluations probe a defendant's understanding of the court process and the roles of the various professionals involved in the legal process. While someone who is cognitively impaired might be able to recite adequately the function of a defense attorney or a judge, the weightier question regarding whether or not the defendant can realistically assist legal counsel in his/her own defense is often assumed based on the defendant's responses to questions about the definitions of legal terminology. Determining accurately whether or not someone can assist counsel in his or her own defense requires careful and detailed mental status examination and in-depth questioning that goes beyond the request for legal definitions. Because of inadequate compensation for competency evaluations, lack of training, or other reasons, many evaluators who specialize in competency assessment do not spend the time and effort required for a thorough assessment of a defendant's capacity to appreciate the nature of the charges that have been brought or the range and nature of possible penalties, to understand the adversary nature of the legal process, to disclose to the defense attorney facts pertinent to the matter, to be able to display appropriate courtroom behavior, and to testify relevantly.

Apart from the matter of competency to stand trial, a ***psychosexual evaluation*** by a forensic psychologist specialized in sexual offender treatment and assessment is often completed at the request of either the prosecutor or the defense attorney. Sometimes, the prosecutor and defense attorney will each request an evaluation from his/her own expert. The purpose of such an evaluation is to inform the court about the defendant's psychosexual functioning. Regardless of the referral source, the primary task in psychosexual evaluation is to sort fact from fiction, determine true deviance from counterfeit deviance, reach accurate conclusions about degree of risk and dangerousness, and make appropriate recommendations for treatment. This is often an extremely difficult process, particularly if the evaluator must rely solely upon the defendant's self-report for information. Moreover, many evaluators are not even aware of the problem of counterfeit deviancy in the case of defendants with CNS impairment. While the evaluation and risk assessment process can be creatively adapted to the specific abilities of the offender, the matter of structuring the evaluation in terms of two competing hypotheses (i.e., sexual deviancy vs. counterfeit deviance) is important in terms of comprehensive assessment and relevant data collection. Also important is the necessity of verifying self-report data through corroboration from sources other than the defendant. While this process is essential in any forensic evaluation, it is particularly important for defendants with cognitive impairments who may fill in memory gaps with false information or provide inaccurate data in order to please the evaluator.

TREATMENT

Mental health professionals who specialize in sexual offender assessment and treatment tend to be reluctant to treat offenders with cognitive deficits because of lack of specialized training and experience. Instead of obtaining such training, many try to integrate cognitively impaired sex offenders into groups of non-impaired individuals. This process not only creates frustration for non-disabled participants as well as group leaders (Demetral, 1994), it also fails in the primary objective of treatment: teaching the disabled offender how to recognize and interrupt the cycle of reoffense. Social skills training and sexual socialization are typically not even considered.

The continuum of treatment resources currently available to sex offenders with CNS deficits includes the following:

- short-term, specialized psychoeducational programs (e.g., relationship classes);
- outpatient sex offender treatment programs;
- day treatment programs for individuals who remain at home, in foster care, in supervised living arrangements, or in residential group homes;
- residential treatment facilities for adolescents and young adults;
- unlocked residential treatment units made secure by staff;
- locked residential treatment facilities;
- secure units in mental health facilities or hospitals;
- prison-based treatment programs; and
- involuntary civil commitment for Sexually Violent Predators.

Unfortunately, with the possible exceptions of short-term psychoeducation programs such as relationship and sex education classes and secure units in mental heath facilities, very few of these resources are specifically designed to meet the special needs of cognitively impaired sex offenders. In general, services for this population tend to be overly restrictive and fragmented at best. However, in order to be effective, treatment methods for individuals with cognitive disabilities need to be practical, efficient, flexible, and individualized. Ideally, treatment programs should provide sufficient structure and supervision to protect the participants with as little restriction of liberty as necessary (Mikkelsen and Stelk, 1997). Cognitive-behavioral approaches involving a combination of cognitive retraining, victim empathy, and relapse prevention training are recognized forms of treatment for sex offenders without cognitive impairment. Adaptation of these methods is not only possible but necessary for effective treatment of those who are cognitively impaired. While there is little outcome research on the efficacy of treatment programs for offenders with cognitive disabilities, available studies and anecdotal reports appear to be favorable (Haaven, Little and Petre-Miller, 1990).

Several authors have published specialized materials on the treatment of cognitively impaired sex offenders (e.g., Haaven and Coleman, 2000; Hingsburger, 1996; Lindsay et al., 1999; Luiselli, 2000). In addition to modification of standard relapse prevention treatment, which emphasizes a self-awareness and self-control model endorsed by the Association for the Treatment of Sexual Abusers (ATSA, 1997), it also is important to tailor instruction methods and group processes to the individual strengths of the offender. In particular, many individuals will have great difficulty understanding basic treatment concepts if the program relies on the verbal processes and written homework assignments that are standard for non-impaired treatment groups. Thus, it is important to determine at the outset of treatment how the individual best learns (i.e., visually, via auditory mechanisms, or kinesthetically) and then tailor treatment delivery to the learning strengths of each individual in order to improve understanding, assimilation, and generalization of treatment concepts.

A primary objective in sex offender treatment is *relapse prevention*. Offenders learn about the sequence of steps that lead of sexual offending and how to intervene early in this process. While sequential thinking is quite difficult for many individuals with cognitive and neurological impairments, such individuals are generally able to learn three- and four-step processes that involve "danger zones" or "high risk situations." For those more significantly impaired, a two-step process can be effectively taught. However, understanding and identifying pre-offense triggers is one matter. Retention and generalization are another -- and often far more difficult -- challenge. Unfortunately, even in programs that do well in tailoring treatment procedures to the special needs of the disabled, the issues of retention and generalization are ignored. Once the individual has learned the basic components in his/her unique cycle of offense behavior, retention and generalization to environments outside the treatment office are assumed despite the fact that persons with CNS impairments often have deficits that directly impede this process (e.g., deficits in memory, cause-and-effect sequencing, inhibition control). Thus, not only is repetition the key to retention, but repetition in a variety of formats and situations is important in terms of generalizing treatment skills to all contexts.

Ideally, the treatment process involves *group treatment* as well as *individual therapy*. Marshall and Barbaree (1990) note that group processes can facilitate new ways of thinking and social interaction that are unavailable in traditional individualized treatment. However, the potential advantages of group therapy should be weighed against the possible disadvantages of negative peer influence, particularly if the cognitively impaired sex offender is integrated into a group of non-impaired offenders.

The essential counterpart to relapse prevention training for sex offenders with cognitive impairments is *sexual socialization*. As noted previously in this chapter, this process involves skill building in a number of areas, including the complex social skills that accompany healthy sexuality and relationship development.

Another consideration in the treatment process for cognitively impaired sex offenders is *collaboration with specialized medical practitioners who are trained and experienced in assessing the medication needs of these special populations of developmentally delayed adolescents or adults,* and are able to prescribe appropriate drugs that can improve self-control and thereby enhance treatment objectives.

For example, some antidepressant medications reduce sexual activity and preoccupation (e.g., Prozac, Zoloft, Luvox). Other medications directly target sexual arousal potential. For example, Depo provera is an anti-androgen that counters male production of testosterone and significantly reduces sex drive. Zyban may be effective for compulsive sexual behavior. For individuals with ADHD, Wellbutrin (which contains the same active ingredient as Zyban) may be an effective medication alone or in combination with other drugs as it appears to reduce impulsivity. Of course, psychostimulants are the drug of choice for ADHD symptoms in general (e.g., Ritalin, Dexedrine, Adderall). Pharmacologically, there is no empirical support for treating sex offenders with cognitive impairment any differently than those without such impairment.

COMMUNITY MANAGEMENT AND SUPERVISION

As previously noted, sex offenders with cognitive impairments are typically incarcerated or released to the community under a wide range of restrictions and conditions. If they are fortunate enough to receive community placement, their troubles are not over. If the individual cannot remain at home or with relatives under strict supervision from supportive but responsible caregivers (perhaps including court-imposed restrictions such as house arrest), the next best option in terms of less restrictive alternatives is residential care with 24-hour supervision from trained staff. In addition to this intensive level of community supervision, sex offenders with cognitive impairments may also need specialized treatment services in addition to sex offender treatment, such as immediate behavioral intervention for anger control problems and/or substance abuse, mental heath services, and specific environmental modifications (Ward et al., 2001). Ideally, the community reintegration process will take into account the cognitively impaired sex offender's right to enjoy a lifestyle that is as independent as is practical given the limits of his cognitive impairments and extent of his sexual offending (Tudiver, 1997) balanced against the community's right to safety.

A community support team composed of key persons in a sex offender's life, as well as paid professional staff, can be an effective method of supporting an offender with cognitive disabilities. Working in collaboration, parents and other family members, friends, church members, probation officers, residential program staff, caseworkers, and therapists all can assist in day-to-day support. According to Blasingame (2000), a primary advantage of a collaborative partnership to support cognitively impaired sex offenders is that the responsibility of community safety and supervision becomes a shared responsibility. Another benefit is more thorough integration of relapse prevention skills across settings. The role of treatment providers is to assess, diagnose, recommend services, and treat the mental health needs as well as sexual health needs of cognitively impaired clients. Service coordinators or case managers representing the regional referral agency might function as the coordinator for information and service flow. Residential program administrators and staff may assume primary responsibility for the day-to-day care and activities of their clients. Job coaches and employers might assist in the structuring of daily work activities and practical skills development as well as social skill development within the work setting. Probation and parole officers may play a key role by supporting clients who are enrolled in such programs and holding them accountable for compliance with court orders and other legal obligations. Family members can participate in family treatment and learn skills to apply within the home setting, such as supporting the relapse prevention process or scheduling supervised social activities where clients can practice the skills they are learning in treatment.

Although specific behavioral guidelines might vary depending upon the individual's specific sexual offense pattern, some variation of the following "safety rules" are found in many *community reintegration contracts:*

Table 3. Safety Contract

1)	The individual is never allowed to be alone or unsupervised with anyone under the age of 18. (This guideline alone reduces reoffense risk significantly as the individual has no access to a large group of potential victims.)
2)	The individual cannot initiate any kind of contact with a child, either in person, by telephone, by letter, or on the Internet.
3)	The individual should be prohibited from going to places in the community where children or teenagers congregate, such as near school grounds, preschools, school buses, playgrounds, fast food restaurants with play areas, afternoon movies, public swimming pools, and beaches. Outings to public parks and neighborhood settings should be carefully supervised to ensure the individual maintains appropriate distance from all children. Literal line-of-sight and within-hearing distance supervision should be maintained whenever the individual is in a public setting where incidental contact with a child or vulnerable person might occur.
4)	Situations should be avoided where accidental contact with children or vulnerable adults could occur, such as unsupervised outings and shopping trips, doctor visits, or family visits. In the case of the latter, the individual should be supervised by a knowledgeable adult when in the presence of anyone who is not knowledgeable about his/her history. In the case of home visits and family gatherings, line-of-sight supervision is essential. When the individual uses the bathroom, the family chaperone should ensure the door to the bathroom is closed, and the door should be monitored continuously to ensure no one enters. Additional special precautions may be necessary for individuals who have sexualized toileting activities.
5)	The individual should never be left unsupervised in the presence of vulnerable adults, including adults with developmental delay and cognitive deficits and adults with restricted mobility.
6)	The individual should not be permitted to discuss sexuality, sex education, or other sexual matters with anyone who is not trained and authorized to discuss such matters with him/her (e.g., therapist).
7)	Unless given permission for specific items that are monitored and approved in advance, the individual should not be permitted access to pornography of any kind, including the Internet. (Access to downloaded pornography and sexual chat rooms has become a frequent problem for this population. Therefore, computer use should be avoided if possible.) If permitted, the individual's use of the computer should be monitored whenever he/she is using it. With regard to television, the individual should not be permitted to view programs containing children in primary roles or adult sexual themes. This requires careful screening and monitoring at all times. Adult videos should be prohibited. Catalogs and print media depicting children and adult magazines also should be prohibited unless advance permission for a specific adult magazine is given by the therapist in support of the therapeutic process (e.g., redirecting someone with a history of inappropriate sexual behaviors with children to adult sexual interests). It should be noted that unless authorized by the therapist for treatment purposes, any media containing examples of fetish material also should be prohibited if the individual has displayed a problem in this area (e.g., catalogs, magazines, and newspapers with child models; photographs of underwear or bras).

Table 3. Safety Contract (Continued)

8)	Family members who wish to chaperone the individual should receive specialized training by the individual's therapist to ensure understanding of line-of-sight supervision and how to enforce a Safety Plan (i.e., intervention).
9)	Someone who has sexually offended should never have any form of contact with his/her victim unless preapproved in writing by the victim's therapist, the probation officer, the service coordinator, and the treating therapist. Clarification and responsibility-taking letters should be processed through the therapist.
10)	There should be no interactions or contact between care providers and their cognitive impaired clients that are sexual in nature, including watching movies with adult sexual themes.
11)	The individual must follow his/her Safety Contract while on home passes, visits, outings in the community or other places where there may be opportunity for contact with vulnerable persons.

While the above guidelines do not ensure that cognitively impaired sex offenders will not sexually offend again, contracts such as this represent a powerful combination of interventions applied at the environmental level as well as the individual level – a combination that may be instrumental in significantly reducing sexual reoffending in this population.

FUTURE DIRECTIONS

At this point in time, what little research exists on the topic of sexuality in special needs populations involves a few isolated prevalence studies. While more prevalence data are needed, particularly studies such as the University of Washington research on FASD pertaining to a specific sub-group within the special needs population, it is especially important to gain knowledge about the *nature* of the sexual misconduct found in persons with cognitive and neurological impairment. It is suspected, given the diminished capacity to form criminal intent in this group, that much if not most of the sexual misconduct in individuals with CNS impairment stems from inadequate sexual socialization rather than sexual deviancy. If this is the case, such a finding should have significant influence on how these individuals are handled when they come into contact with the legal system. Most importantly, knowing that inadequate sexual socialization underlies a major proportion of the sexual misconduct in this population, there is much that could be done at an early stage by caregivers to prevent the kind of scenario described in the opening paragraphs of this chapter.

REFERENCES

American Psychiatric Association (2000). *Diagnostic and statistical manual of mental disorders* (4th ed., Text Revision). Washington, DC: Author.

Arnold, L.E., and Jensen, P.S. (1995). Attention0deficit disorders, In Sadock, B.J. and Yudofsky, S.C. (Eds.). *Comprehensive textbook of psychiatry, Sixth Ed.* Washington, DC: American Psychiatric Press, pp. 2295-2310.

Association for the Treatment of Sexual Abusers (1997). Beaverton, OR.

Barkley, R.A. (1985). The social interactions of hyperactive children: Developmental changes, drug effects, and situational variation. In R. McMahon and R. Peters (Eds.), *Childhood disorders: Behavioral-developmental approaches* (pp. 218-243). New York: Brunner/Mazel.

Barkley, R.A. (1990). *Attention-Deficit Hyperactivity Disorder: A handbook for diagnosis and treatment.* New York: Guilford Press.

Barkley, R.A. (1997). *ADHD and the nature of self-control.* New York: Guilford.

Barkley, R.A., DuPaul, G.J., and McMurray, M.B. (1990). A comprehensive evaluation of Attention Deficit Disorder with and without Hyperactivity. *Journal of Consulting and Clinical Psychology, 58,* 775-789.

Barkley, R.A., Fischer, M., Edelbrock, C.S., and Smallish, L. (1990). The adolescent outcome of hyperactive children diagnosed by research criteria: I. An 8 year prospective follow-up study. *Journal of the American Academy of Child and Adolescent Psychiatry, 29,* 546-557.

Barkley, R.A., Grodzinsky, D.G., and DuPaul, G. (1992). Frontal lobe functions in Attention Deficit Disorder with and without Hyperactivity: A review and research report. *Journal of Abnormal Child Psychology, 20,* 163-188.

Baumbach, J. (2002). Some implications of prenatal alcohol exposure for the treatment of adolescents with sexual offending behaviors. Sexual Abuse 14 (4), 313-327.

Bennett, L.A., Wolin, S.J., and Reiss, D. (1988). Cognitive, behavioral, and emotional problems among school-age children of alcoholic parents. *American Journal of Psychiatry, 145,* 185-190.

Berk, L.E., and Potts, M.K. (1991). Development and functional significance of private speech among Attention-Deficit Hyperactivity Disorder and normal boys. *Journal of Abnormal Child Psychology, 19,* 357-377.

Biederman, J., Faaone, S.V., Millberger, S., Curtis, S., Chen, L., Marrs, A., Ouellette, C., Moore, P., and Spencer, T. (1996). Predictors of persistence and remission of ADHD into adolescence: Results from a four-year prospective follow-up study. *Journal of the American Academy of Child and Adolescent Psychiatry, 35,* 343-351.

Blasingame, G. (2000). *Developmentally disabled persons with sexual behavior problems.* Oklahoma, OK: Wood 'N' Barnes Books.

Bonner, B.L., Walker, C.E., and Berliner, L. (1999). *Children with sexual behavior problems: Assessment and treatment.* Final Report, National Center on Child Abuse and Neglect, Department of Health and Human Services.

Bookstein, F.L., Streissguth, A.P., Sampson, P.D., Connor, P.D., and Barr, H.M. (2002). Corpus callosum shape and neuropsychological deficits in adult males with heavy fetal alcohol exposure. *NeuroImage, 15,* 233-251.

Breer, W. (1987). *The adolescent molester.* Springfield, IL: Charles C. Thomas.

Cantwell, D.P ., and Satterfield, J.H. (1978). The prevalence of academic underachievement in hyperactive children. *Journal of Pediatric Psychology, 3,* 168-171.

Carmichael Olson, H., Feldman, J.J., Streissguth, A.P., and Gonzales, R.D. (1992). Neuropsychological deficits and life adjustment in adolescents and young adults with fetal alcohol syndrome. *Alcoholism: Clinical and Experimental Research, 16,* 380.

Castellanos, F.X., Giedd, J.N., Eckburg, P., Marsh, W.L., Vaituzis, C., Kaysen, D., Hamburger, S.D., and Rapoport, J.L. (1994). Quantitative morphology of the caudate nucleus in Attention Deficit Hyperactivity Disorder. *American Journal of Psychiatry, 151,* 1791-1796.

Chess, S.D. (1960). Diagnosis and treatment of the hyperactive child. *New York State Journal of Medicine, 60,* 2379-2385.

Children's Bureau, Department of Health and Human Services (2002). *Child Maltreatment 2002.* Washington, DC: National Clearinghouse on Child Abuse and Neglect Information.

Clements, S.D. (1966). *Task force one: Minimal brain dysfunction in children* (National Institute of Neurological Diseases and Blindness, Monograph No. 3). Washington, DC: U.S. Department of Health, Education and Welfare.

Cockram, J., Jackson, R., and Underwood, R. (1998). People with an intellectual disability in the criminal justice system: The family perspective. *Journal of Intellectual and Developmental Disability, 23,* 41-55.

Copeland, A.P. (1979). Types of private speech produced by hyperactive and nonhyperactive boys. *Journal of Abnormal Child Psychology, 7,* 169-177.

Curran, S., and Fitzgerald, M. (1999). Attention deficit hyperactivity disorder in the prison population. *American Journal of Psychiatry,* 156 1664-1665.

Cyr, M. and Brown, C.S. (1998). Current drug therapy recommendations for the treatment of ADHD. *Drug, 56,* 215-222.

Day, K. (1994). Male mentally handicapped sex offenders. *British Journal of Psychiatry, 165,* 630-639.

Day, K. (1997). Clinical features and offense behavior of mentally retarded sex offenders: A review of research. The NADD Newsletter, 14 86-89.

Demetral, G.D. (1994). A training methodology for establishing reliable self-monitoring with the sex offender who is developmentally disabled. *The Habilitative Mental Healthcare Newsletter, 13,* 57-60.

Douglas, V.I. (1972). Stop, look, and listen: The problem of sustained attention and impulse control in hyperactive and normal children. *Canadian Journal of Behavioural Science, 4,* 259-282.

Douglas, V.I. (1980). Higher mental processes in hyperactive children: implications for training In R. Knights and D. Bakkes (Eds.) *Treatment of hyperactive and learning disordered children* (pp. 65-92). Baltimore: University Park Press.

Douglas, V.I. (1983). Attentional and cognitive problems. In Rutter, M. (Ed.), *Developmental Neuropsychiatry.* (pp. 280-329). New York: Guilford Press.

Everington, C., and Fulero, S.M. (1999). Competence to confess: Measuring understanding and suggestibility of defendants with mental retardation. *Mental Retardation, 37,* 212-220.

Eyestone, LL, Howell, RJ (1994). An epidemiological study of attention-deficit hyperactivity disorder and major depression in a male prison population. Bulletin of the American Academy of Psychiatry and the Law, 22, 181-193.

Finkelhor, D. (1983). *Childhood sexual experiences: A retrospective survey.* Durham, NH: University of NH.

Finkelhor, D., and Strapko, N. (1992). Sexual abuse prevention education: A review of evaluation studies. In Willis, D.J., Holder, E.W., and Rosenberg, M. (Eds.), *Prevention of Child Maltreatment.* New York: Wiley.

Friedrich, W.N. (1994). *Psychological assessment of sexually abused children: The case for abuse-specific measures.* Paper presented at American Psychological Association Annual Convention, Los Angeles, CA, August 12.

Friedrich, W., Beilke, R ., and Urquiza, A. (1987). Children from sexually abusive families: A behavioral comparison. *Journal of Interpersonal Violence, 2,* 391-402.

Friedrich, W.N ., and Luecke, W.J. (1988). Young school-age sexually aggressive children. *Professional Psychology Research and Practice, 19,* 155-164.

Gil, E., and Johnson, T.C. (1993). Sexualized children: *Assessment and treatment of Sexualized Children and Children Who Molest.* Rockvile, MD: Launch Press.

Gilby, R., Wolf, L., and Goldberg, B. (1989). Mentally retarded adolescent sex offenders: A survey and pilot study. *Canadian Journal of Psychiatry, 34(6),* 542-548.

Gillespie, R.A., Eriksen, J., Hao, H.L., and Druse, M.J. (1997) . Effects of maternal ethanol consumption and buspirone treatment on dopamine and norepinephrine reuptake sites and DI receptors in offspring. *Alcohol Clinical Experience and Research, 21,* 452-458.

Goldman, R., and Goldman, J. (1988). *Show me yours: Understanding children's sexuality.* New York: Penguin.

Griffiths, D., Hingsburger, D., and Christian, R. (1985). Treating developmentally handicapped sex offenders: The York Behavior Management Services Treatment Program. *Psychiatric Aspects of Mental Retardation Reviews, 4,* 49-53.

Grodzinsky, G.M., and Diamond, R. (1992). Frontal lobe functioning in boys with Attention-Deficit Hyperactivity Disorder. *Developmental Neuropsychology, 8,* 427-445.

Gross, G. (1985). Activities of the developmental disabilities adult offender project. Olympia: Washington State Developmental Disability Planning Council.

Groth, A.N. (1979). Sexual trauma in the life histories of rapists and child molesters. *Victimology, 4,* 10-16.

Haaven, J., and Coleman, E. (2000). Treatment of the developmentally disabled sex offender. In D.M. Laws, S.M. Hudson, and T. Ward (Eds.), *Remaking relapse prevention with sex offenders: A sourcebook* (pp. 369-38). London: Sage.

Haaven, J., Little, R., and Petre-Miller, D. (1990). *Treating intellectually disabled sex offenders.* Orwell, VT: Safer Society Press.

Hallowell, E.M., and Ratey, J.J. (1994). *Driven to distraction: Recognizing and coping with attention-deficit disorder from childhood through adulthood.* NY: Simon and Schuster.

Hanson, R.K. and Bussiere, M.T. (1998). Predicting relapse: A meta-analysis of sexual offender recidivism studies. *Journal of Consulting and Clinical Psychology, 66 (2),* 348-362.

Hamlet, K.W., Pellegrini, D.S., and Conners, C.K. (1987).An investigation of executive processes in the problem-solving of Attention Deficit Disorder-Hyperactive children. *Journal of Pediatric Psychology, 12,* 227-240.

Hanson, R.K., and Morton-Bourgon, K. (2004). Predictors of sexual recidivism: An updated meta-analysis. Public Safety and Emergency Preparedness Canada.

Hare, R.D. (1991). *The Hare Psychopathy Checklist-Revised.* Toronto: Multihealth Systems.

Hart, E.L., Lahey, B.B., Loeber, R., Applegate, B., Green, S., and Frick, P.J. (1996). Developmental change in Attention-Deficit Hyperactivity Disorder in boys: A four-year longitudinal study. *Journal of Abnormal Child Psychology, 23,* 729-750.

Haugaard, J., and Tilly, C. (1988). Characteristics predicting children's responses to sexual encounters with other children. *Child Abuse and Neglect, 12,* 209-218.

Hayes, S.C. (1997). Prevalence of intellectual disability and local courts. *Journal of Intellectual and Developmental Disability, 22,* 71-85.

Hingsburger, D. (1996). Counseling strategies: Some adaptations for sex offenders with developmental disabilities. *Canadian Journal of Human Sexuality, 5,* 48-54.

Hingsburger, D., Griffiths, D., and Quinsey, V. (1991a).Are sex offenders treatable? A research overview. *Psychiatric Services, 50,* 349-361.

Hingsburger, D., Griffiths, D., and Quinsey, V. (1991b). Detecting counterfeit deviance: Differentiating sexual deviance from sexual inappropriateness. *The Habilitative Mental Healthcare Newsletter, 10* (9).

Hingsburger, D., and Tough, S. (1997). Hey!! Watch your mouth! A response to clinical features and offence behaviour of mentally retarded sex offenders: A review of the research. *NADD Newsletter, 14* (6), 86-90.

Huebert, K., and Raftis C. (1996). *Fetal alcohol syndrome and other alcohol-related birth defects* (2nd Ed.). Alberta Alcohol and Drug Abuse Commission.

Hynd, G.W., Hern, K.., Novey, E.S., Eliopulos, D., Marshall, R., Gonzalez, J.J., and Voeller, K.K. (1993). Attention-Deficit Hyperactivity Disorder and asymmetry of the caudate nucleus. *Journal of Child Neurology, 8,* 339-347.

Ikonomidou, C., Bittigau, P., Ishimaru, M.J., Wozniak, D.F., Koch, C., Genz, K., et al. (2000). Ethanol-induced apoptotic neurodegeneration and fetal alcohol syndrome. *Science, 287,* 1056-1060.

Institute of Medicine. Stratton, K.R., Howe, C.J., and Battaglia, F.C. (Eds.). (1996). *Fetal alcohol syndrome: Diagnosis, epidemiology, prevention, and treatment.* Washington, D.C.: National Academy Press.

Johnston, C., Pelham, W.E., and Murphy, H.A. (1985). Peer relationships in ADHD and normal children: A developmental analysis of peer and teacher ratings. *Journal of Abnormal Child Psychology, 13,* 89-100.

Jones, K.L., and Smith, D.W. (1973). Recognition of the Fetal Alcohol Syndrome in early infancy. *Lancet, 2,* 999-1001.

Knight, R.A. (1989). An assessment of the concurrent validity of a child molester typology. *Journal of Interpersonal Violence, 14,* 303-330.

Knight, R.A. and Prentky, R.A. (1990). Classifying sexual offenders: The development and corroboration of taxonomic models. In W.L. Marshall, D.R. Laws and H.E. Barbaree (Eds.), *The handbook of sexual assault: Issues, theories, and treatment of the offender* (pp. 27-52). New York: Plenum Press.

LaDue, R. and Dunne, T. (1997). Legal issues and FAS. In A. Streissguth and J. Kanter (Eds.), *The challenge of Fetal Alcohol Syndrome: Overcoming secondary disabilities.* Seattle, WA: University of Washington Press.

LaDue, R.A., Streissguth, A.P., and Randels, S.P. (1992). Clinical considerations pertaining to adolescents and adults with Fetal Alcohol Syndrome. In T.B. Sonderegger (Ed.), *Perinatal Substance Abuse: Research Findings and Clinical Implications* (pp. 104-131). Baltimore, MD: The Johns Hopkins University Press.

Lindsay, W.R., Olley, S., Baillie, N., and Smith, A.H.W. (1999). Treatment of adolescent sex offenders with intellectual disabilities. Mental Retardation, 17, 201-211.

Loeber, R., Green, S.M., Lahey, B.B., Christ, M.A.G., and Frick, P.J. (1992). Developmental sequences in the age of onset of disruptive child behaviors. *Journal of Child and Family Studies, 1,* 21-41.

Longo, R.F. (1986). Sexual learning and experience among adolescent sexual offenders. *International Journal of Offender Therapy and Comparative Criminology, 26,* 235-241.

Luiselli, J.R. (Ed.). (2000). Diagnosis , assessment, and treatment of sexual deviance and sexually offending behavior in people with developmental disabilities (Special issue). *Mental Health Aspects of Developmental Disabilities, 3(2).*

Manuzza S., Kein, RG, Konig, PH, Giampino, TL (1989). Hyperactive boys almost grown up, IV: Criminality and its relationship to psychiatric status. Archives of General Psychiatry, 46, 1073-1079.)

Manuzza, S., Gittelman-Klein, R., Bessler, A., Malloy, P., and LaPadula, M. (1993). Adult outcome of hyperactive boys: Educational achievement, occupational rank and psychiatric status. *Archives of General Psychiatry, 50,* 565-576.

Mariani, M., and Barkley, R.A. (1997). Neuropsychological and academic functioning in preschool children with Attention Deficit Hyperactivity Disorder. *Developmental Neuropsychology, 13,* 111-129.

Marshall, W.L., and Barbaree, H.E. (1990). Outcome of comprehensive cognitive-behavioral treatment programs. In *Handbook of Sexual Assault: Issues, Theories, and Treatment of the Offender.* Marshall, W.L., Laws, D.R., and Barbaree, H.E. (Eds.), New York: Plenum Press.

Mikkelsen, E.J., and Stelk, W.J. (1997). Assessment of risk in criminal offenders with mental retardation. *The NADD Newsletter, 14,* 91-95.

Mrazek, P., and Mrazek, D. (1987). Resilience in child maltreatment victims: A conceptual exploration. *Child Abuse and Neglect, 11,* 357-366.

Murphy, W., Coleman, E., and Hanes, M. (1983). Treatment and evaluation issues with the mentally retarded sex offender. In J.G. Greer and I.R. Stuart (Eds.), The sexual aggressor: Current perspectives on treatment (pp. 22-41). New York: Van Nostrand Reinhold.

Nanson, J.L. (1990). Behavior in children with Fetal Alcohol Syndrome. In W.I. Fraser (Ed.) *Key Issues in Mental Retardation Research.* London: Blackwell.

Nanson, J.L., and Hiscock, M. (1990). Attention deficits in children exposed to alcohol prenatally. *Alcoholism: Clinical and Experimental Research, 14,* 656-661.

Niccols, G.A. (1994). Fetal alcohol syndrome: Implications for psychologists. *Clinical Psychology Review, 14,* 91-111.

Nichols, P.L., and Chen, T.C. (1981). *Minimal brain dysfunction: A prospective study.* Hillsdale, NJ: Erlbaum.

Novick, N (1997). FAS: Preventing and treating sexual deviancy. In A.P. Streissguth and J. Kanter (Eds.). *The challenge of fetal alcohol syndrome: Overcoming secondary disabilities,* Seattle, University of Washington Press, (pp.162-170).

Nucci, L.P., and Herman, S. (1982). Behavioral disordered children's conceptions of moral, conventional, and personal issues. *Journal of Abnormal Child Psychology, 10,* 411-426.

O'Malley, K.D., and Nansun, J. (2002). Clinical implications of a link between fetal alcohol spectrum disorder and attention-deficit hyperactivity disorder. *Canadian Journal of Psychiatry, 47(4),* 349-354.

Paternite, C., and Loney, J. (1980). Childhood hyperkinesis: Relationships between symptomatology and home environment. In C.K. Whalen and B. Henker (Eds), Hyperactive children: The social ecology of identification and treatment (pp. 105-141). New York: Academic Press.

Pelham, W.E., and Bender, M.E. (1982). Peer relationships in hyperactive children: Description and treatment. In K.D. Gadow and I. Bialer (Eds.), *Advances in learning and behavioral disabilities* (Vol. I, pp. 365-436). Greenwich, CT: JAI Press.

Perske, R. (1991). *Unequal justice? What can happen when persons with retardation or other developmental disabilities encounter the criminal justice system.* Nashville: Abingdon Press.

Pliszka, S.R., McCracken, J.T., and Maas, J.W. (1996). Catecholamines in attention deficit hyperactivity disorder, current perspectives. *Journal of the American Academy of Child and Adolescent Psychiatry, 35, 264-272.*

Prentky, R.A., Knight, R.A., Lee, A.S., and Cerce, D.D. (1995). Predictive validity of lifestyle impulsivity for rapists. *Criminal Justice and Behavior, 22,* 106-128.

Rapoport, J.L. (1996). *Anatomic magnetic resonance imaging in Attention Deficit Hyperactivity Disorder.* Paper presented at the annual meeting of the International Society for Research in Child and Adolescent Psychopathology. Santa Monica, CA.

Rasmussen, K., Almvik, R ., and Levander, S (2001). Attention deficit hyperactivity disorder, reading disability, and personality disorders in a prison population. Journal of the American Academy of Psychiatry and the Law, 29, 186-193.

Roberts, M.A. (1990). A behavioral observation method for differentiating hyperactive and aggressive boys. *Journal of Abnormal Child Psychology, 18,* 131-142.

Sampson, P.D., Streissguth, A.P. Bookstein, F.L., Little, R.E., Clarren, S.K., Dehaene, P., Hanson, J.W., and Graham Jr., J.M. (1997). Incidence of fetal alcohol syndrome and prevalence of alcohol-related neurodevelopmental disorder. *Teratology, 56,* 317-326.

Santamour, M. (1986). The offender with mental retardation. *The Prison Journal, 66* (7), 3-18.

Simmel, C ., and Hinshaw, S.P. (1993) . *Moral reasoning and antisocial behavior in boys with ADHD.* Poster presented at the biennial meeting of the Society for Research in Child Development, New Orleans.

Snyder, J., Nanson, J., Snyder, R., and Block, G. (1997). A study of stimulant mediation in children with FAS. In A. P. Streissguth and J.U. Kanter (Eds.), *The challenge of fetal alcohol syndrome: Overcoming secondary disabilities* (pp. 25-39). Seattle, WA: University of Washington Press.

Still, G.F. (1902). Some abnormal psychical conditions in children. *Lancet, i,* 1008-1012, 1077-1082, 1163-1168.

Stratton, K.R., Howe, C.J., and Battaglia, F.C. (1996). *Fetal alcohol syndrome: Diagnosis, epidemiology, prevention and treatment.* In: Institute of Medicine, eds. Washington (DC): National Academy Press, 1996.

Strauss, A.A., and Lehtinen, L.E. (1947). *Psychopathology and education of the brain-injured child.* New York: Grune and Stratton.

Streissguth, A.P. (1997). *Fetal Alcohol Syndrome: A Guide for Families and Communities.* Baltimore, MD: Paul H. Brookes Publishing Co.

Streissguth, A.P., Martin, D.C., Barr, H.M., Sandman, B.M., Kirschner, G.L., and Darby, B.L. (1984). Intrauterine alcohol and nicotine exposure: Attention and reaction time in 4 year old children. *Developmental Psychology, 20,* 541-553.

Streissguth, A.P., Barr, H.M., Kogan, J., and Bookstein, F. (1997). Primary and secondary disabilities in fetal alcohol syndrome. In A. P. Streissguth and J.U. Kanter (Eds.), *The challenge of fetal alcohol syndrome: Overcoming secondary disabilities* (pp. 25-39). Seattle, WA: University of Washington Press.

Streissguth, A.P., Bookstein, F.L., Barr, H.M., Sampson, P.D., O'Malley, K., and Kogan Young, J. (2004). Risk factors for adverse life outcomes in Fetal Alcohol Syndrome and Fetal Alcohol Effects. *Developmental and Behavioral Pediatrics, 25(4),* 228-238.

Swanson, C.K., and Garwick, G.B. (1990). Treatment for low-functioning sex offenders: Group therapy and interagency coordination. *Mental Retardation, 28,* 155-161.

Thomas, A., and Chess, S. (1977). *Temperament and development.* NY: Brunner Mazel.

Tudiver, J., Broekstra, S., Josselyn, S., and Barbaree, H. (1997). *Addressing the needs of developmentally delayed sex offenders.* Health Canada, Family Violence Prevention Division.

Voelker, S.L., Carter, R.A., Sprague, D.J., Gdowski, C.L., and Lachar, D. (1989). Developmental trends in memory and metamemory in children with Attention Deficit Disorder. *Journal of Pediatric Psychology, 14,* 75-88.

Ward, K., Trigler, J., and Pfeiffer, K. (2001). Community services, issues, and service gaps for individuals with developmental disabilities who exhibit inappropriate sexual behaviors. *Mental Retardation, 39* (1), 11-19.

Wittenberg, J.V. (2001). Regulatory disorders: A new diagnostic classification for difficult infants and toddlers. *Canadian Journal of Diagnosis,* 111-123.

Yates, A. (1982). Children eroticized by incest. *American Journal of Psychiatry, 139,* 482-485.

Yates, A. (1987). Psychological damage associated with extreme eroticism in young children. *Psychiatric Annals, 17,* 257-261.

Yates, A. (1990). Eroticized children. In M.E. Perry (Ed.), *Handbook of sexology: Childhood and adolescent sexology.* New York, NY: Elsevier Science Publishers.

Zentall, S.S. (1988). Production deficiencies in elicited language but not in the spontaneous verbalizations of hyperactive children. *Journal of Abnormal Child Psychology, 16,* 657-673.

Zentall, S.S., and Smith, Y.S. (1993). Mathematical performance and behaviour of children with hyperactivity with and without coexisting aggression. *Behaviour Research and Therapy, 31,* 701-710.

In: ADHD and Fetal Alcohol Spectrum Disorders (FASD)   ISBN: 1-59454-573-1
Editor: Kieran D. O'Malley, pp. 161-178   © 2008 Nova Science Publishers, Inc.

Chapter 9

IDENTIFYING AND TREATING SOCIAL COMMUNICATION DEFICITS IN SCHOOL-AGE CHILDREN WITH FETAL ALCOHOL SPECTRUM DISORDERS

Truman E. Coggins[·1]*, Geralyn R. Timler*[2] *and Lesley B. Olswang*[3]

[1] Center on Human Development and Disability; University of Washington
[2] Department of Communicative Disorders and Sciences; University at Buffalo
[3] Department of Speech and Hearing Sciences; University of Washington

ABSTRACT

Children with fetal alcohol spectrum disorders (FASD) have functional deficits that compromise their ability to use language in socially appropriate ways. An interpretive framework conceptualizing social communicative competence is presented. The framework provides experienced clinicians and educators with new ways of thinking about and treating the social communication problems of school-age children with FASD.

Fetal Alcohol Syndrome (FAS) is a birth defect characterized by growth deficiency, a cluster of minor facial anomalies and central nervous system damage in the presence of confirmed prenatal alcohol exposure (Astley and Clarren, 2000; Jones, Smith, Ulleland and Streissguth, 1970). A large body of descriptive and experimental research underscores the broad range of harmful effects teratogenic alcohol exposure exerts on growth and development (Astley and Clarren, 2000; Mattson and Riley, 1998; Thomas, Kelly, Mattson, and Riley, 1998). The term fetal alcohol spectrum disorders (FASD) describes the range of effects that can occur in an individual whose mother drank alcohol during pregnancy (O'Malley and Hagerman, 1998). Much of the clinical research over the last decade for

[*] Please address correspondences to: Truman E. Coggins, Ph.D. Head, Speech-Language Pathology; Center on Human Development and Disability; University of Washington; Seattle, WA 98195; USA; Office Phone: 206-685-2999; Email: tec@u.washington.edu

children with FASD has focused on refining identification criteria (Astley, 2004; Astley and Clarren, 1996; Clarren, Carmichael Olson, Clarren and Astley, 2000) and/or increasing access to related services (Streissguth, 1997).

Children with FASD present complex clinical profiles. They often show problems learning from experience, following directions and understanding logical consequences (Carmichael Olson, Morse and Huffine, 1998). They are frequently unfocused and impulsive, have recurring difficulties adapting to routine school activities, and interacting with peers (Coles, Platzman, Raskind-Hood, Brown, Falek and Smith, 1997; Kleinfeld, and Wescott, 1993; Mattson and Riley, 1998 Streissguth, 1997). The social and behavioral problems often associated with FASD become more pronounced during the school years and coincide with problems in adaptive behavior and secondary disabilities (Streissguth, 1977). It is, therefore, not particularly surprising to find that many school-age children with histories of significant prenatal alcohol exposure have also been diagnosed as having a learning disability and/or an attention deficit hyperactivity disorder (Oesterheld and O'Malley, 1999).

Of particular interest for speech-language pathologists is the impressive number of alcohol-exposed youngsters who exhibit social problems, as revealed during verbal interactions with peers (Coggins, Olswang, Carmichael Olson and Timler, 2003; Spohr, and Steinhausen, 1993; Olswang, Coggins and Timler, 2001; Thomas, Kelly, Mattson, and Riley, 1998; Timler, Olswang and Coggins, 2005). Interestingly, the majority of these youngsters do not typically have debilitating conduct disorders of serious social-emotional problems if they experience supportive environments and appropriate expectations. Moreover, even though they exhibit processing limitations and learning difficulties, their intellectual abilities are often found to be broadly within the normal range (Kerns, Don, Mateer and Streissguth, 1997).

What sets these children apart from their school-age peers is their difficulty using language in more sophisticated social contexts. They lack the pivotal communicative abilities to enter peer groups, resolve conflicts, negotiate compromises, and maintain friendships. While interdisciplinary assessment teams are becoming increasingly effective in diagnosing the spectrum of disabilities associated with FASD (Clarren, Carmichael Olson, Clarren and Astley, 2000), few professionals have the necessary information for treating children with social communication problems

The purpose of this paper is to present an interpretive framework for understanding communicative deficits in school-age children with FASD. To this end, we build an argument that the complex array of deficits in this clinical population creates special problems in social aspects of language use. Based on this argument, we present a model for conceptualizing social communication competence. We believe this framework offers practitioners a rational basis for selecting functional objectives and designing effective interventions for children who have do not use language to communicate appropriately.

A SOCIAL COMMUNICATIVE FRAMEWORK

Those who have studied developmental outcomes in children with FASD report that high levels of prenatal alcohol exposure disrupt the development and use of language (Dorris, 1989; Huffine, 1998; Kleinfeld and Wescott, 1993; Streissguth, 1997; Streissguth, and

Kanter, 1997). This is not an unexpected finding since alcohol is a teratogen that can alter brain structure and/or chemistry and communicative development is highly correlated with brain maturation. Evidence from parental reports (e. g., Caldwell, 1993; Wright, 1992), feasibility studies (e.g., Thorne, Coggins, Carmichael Olson and Astley, accepted; Timler, Olswang and Coggins, 2005) and controlled clinical investigations (e.g., Becker, Warr-Leeper and Leeper, 1990); Weienberg, 1997), have revealed an array of performance profiles, but no identifiable pattern of deficits.

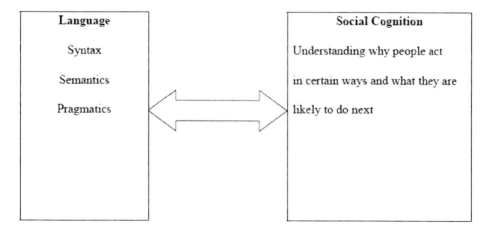

Social Communicative Competence

Using language in interpersonally appropriate ways to successfully influence people and interpret events

Social Communicative Behaviors

Words and observable, nonverbal behaviors that competent communicators use in specific situations to resolve social dilemmas

Higher-Order Executive Functions

Decision-making and strategic planning processes

Language

Syntax

Semantics

Pragmatics

Social Cognition

Understanding why people act in certain ways and what they are likely to do next

Figure 1. A framework of social communication competence.

A group of clinical researchers at the University of Washington has embraced a more functional approach to describe the language and communication problems faced by children with complex behavioral profiles like FASD (Coggins, Friet and Morgan, 1998; Hamilton, 1981; Thorne, Coggins, Carmichael Olson and Astley, 2006; Timler, Olswang and Coggins,

2005). This research cadre has been interested in the ability of school-age children to use their language effectively in achieving important communicative goals. To this end, a promising framework has been proposed for assessing and treating children with complicated and diverse etiologies who exhibit compromises in social communication.

Figure 1 presents a conceptual framework of social communicative competence. The model is an attempt to understand underlying factors that interact and influence children's communication during social interactions. The model reflects the social information processing paradigm proposed by Crick and Dodge (1994), the social behavior construct advanced by Campbell and Siperstein (1994) and Guralnick's (1999) model of peer-related social competence. We believe this conceptual framework is a useful basis for revealing how children with prenatal alcohol exposure may share characteristics with other children with impaired functioning, especially those with ADHD.

Three developmental processes anchor this conceptual framework. These underlying processes include language, social cognition and higher-order executive functions. Because these processes ultimately determine children's social communicative behaviors, they are pivotal to social communicative competence. A disruption in one or more of the processes is likely to yield a less capable, if not impaired ability to use language appropriately during social interactions. Because the extent and nature of these disruptions are likely to vary across children, social communicative abilities are also variable.

The framework in Figure 1 is an attempt to sort through the complexities of social communication in order to offer a construct for meaningful intervention. It serves to focus our attention on behaviors of concern, followed by the skills that are necessary for optimum performance, and the underlying cognitive operations that support these skills and behaviors. While the underlying processes are presented and discussed as separate components, they are, in reality, dynamic and overlapping.

Language

Social communication is predicated on linguistic competence. Language competence reflects what a child is able to do with language. Competence may be best described by considering its three functional components: form (syntax, morphology and phonology), content (semantics), and use (pragmatic or language use within a communicative context).

By the time they begin school, most typically developing children demonstrate impressive syntactic, semantic and pragmatic knowledge. They use this knowledge to achieve important communicative goals, for example providing sufficient information to the listener, maintaining the topic of discussion, insuring utterances are appropriate in style and tone to the situation and, providing timely responses during discourse (Damico, Oller and Tetnowski, 1999). DeVilliers, Roper and deVilliers (1999) have identified core communicative skills that children need as they enter school. These skills include:

1. Mapping questions and answers (asking and answering the right questions for specific information i.e., double wh-questions-"Who is wearing what"?)
2. Uniquely specifying references (which X am I talking about -i.e., relative clauses)
3. Linking meaning across referents and events (discourse cohesion in extended turns-I i.e., temporal and causal links specified between events)

4. Recognizing different points of view (taking on more than one perspective on events-i.e., verbs of cognitive state, as thinking, believing, and knowing).

Recent experimental evidence suggests that school-age children with FASD have meaningful compromises in using language to manage longer units of discourse during narratives. Thorne and colleagues (accepted) examined two independent parameters of narrative production in 16 school-age children with FASD and 16 age and gender matched counterparts with normal language peers. Narrative samples were coded for semantic elaboration of verbal and nominal concepts, and the degree to which unambiguous reference of nominal concepts was maintained as the story progressed. Results showed that both typically developing children and those with a diagnosis of FASD varied widely in the degree of semantic elaboration they included in their stories. However, the children with FASD were significantly more likely to use pragmatically inappropriate strategies for establishing and maintaining unambiguous reference in their stories than were their typically developing peers. In particular, the children in the FASD group were more likely to inappropriately distinguish between shared information and new information in their stories resulting in greater ambiguity.

Social Cognition

Because language is learned in dynamic social interactions, children are naturally curious about the people around them. They try to make sense of social situations by figuring out why people act in particular ways and what they are likely to do next. The social cognitive component is, therefore, concerned with how children conceptualize and think about their social world – the people they observe, the relations between people, and the groups in which they participate.

Crick and Dodge (1994) have postulated six social cognitive processes that operate while children try and interpret social interactions. The dynamic integration of these processes provides an important influence on social communication behaviors. The six processes include:

1. *Encoding external and internal cues*: Attending to and recognizing the cues present in a social situation, including who/what is in the context, and what the participants are doing and saying.
2. *Interpreting and representing cues*: Appraising and understanding the contextual cues, including what the participants know, believe, think, desire, etc. and what would be appropriate in that context.
3. *Clarifying or selecting a goal*: Identifying one's social communication goal (e.g., wanting to enter a group) that is the desired social outcome for the situation
4. *Response access or construction*: Identifying the possible strategies to reach the selected goal (e.g., approaching the group and asking to join in)
5. *Response decision*: Evaluating the possible consequences of the previously accessed (or constructed) responses, and selecting the most appropriate one for the situation.
6. *Behavioral enactment*: Monitoring effectiveness of the selected strategies and goals, including others reactions/feedback, personal feedback, and goal achievement.

A breakdown in one or more of these processes could conceivably compromise a child's ability to perform in a socially competent manner.

Another important area of social cognitive research is theory of mind (TOM). The primary focus of TOM is knowledge of mental states or how individuals learn to appreciate, imagine or represent states of mind in themselves and other people in order to make sense of social interactions, and behave competently in social situations. Since communication is the vehicle for social interaction, school-age children need a well-defined TOM in order to exchange information, initiate and develop satisfying social relationships, cope with changing environmental demands and appropriately assert their needs, desires and preferences.

Caregivers and clinical researchers have consistently reported that school-age children with FASD seem unable to empathize and have genuine difficulty anticipating the consequences of their actions in social situations. Hinde's (1993) observations led her to argue that this heterogeneous clinical population does not understand "what is going on in social life and how they should behave in different situations" (p. 139). Clinical studies have produced preliminary evidence suggesting that school-age children with FASD have limited ability to make inferences about what other persons believe in specific situations. Timler, Olswang and Coggins (2005) have suggested that this difficulty may, in part, be due to compromises these children have in using mental state words to reference another person's perspective. Since effective use of these cognitive verbs is a critical measure of a child's ability to represent states of mind in themselves and others, they may not use language to describe what others may think or know during social interactions

The social cognitive processes children use to try and interpret social interactions clearly depend on linguistic competence. For example, children's ability to selectively attend and encode particular situation and internal cues depend on their knowledge of language (i.e., syntactic, semantic, pragmatic variables used by the speaker) and their understanding of extra-linguistic elements (e.g., body posture, eye contact, etc.). Similarly, language competence is influenced by social processing. For example, the pragmatic skill of selecting and the using the appropriate tone in talking with a teacher requires encoding and interpreting cues, and identifying and selecting goals and strategies for a response. Thus, the enactment of social communication behaviors is viewed, in part, as the culmination of the interaction between social processing and language competence.

Higher-Order Executive Functions

Executive functions are higher-order, decision-making and planning processes invoked at the outset of a task and in the face of novel challenges (Singer and Bashir, 1999). Such processes permit children to disengage from the immediate context and reason about interpersonal goals. We have nested language and social cognition within higher-order executive functions because socially competent communicators must integrate and/or modify their language and social cognitive abilities in accordance with the demands of particular situations.

Executive functions incorporate an array of crucial functions. These functions include planning and employing flexible cognitive strategies, using organized search strategies, inhibiting responses, and manipulating information in working memory. Executive functioning also includes the ability to take into account another person's perspective, and to infer the knowledge, ideas, and beliefs of others.

Findings from a growing number of executive function investigations reveal that children with FASD have deficits in these critical functions (Jacobson and Jacobson, 1997; Kopara-Frye, Dehaene and Streissguth, 1996; Mattson, Goodman, Caine, Delis and Riley, 1999). Furthermore, executive function deficits appear to constrain the amount of information children with high prenatal alcohol can process when confronted with more complex challenges (Carmichael Olson, Feldman, Streissguth, Sampson and Bookstein, 1998; Kerns, Don, Mateer and Streissguth, 1997; Kodituwakku, Handmaker, Cuttler, Weathersby and Handmaker, 1995). Thus, it is not a leap of faith to suggest that processing deficits are likely to interfere with social performance and/or use of complex language.

Social Communicative Behaviors

Sitting atop the framework are social communicative behaviors. These behaviors (generally occurring in combinations) are observed when a child interacts with others for example while entering peer groups, negotiating and resolving conflicts or during discourse narratives. These are the actions often reported by parents, teachers and clinicians as problematic during daily social interactions.

Language, social cognition, and executive functions support social communication behaviors. These components reflect the necessary skills or abilities a child must control to execute social communication behaviors; in essence, they are the substance of the observable behaviors. To our way of thinking, these neuropsychological operations enable a child to utilize and manipulate existing knowledge, organize, manage and deploy information from social processing and language competence in the service of social communication

SIMILARITIES TO OTHER CLINICAL POPULATIONS

As we consider the social communication problems of children with FASD, we cannot help but appreciate similarities to other clinical populations, particularly those with ADHD. Children with ADHD often have problems with social behaviors, as do children with FASD. These include such difficulties as participating appropriately in groups, collaborating, negotiating, and waiting a turn

Children with ADHD can also have difficulty with social processing and language. For example, it has been reported that children with ADHD have deficits with respect to appraising situations, deciding how to behave, and evaluating their actions. Furthermore, a high proportion of children with ADHD have also been found to exhibit deficits in their pragmatic uses of language (Tannock and Schachar, 1996). Specifically, they demonstrate difficulties with story telling (Tannock, Purvis, and Schachar, 1993) and adjusting language to their listener (Landau and Milich, 1988).

Several authors have argued that impairment in social skills and social communication behaviors reflect underlying deficits in executive functions among children with ADHD (see Tannock and Schachar, 1996). Indeed, children with these neurodevelopmental disabilities show compromises in their ability to plan future actions, hold plans and action sequences in working memory until they are executed, and inhibit irrelevant actions (Pennington and Ozonoff, 1996).

We do *not* intend to argue that children with ADHD and FASD constitute distinct clinical populations. Rather, our point is that heterogeneous children, representing different etiologies, may have similar deficits in social communicative behaviors, similar impairments in social processing and language, and similar underlying difficulties in higher order executive function. This remarkable degree of overlap gives us license as clinical researchers to draw on what we know about other populations of atypical children in conceptualize treatment approaches for children with prenatal alcohol exposure.

IMPLICATIONS FOR TREATMENT

In this paper, we have argued that children's knowledge about their social world, and the language they use to represent it, is a product of three interrelated processes: language, social cognition and higher-order executive functions. We have also argued that a disruption in one or more of these fundamental processes places school-age children at considerable risk for social communication impairments. Earlier we presented a conceptual framework for better understanding how these processes might interact and influence children's communication during social interactions. In Table 1, we now consider this framework as a guide for selecting treatment objectives to improve social communication since we believe in the wisdom of selecting objectives that directly address social communication behaviors and processes.

What to Treat?

Targeting social behaviors means focusing treatment on specific observable actions that are missing or problematic. These are the behaviors listed in the upper panel of Table 1. Productive social communicative behaviors rely on effective underlying social cognitive abilities. Learning how to use language to appropriately resolve a social conflict is predicated, in part, on knowing how to encode and interpret cues, identifying and selecting goals and strategies, evaluating possible outcomes, and monitoring one's performance. Likewise, intervention needs to target questionable syntactic, semantic, and pragmatic skills that are ineffective during social exchanges, and thus contribute to problematic social communication behaviors.

School-aged children need to function appropriately in a variety of social situations, rather than learning an assortment of isolated social communication behaviors. From this perspective, social cognitive and advanced linguistic knowledge become *pivotal* abilities that children need become competent social communicators. Pivotal abilities are core to learning subsequent behaviors. They appear to be generative and facilitate functional change (Koegel, Koegel and Dunlap, 1996). Thus, treatment objectives should target social processing and language competence along with social communication behaviors.

Table 1. An interpretative framework for conceptualizing social communication in school-aged children (based on Campbell & Siperstein, 1994, and Crick & Dodge, 1994)

Social Communication Behaviors	
Specific observable actions that occur in isolation or are linked together, which reflect the child's understanding of his/her own and others' beliefs, desires, and intentions. At school age these include: Problems appropriately entering groups, working cooperatively with others, resolving conflicts, providing explanations about their own behavior, producing narratives, knowing when to ask for help, telling the truth, negotiating interactions, etc.	
Social Cognition	**Language Competence**
Problem-solving abilities that include: Encoding external and internal cues Interpreting the cues-understanding the present situation, including the participants, their roles, their knowledge Identifying and selecting personal goals based upon recalling previous situations Considering and selecting possible strategies or responses Evaluating the possible consequences associated with the goals and responses Following enactment, monitoring and evaluating the effectiveness of the strategies based upon feedback from others, from one's self, and goal achievement	Pragmatic skills and related semantic and syntactic forms that children need as they enter school. These include a variety of illocutionary acts (Damico, Oller & Tetnowski, 1999): Constatives Directives Commissives Acknowledgements Attending Verbal conversational skills (Damico, Oller & Tetnowksi, 1999): Providing significant information to the listener, topic maintenance, situational appropriateness, appropriate speech style, timing, etc. And pragmatic acts with accompany syntactic and semantic forms (deVilliers, Roper & deVilliers, 1999): Mapping questions and answers (asking and answering the right questions for specific information, e.g., double wh-questions-"Who is wearing what"?), Uniquely specifying references (which X am I talking about-e.g., relative clauses), Linking meaning across referents and events (discourse cohesion in extended turns-e.g., temporal and causal links specified between events), and Recognizing different points of view (taking on more than one perspective on events-e.g., verbs of cognitive state, as thinking, believing, and knowing).
Higher-Order Executive Functions	
Basic cognitive operations that include (Korkman et al., 1998): Attending and using working memory Planning and flexible strategy employment The ability to adopt, maintain, and shift cognitive set The ability to use organized search strategies, and to monitor performance and correct errors The ability to resist or inhibit the impulse to respond to salient but irrelevant aspects of a task Inferring the knowledge, beliefs, and ideas of other (e.g., theory of mind).	

What about children who demonstrate compromises in executive functions? Should this basic component be targeted in treatment? Attempting to change executive function through direct treatment is, at best, a formidable challenge. Even if executive functions could be enhanced, social processing, language skills, and social communication behaviors would still need to be taught, because altering executive function does not necessarily result in the change of functional behaviors. The more logical approach to treatment would be to take executive function problems into account, recognize their burden on the process of participating appropriately in social situations, and devise ways to minimize their impact.

In summary, the desired goal of intervention is to change inappropriate social communicative behaviors in children who exhibit social problems. To reach this goal, treatment objectives should focus on social processing along with language competence in the context of social communication behaviors, while recognizing and working with the executive function deficits. With such goals and objectives in mind, what would such an intervention look like?

How to Treat?

An effective intervention attempts to change performance by teaching pertinent and relevant skills. In this phase of treatment, professionals would attempt to actually change social communication performance by directly teaching children appropriate behaviors, and by improving social processing and language competence. Treatment would directly teach the behaviors, skills and processes listed in Table 1.

At the same time, intervention must provide compensatory strategies to support learning and performance in children with specific cognitive deficits. The assumption is that underlying brain dysfunction may impede the learning, generalization, and maintenance of the interrelated skills necessary to become a competent communicator. Thus, environmental supports are provided that help children to compensate for neurological limitations that may interfere with direct treatment. Treatment shapes and alters the environment to accommodate the child's deficits in attention, memory, organizing and planning. Environmental prompts and cues provide assistance to performance of social communication behaviors, social processing, and language competence. Further, treatment is designed to change the expectations of others so that they learn to accept the child's weaknesses, and encourage the child's strengths in social situations. The ideal treatment for children with FASD capitalizes on this -pronged approach.

A growing and informative body of intervention literature has accumulated regarding treatment ideas and techniques for children with complex cognitive and behavioral profiles (Carmichael Olson, 1994; Clarren, 2004; Connor and Streissguth, 1996; Kleinfeld and Wescott, 1993; Morse and Weiner, 1996; Streissguth, 1997; Timler, Olswang and Coggins, 2005). The literature describes innovative programs that not only teach children socially important behaviors and skills but also include environmental accommodations and cues that shape the environment. The components to these programs are important to consider prior to presenting specific guidelines for treating social communication.

Treating Children with FASD

Parents have repeatedly stressed structure and consistency when treating children with FASD. Malbin (1993) reported one family's story of finally recognizing the child's inability to "deduce, make connections, and transfer learning from one situation to another." This family subsequently devised a checklist to help their 11-year-old son remember to do his chores and stay on task. Vigilance and repeated exposure to learning material within a structured, supportive environment enhance successful learning.

Clinical observation and research also underscore the importance of structured environment is facilitating learning. For example, children with FASD appear more successful when they are involved in routines, when they can predict what will happen next, and when they know what is expected of them. They seem to learn best when difficult tasks are broken down into manageable parts. Task analysis, which involves teaching and rewarding small steps, may prove valuable for children with FASD (Hinde, 1993). In addition, their learning appears enhanced by multi-modality cues, particularly visual prompts (e.g., pictures), which heighten the saliency of critical target features (Tanner-Halverson, 1993). Rehearsal and meaningful repetitions seem to be an important part of most teaching efforts for children affected by alcohol (Tanner-Halverson, 1993). Structure that includes focusing a child's attention, providing demonstrations with multi-modality prompts and cues, and systematically guiding a child through sequential learning seems to create a positive learning environment.

GUIDING PRINCIPLES FOR TREATING SOCIAL COMMUNICATION PROBLEMS

Problematic social communication behaviors should serve as treatment targets. The emphasis in treatment will be teaching the children how to use their social processing and linguistic abilities to enable them to produce appropriate and adequate social communication behaviors. Because of executive function problems, the children will need assistance in attending to the individual components of social processing: encoding and interpreting cues, identifying and selecting goals and strategies, and evaluating the consequences of their selections and their performance. Further, they may need support in using the most appropriate language forms.

An informative literature is available for those interested in teaching social behaviors (Campbell, and Siperstein, 1994; Crick and Dodge, 1994; Gresham, 1998; McFadyen-Ketchum, and Dodge, 1998). Analog or hypothetical situations that simulate social communication can be used to elicit social behaviors, such as peer entry, negotiating, problem solving, and to teach and practice the steps of social processing and language skills (Gresham, 1998). These situations are appropriately implemented in peer groups with children who do and do not have social problems.

Within the context of the group, analog situations can be presented in scenarios utilizing joint-action routines. Joint-action routines are predictable events that provide "scripts" for all of the participants. These highly structured interactions allow children to know exactly what is expected of them. The children learn their roles and their response options as they participate with others in the scenarios. For example, joint-action routines can include common everyday scenarios, as mealtime, shopping, or recess, which are structured to elicit specific behaviors. The routine is defined by a structure of individual events in a predictable sequence. Because the events are routine and anticipated, the children know what is expected of them; it is as though they have a "script' for how to perform. Thus, the joint-action routines can provide structured opportunities to explicitly proceed through the steps of social processing, which in turn allows for opportunities to produce a variety of language forms for different social communication behaviors.

Utilizing this type of teaching environment in a group will necessitate the use of different teaching techniques, including modeling, role-playing, behavioral rehearsal, coaching, and discussions. Modeling has been shown to be an effective technique for teaching social behaviors and processing (Campbell and Siperstein, 1994; Gresham, 1998) and language skills (Camarata et al., 1994; Warren, and Kaiser, 1986; Weismer et al., 1989). Other children in the group can serve as appropriate models, which become a powerful learning tool. If children with social problems are included, inappropriate models can be used to discuss ways in which not to behave.

Along with modeling, role-playing can be an effective technique for isolating specific target skills. For example, role-playing can be valuable in demonstrating the various perspectives of a social conflict (e.g., the child's view, the parent's view, the friend's view) and using a variety of mental state words (e.g., "I *know*", "he *believes*", "she *thinks*"). Through role-playing and modeling, children learn how to behave and what language to use when they are in different social situations, and when they are in different roles. Different roles can be identified for the children, with the analog situations enacted several times. As the situations are reenacted, children can play different roles and offer different solutions for the conflict that occurs (Timler, Olswang and Coggins, 2005).

'Behavioral rehearsal' has also become an important teaching technique. Behavioral rehearsal involves repeatedly practicing newly learned behaviors in structured, protected situations (Gresham, 1998). This repetition allows for proceeding through the steps of social processing several times, with each exposure presented from a different perspective. The repeated practice, and the varying perspectives, has been shown to enhance learning (Gresham, 1998).

Coaching and discussions are useful techniques to teach social behavior. These techniques enlist an adult "coach" who can prompt a child with respect to what they might do or say as while participating in the analog social situations (Campbell and Siperstein, 1994; Gresham, 1998). Coaching provides explicit opportunities for discussing options regarding social processing decisions and language forms. Through coaching and follow-up discussions, children can consider their perceptions of a situation, the perceptions of others, options for how to proceed and what to say, and the possible consequences of each option.

Optimum coaching leads to discussion, and discussion encourages the process of problem- solving. With respect to children with FASD, coaching and discussions provide an opportunity for these individuals to use their language in assisting thinking. Since most children with FASD have basic semantic and syntactic language skills, they can use these skills to facilitate their problem-solving. Further, they can build on these skills to learn more complex, sophisticated forms. In this way, language and social processing can be simultaneously targeted and taught. Campbell and Siperstein (1994) provide specific suggestions regarding how to implement coaching and discussions. Table 2 presents a summary of the treatment guidelines for teaching social competence while Table 3 presents an example of two social communication analog situations.

Table 2. Summary of treatment guidelines for teaching social communication competence to school-aged children with FASD

Context For Treatment	
Social communication analog situations presented via joint action routines in group therapy. Natural social communication situations in the classroom.	
Treatment Techniques for Direct Teaching	**Compensatory Strategies for Environmental Support**
Modeling	
Role-Playing	Multi-modality Reminders:
Behavioral Rehearsal	Visual Prompts
Coaching	Checklists
Discussions	Schedules

Table 3. Social communication analog situations to be enacted in joint-action routines

Scenario: Going to the movies   Social Behavior: Negotiating **You and your friend Tom are at the movie theater. You see that both Independence Day and Starship Troopers are playing. You and Tom talk and decide you really want to see Independence Day. Your friend Brian is not here yet; you do not know which movie Brian wants to see. Brian finally comes to meet you. He says, "well let's talk about which movie to see."** *Prompt the child, What do you do now? What do you think will happen?* **Brian goes on to say, "I really want to see Scream."** *Prompt the child, What do you do now? What do you think will happen?* You tell Brian you and Tom want to see Independence Day. Brian gets really mad. He says, "Tom, you know I don't want to see Independence Day." Tom did not tell you, but Brian saw Independence Day yesterday with Tom's brother. *Prompt the child,* *What do you do now? What do you think Tom will do? Brian will do?* *Do you know why Brian does not want to see Independence Day?* *Does Tom know why Brian does not want to see Independence Day?* *Does Brian know that Tom knows he does not want to see Independence Day?* *Does Brian know that you don't know why he does not want to see Independence Day?* *What will you say to Brian?* **Scenario: Joining a group   Social Behavior: Peer Entry** Your science teacher tells everyone to find two other students for a group project. She says you will be doing a science experiment in your group of three for the next several days. You see two students, John and Sue, sitting at a table together. You want to join their science group. *Prompt the child, What do you do? What do you think will happen?* You say to John and Sue, "Can I be in your science group"? Sue says, "I want my friend Lisa to be in our group". Lisa is not in class today. *Prompt the child, what do you do now? What do you think will happen?* You say to Sue, "Where is Lisa"? Sue tells you, "Lisa is at the dentist, but she will be back tomorrow for science class". Sue says, "Let's go over to Bill and ask him if you can be in his group". You go over to Bill and ask him if you can be in his science group. Bill says, "No, you can only be in one group and you are already working with John and Sue". *Prompt the child, What do you do now? What do you think will happen?* *Do you know why you aren't working with John and Sue?* *Does Bill know why you aren't working with John and Sue?* *Does Sue know why you aren't working with her and John?* *Does Bill know that Sue knows you aren't working with Sue and John?* *Why does Bill say what he says?* *What could you say to John and Sue?*

Since executive function compromises are not unexpected in children with FASD, treatment should include compensatory strategies for problems in attention, memory, planning, response inhibition and inferencing. Compensatory strategies serve as a valuable heuristic that can increasing accuracy and consistency of performance by supplementing cognitive processing deficits (Mateer, Kerns, and Eso, 1996). Multi-modality reminders, such as checklists, schedules, or other devices that serve to cue the child, have been effective in clinical populations with diverse etiologies (Hodgdon, 2001). Visual prompts and cues can be used during the role-playing activities to assist the children in remembering the various steps of social processing. Treatment needs to include procedures for learning how to use the compensatory strategies, and for practicing their use in a variety of situations. In essence, multi-modality strategies become the means by which children compensate for their limited executive functions.

To insure generalization, treatment must include a variety of relevant socials contexts and socially relevant communicative partners. By systematically shifting treatment towards natural contexts, a child gains meaningful experience with everyday social situations, with people who matter, at important times during the day. Most importantly, generalizing treatment provides the opportunity for a child to utilize newly acquired behaviors in a context of competing stimuli (Gresham, 1998). When a child enters a situation with strong, competing stimuli, the situation may elicit potent, undesirable behaviors. In such situations, "the newly taught behaviors are masked or overpowered by older, stronger behaviors" (Gresham, 1998, p. 493). Within a treatment program, it becomes paramount to build the strength and fluency of new behaviors and skills in order to decrease interfering behaviors. In these situations, a child learns the value of compensatory strategies in minimizing the negative consequences of impaired decision-making processes.

The intervention guidelines presented above are based on existing literature addressing social competence and our clinical experience with children who exhibit complex behavioral profiles. The social problems and co-occurring language and communication problems in children with FASD are often frustrating and stressful for both child and family, especially since their developmental course can be erratic and their response to treatment inconsistent. However, the final guideline we offer centers on loss and disruption. Many children with FASD have been separated from birth families and/or have experienced multiple home placements. In some cases where children remain with birth parents, continued alcoholism creates home environments that are not safe, not predictable and not stimulating or responsive. The interventionist must be aware of these confounding issues, and prepare for them.

We believe that an interdisciplinary team, which can readily integrate and synthesize information from numerous disciplines, is a powerful intervention tool for adequately addressing and supporting the complex needs of children with FASD and their families and, most importantly, to offer support and encouragement to the interventionists themselves.

CONCLUSION

The ultimate goal of intervention for children with complex clinical profiles is to prevent the emergence of secondary disabilities, such as mental health problems or disruptions in the school setting. Such secondary disabilities are most likely to occur when appropriate interventions are absent. The findings from several recent studies at the University of Washington suggest that children with significant prenatal alcohol exposure have limitations in their interpersonal uses of language, particularly when confronted with the demands associated with more sophisticated social interactions (Coggins, Friet and Morgan, 1998; Coggins, Olswang, Carmichael Olson and Timler, 2003; Olswang, Coggins and Timler, 2001; Timler, Olswang and Coggins, 2005; Thorne, Coggins, Carmichael Olsen and Astley, accepted). These limitations appear to be the result of an array of subtle, but substantial deficits in language, social cognitive higher-order executive functions. The outcome is a decided lack of social savvy and difficulty performing adequately in socially demanding situations. This has provided guidelines for developing an intervention program that takes into account both the behaviors and skills that need to be taught directly to these children as well as environmental support that are needed for ultimate success. Clinical research to document the areas of deficit and effectiveness of intervention programs remains a pressing need. Until such research is available, we offer this framework for thinking about and treating the social communication problems of school-age children with FASD.

REFERENCES

Astely, S. (2004). Fetal alcohol syndrome prevention in Washington State: Evidence of success. *Paediatric and Perinatal Epidemiology*, 18, 344-351.

Astley, S. and Clarren, S. (1996). *Diagnostic guide for fetal alcohol syndrome and related conditions: the 4-digit diagnostic code*. Seattle, WA: FAS Diagnostic and Prevention Network, University of Washington.

Astley, S. and Clarren, S. (2000). Diagnosing the full spectrum of fetal alcohol exposed individuals: Introducing the 4-digit diagnostic code. *Alcohol and Alcoholism*, 35, 400-410.

Calculator, S.and Jorgensen, C. (1994). *Including students with severe disabilities in schools: fostering communication, interaction, and participation*. Baltimore, MD: Paul H. Brookes Publishing Co.

Caldwell, S. (1993). Nurturing the delicate rose. In J. Kleinfeld. and S. Wescott (Eds.), *Fantastic Antone Succeeds! Experiences in education children with Fetal Alcohol Syndrome*. Anchorage, AK: University of Alaska Press.

Camarata, S., Nelson, K. and Camarata, M. (1994). Comparison of conversational-recasting and imitative procedures for training grammatical structures in children with specific language impairment. *Journal of Speech and Hearing Research* 37, 1414-1423.

Campbell, P. and Siperstein, G. (1994). *Improving social competence*. Allyn and Bacon Publishing.

Carmichael Olson, H. (1994). The effects of prenatal alcohol exposure on child development. *Infants and Young Children: An Interdisciplinary Journal of Special Care Practices* 6, 10-25.

Carmichael Olson, H., Morse, B.A., and Huffine, C. (1998). Development and psychopathology: FAS and related conditions. *Seminars in Clinical Neuropsychiatry*, 3, 262-284.

Clarren, S. (2004). Teaching students with fetal alcohol spectrum disorder: Programming for students with special needs. Edmonton, Alberta: Alberta Learning Special Programs.

Clarren, S., Carmichael Olson, H., Clarren, S. and Astley, S. (2000). A child with fetal alcohol syndrome. In M. Guralnick (Ed.), *Interdisciplinary clinical assessment of young children with developmental disabilities*. Baltimore. MD.: Paul H. Brookes Co. ,307-326.

Coggins, T., Friet, T. and Morgan, T. (1998). Analyzing narrative productions in older school-age children and adolescents with fetal alcohol syndrome: An experimental tool for clinical applications. *Clinical Linguistics and Phonetics,* 12, 221-236.

Coggins, T., Olswang, L. Carmichael Olson, H. and Timler, G. (2003). On becoming socially competent communicators: The challenge for children with fetal alcohol exposure. *International Review of Research in Mental Retardation,* 27, 121-150.

Coles, C.D., Platzman, K.A., Raskind-Hood, C.L., Brown, R.T., Falek, A. and Smith, I.E. (1997). A comparison of children affected by prenatal alcohol exposure and attention deficit, hyperactivity disorder. *Alcoholism: Clinical and Experimental Research,* 21, 150-161.

Connor, P. and Streissguth, A. (1996). Effects of prenatal exposure to alcohol across the lifespan. *Alcohol Health and Research World ,* 20, 170-174.

Crick, N. and Dodge, K. (1994). A review and reformulation of social information-processing mechanisms in children's social adjustment. *Psychological Bulletin,* 11, 74-101.

Damico, J., Oller, J. and Tetnowski, J. (1999). Investigating the interobserver reliability of a direct observational language assessment technique. *Advances in Speech-Language Pathology,* 1, 77-94.

De Villiers, P., Roeper, T. and DeVilliers, J. (1999). What every 5-year-old should know: syntax, semantics, and pragmatics. American Speech-Language-Hearing Association Annual Convention, San Francisco, CA. November, 1999.

Dorris, M. (1989). *The broken cord.* New York, NY: Harper Perennial.

Gresham, F. (1998). Skills training with children: social learning and applied behavioral analytic approaches. In T. Watson and F. Gresham (Eds.), *Handbook of Child Behavior Therapy.* New York: Plenum Press.

Hinde, J. (1993). Early intervention for alcohol-affected children. In J. Kleinfeld, J. and S. Wescott (Eds.), *Fantastic Antone Succeeds! Experiences in education children with Fetal Alcohol Syndrome.* Anchorage, AK: University of Alaska Press.

Hodgdon, L. (1995). *Visual strategies for improving communication: Practical supports for school and home.* Troy: MI: Quirk Roberts Publishing.

Huffine, C. (1998). Sorting out adolescence and the effects of fetal alcohol exposure. *Iceberg* 8, 1-3.

Jones, K., Smith, D., Ulleland, C. and Streissguth, A. (1973). Pattern of malformation in offspring of chronic alcoholic mothers. *Lancet,* 1, 1267-1271

Kehle, T.J., Clark, E., and Jenson, W.R. (1996). Interventions for students with traumatic brain injury: Managing behavioral disturbances. *Journal of Learning Disabilities* 29, 633-642.

Koegel, L., Koegel, R. and Dunlap, G. (1996). Positive behavioral support. Baltimore, MD: Paul H. Brookes Publishing Co.

Kleinfeld, J. and Wescott, S. (1993). *Fantastic Antone Succeeds! Experiences in educating children with Fetal Alcohol Syndrome.* Anchorage, AK: University of Alaska Press.

Malbin, D. (1993). A poor fit: Treating FAS with non-FAS methods. *Iceberg ,* 7, 1-2.

Mateer, C., Kerns, K. and Eso, K. (1996). Management of attention and memory disorders following traumatic brain injury. *Journal of Learning Disabilities*, 29, 618-632.

Mattson, S.N., Goodman, A.M., Caine, C., Delis, D.C. and Riley, E.P. (1999). Executive functioning in children with heavy prenatal alcohol exposure. *Alcoholism: Clinical and Experimental Research, 23*, 1808-1815.

Mattson, S.N.and Riley, E.P. (1998). A review of the neurobehavioral deficits in children with fetal alcohol syndrome or prenatal exposure to alcohol. *Alcoholism: Clinical and Experimental Research, 22*, 279-294.

McFadyen-Ketchum, S. and Dodge, K. (1998). Problems in social relationships. In E. Mash, and R. Barkley (Eds.), *Treatment of childhood disorders*. New York: NY: Guilford Press.

Morse, B.A. and Weiner, L. (1996). Rehabilitation approaches for fetal alcohol syndrome. In H. Spohr and H. Steinhausen Eds.), *Alcohol, pregnancy and the developing child.* Cambridge, England: Cambridge University Press..

Oesterheld, J. and O'Malley, K. 1999: Are ADHD and FAS really that similar? *Iceberg, 9, 1-7.*

Olswang, L., Coggins, T., and Timler, G. (2001). Outcome measures for school-age children with social communication problems. *Topics in Language Disorders, 22*, 50-73.

O'Malley, K. and Hagerman, R. (1998). Developing Clinical Practice Guidelines for Pharmacological Interventions in Alcohol-Affected Children. In K. O'Malley and R. Hagerman (eds.), *Intervening with Children Affected by Prenatal Alcohol Exposure .* Monograph from the Interagency Coordinating Committee on Fetal Alcohol Syndrome Special Focus Session. Chevy Chase, MD: Centers for Disease Control and Prevention.

Pennington, B. and Ozonoff, S.(1996). Executive functions and developmental psychopathology. *Journal of Child Psychology and Psychiatry, 37*, 51-87.

Singer, B. and Bashir, A. (1999). What are executive functions and self-regulation and what do they have to do with language-learning disorders? *Language, Speech, and Hearing Services in Schools, 30*, 265-273.

Spohr, J-L., Willms, J. and Steinhausen, J-C. 1993: Prenatal alcohol exposure and long-term developmental consequences. *Lancet, 341*, 907-910.

Spohr, J, Willms, J. and Steinhausen, J. (1994). The fetal alcohol syndrome in adolescence. *Acta Paediatrica, 83*, 19-26.

Steinhausen, H., Willms, J. and Spohr, H. (1993). Long-term psychopathological and cognitive outcome of children with fetal alcohol syndrome. *Journal of the American Academy of Child and Adolescent Psychiatry, 32*, 990-994.

Strain, P., Kohler, F., Storey, K. and Danko, C. (1994). Teaching preschoolers with autism to self-monitor their social interactions: An analysis of results in home and school settings. *Journal of Emotional and Behavioral Disorders, 2*, 78-88.

Streissguth, A. (1997). *Fetal alcohol syndrome: A guide for families and communities.* Baltimore: Paul H. Brookes Publishing Co.

Streissguth, A., Barr, H., Kogan, J. and Bookstein, F. (1996). *Understanding the occurrence of secondary disabilities in clients with fetal alcohol syndrome (FAS) and fetal alcohol effects (FAE): Final report to the Centers for Disease Control and Prevention on Grant No. R04/CCR008515* (Tech. Report No. 96060). Seattle: University of Washington Fetal Alcohol and Drug Unit.

Streissguth, A., Barr, J., Kogan, J., and Bookstein, F. (1997). Primary and secondary disabilities in fetal alcohol syndrome. In A. Stressguth, and J., Kanter (Eds.), *The challenge of fetal alcohol syndrome: overcoming secondary disabilities* Seattle, WA: University of Washington Press, 25-39.

Stressguth, A. and Kanter, J. (1997). *The challenge of fetal alcohol syndrome: overcoming secondary disabilities.* Seattle, WA: University of Washington Press.

Swettenham, J., Baron-Cohen, S., Gomez, J-C. and Walsh, S. (1996) What's inside someone's head? Conceiving of the mind as a camera helps children with autism acquire an alternative to a theory of mind. *Cognitive Neuropsychiatry, 1,* 73-88.

Tannock, R. and Schachar, R.(1996). Executive dysfunction as an underlying mechanism of behavior and language problems in attention deficit hyperactivity disorder. In J. Bleitchman, N. Cohen, M. Konstantareas and R. Tannock, R. (Eds.), *Language, learning, and behavior disorders.* Cambridge, UK: Cambridge University Press.

Tannock, R., Purvis, K. and Schachar, R. (1993). Narrative abilities in children with Attention Deficit Hyperactivity Disorder and normal peers. *Journal of Abnormal Child Psychology, 21,* 103-117.

Tanner-Halverson, P. (1993). Snagging the kite string. In J. Kleinfeld and S. Wescott (Eds.), *Fantastic Antone Succeeds! Experiences in education children with Fetal Alcohol Syndrome.* Anchorage, AK: University of Alaska Press

Thorp, D., Stahmer, A. and Schreibman, L. (1995). Effects of sociodramatic play training on children with autism. *Journal of Autism and Developmental Disorders, 25,* 265-282.

Thorne, J., Coggins, T., Carmichael-Olson, H. and Astley, S. (accepted). Exploring the utility of narrative analysis in diagnostic decision-making: Elaboration, reference strategy, and fetal alcohol spectrum disorders. Re-submitted to *Journal of Speech-Language-Hearing Research,* March 2006.

Timler, G. (1997). Social problem solving and social communication skills in children with Fetal Alcohol Syndrome. Presentation of Trainee Leadership Projects, Center for Human Develop and Disabilities, University of Washington, June10, 1997

Timler, G. (2000). Investigation of social communication skills during peer conflict tasks in school-age children with alcohol-related disabilities. Unpublished doctoral dissertation. Seattle, Washington. University of Washington.

Timler, G., Olswang, L. and Coggins, T. (2005). "Do I know what I need to do?": A social communication intervention for children with complex clinical profiles. *Language, Speech, and Hearing Services in Schools, 36,* 73-84.

Thomas, S., Kelly, S., Mattson, S. and Riley, E. (1998). Comparison of social abilities of children with fetal alcohol syndrome to those of children with similar IQ scores and normal controls. *Alcoholism: Clinical and Experimental Research, 22,* 528-533.

Warren, S. and Kaiser, A. (1986). Incidental language teaching: a critical review. *Journal of Speech and Hearing Disorders, 51,* 291-299.

Weismer, S. and Murray-Branch, J. (1989). Modeling versus modeling plus evoked production training: A comparison of two language intervention methods. *Journal of Speech and Hearing Disorders, 54,* 269-281.

Wright, R. (1992). One step forward: Using information about FAE to help my son. *Iceberg, 1,* 3-4.

In: ADHD and Fetal Alcohol Spectrum Disorders (FASD)   ISBN: 1-59454-573-1
Editor: Kieran D. O'Malley, pp. 179-198   © 2008 Nova Science Publishers, Inc.

Chapter 10

FASD AND ADHD: THE NUTS AND BOLTS OF DIAGNOSIS AND TREATMENT IN THE REAL WORLD

Phil Mattheis[*]

INTRODUCTION

The preceding sections of this book have discussed the combination of ADHD with FASD from a variety of perspectives. This chapter describes a clinical model used to provide diagnosis and treatment for a population at high risk for Fetal Alcohol Spectrum Disorders in Alaska, where logistic problems of distance, isolation, and scarce resources compound the already complicated process.

ADHD defines a symptom complex with high comorbidity of cognitive, behavioral, neurologic, and environmental problems (Furman 2005). Within the population given this diagnosis, there is a subset with no other symptoms beyond the hyperactivity, impulsivity and distractibility of the accepted criteria (often with a strong familial component). The majority with ADHD, however, present with additional problems of cognition, behavior, neurologic function, or medical conditions, as well as a variety of issues related to environmental complications. In this latter group, treatment efficacy often is driven by identification of those comorbid features, and successful outcomes often depend on very broadbased supports in school, home and community (Klassen, Miller and Fine 2004)

Fetal exposure to alcohol (and other teratogens and neurotoxins) disrupts normal development of the brain and other neurologic structures, with a wide variety of consequences. O'Malley and Nanson (2002) discuss ADHD in patients with FASD compared to the non-exposed population, and describe clinical features that differ in timing and inattentive subtype, as well as the high frequency of comorbidity. These clinical distinctions certainly impact treatment planning and efficacy, further complicated by brain injury mediated unpredictable responses to medication.

---

[*] Phil Matheis, Alaska Psychiatrc Institute, Anchorage, Alaska, U.S.A.

Regardless of the degree of brain injury due to fetal toxin exposure, the surviving individual is then (far too often) born into a world of trouble, adding further chaotic insult to the prenatal injury. Early neglect (with or without abuse) can result in the 'miss-programming' of Reactive Attachment Disorder (RAD). For many, RAD presents as social and interpersonal dysfunction on a physiologic basis that is as permanent and varied as that caused by prenatal toxins. As Perry (2006) states with blunt simplicity: "Chaos, threat, traumatic stress, abuse, and neglect are bad for children." Precortical associations are formed in early childhood - and can be permanent - while remaining beyond conscious awareness. Meanwhile the abnormal stressors of chaotic or abusive parenting may drive development of reactive behavioral and physiologic pathways that are intrinsically dysfunctional in a world of more normal nurturance and personal interaction.

Neglect, abuse and other emotional traumas that occur later in childhood frequently result in long term Post-Traumatic Stress Disorder (PTSD). PTSD can be overlooked in the presence of more obvious problems, or missed entirely in the short term due to the child's capacity to dissociate and 'lose' memories of the events. Models of therapy to address RAD and PTSD in children are gaining sophistication and wider availability. Perry and others have written extensively with evolving recognition of the implications of these changes - the cited article (Perry 2006) provides a current summary of understanding of developmental differences driven by trauma in childhood. Effective treatment may require a rethinking of the child's world of experiences, and include intensive and consistent interventions that attempt to reset the inappropriate programming and reactivity that intrudes on normal relationships and social function.

Among comorbid conditions in ADHD, specific learning deficits are common, and may be obvious early on in the child's school career. However, cognitive effects of 'milder' brain injury in FASD (or by any cause) may also be subtle; and hidden behind more dramatic behaviors. Language delays are common in children exposed to fetal alcohol, and may include a persistent mixed expressive-receptive language disorder that can be missed due to superficial expressive language output that masks comprehension deficits (Kapp, O'Malley 2001, Coggins etal 1998). Higher levels of cognition can be impacted in isolation, with consequences for learning, judgment, and peer interactions not apparent until academic and social challenges become more sophisticated later in childhood or adolescence. , An unfortunately common consequence of this mixed cognitive function/dysfunction can combine an intact capacity for rote memorization of the rules and expectations that govern appropriate behavior, with an executive-function deficit in deductive reasoning that severely restricts the capacity to act on that apparent knowledge of cause and effect relations (O'Malley 2002). This combination is often labeled as 'antisocial personality disorder' or 'criminalized' behavior, with low or no expectation of change via rehabilitation.

Finally, the effects of prior treatment can add additional baggage to the diagnostic process. This can include childhoods disrupted by 'abuse by system' through multiple foster placements (sometimes with additional real abuse/neglect). Family ties and identity may be disrupted or destroyed, with loss of the potential support of extended family networks. Missed diagnosis of brain injury, complicated by the adverse effects of polypharmacy targeting multiple Axis I diagnoses is extremely common in Alaska, and presents a mess of diagnostic, medical, and mental health complications beyond the scope of this chapter. Other defining characters of clinical treatment of ADHD/FASD in Alaska include scarce and poorly distributed community mental health, medical, and educational resources, combined with the problems of weather, distance, and limited access by road system that impact travel and service delivery.

ALCOHOL IN ALASKA

Alcohol use and abuse has played a prominent historic role in the lifestyle and culture of nonnative migration in the western US; this is especially true in the settlement of Alaska. In an annotated bibliography, Thayne Anderson cites numerous historic examples and further sources (Anderson, 1988). Immigration patterns to the region have historically included a heavy proportion of individuals loosely tied to their previous homes and families, who were free to travel the tremendous distances necessary. Alcoholic beverages have long history as portable, high-value trade goods; alcohol use has also dominated social settings and activities through much of the state's recent history. Native populations have been overwhelmed by the effects of alcohol abuse since first contact with Russian fur traders 300 years ago. Generations of alcohol abuse in Alaska by natives and non-natives have decimated many rural and remote communities, and contributed to endemic levels of FASD across the state and region (refs of prevalence studies).

HISTORY OF DIAGNOSTIC CLASSIFICATION

Fetal Alcohol Spectrum Disorder (FASD) is the current term used to refer to that range of conditions expressed by individuals affected by fetal exposure to alcohol. There are no 'gold standards' of clinical findings or test results to confirm or rule out the diagnosis. This umbrella term covers the range of conditions comprising the Institute of Medicine classification scheme (Stratton 1996), including Fetal Alcohol Syndrome (FAS), partial FAS, FAS without confirmed fetal exposure, and Alcohol Related Birth Defects (ARBD).

Hoyme, etal (2005) recently produced clarification of the 1996 Institute of Medicine criteria (that publication has been made broadly available by the National Institute of Health). The original criteria suffered from vague parameters to the diagnostic categories, and lacked guidelines for "the complex pattern of behavioral or cognitive difficulties". Several of the categories (ARBD and ARND) were comprised of individuals with less obvious involvement, but the categorical definitions did not allow easy clinical application.

The term 'ARBD' has been used in the presence of one or more congenital physiologic defects known to be increased during fetal exposure to alcohol, when that exposure has been confirmed. Typically this term was limited to those with medical complications associated with fetal alcohol exposure, but without apparent functional brain deficits. All other conditions under the FASD umbrella include brain deficits as part of the symptom complex. FAS is the most completely defined, with significant differences in each physiologic parameter combined with certainty of fetal exposure to alcohol. Clinical criteria for these conditions address evidence of fetal exposure and indications of brain injury, as well as growth measurements and facial characteristics. However, the boundaries of each of these parameters remained vaguely defined, particularly for ARBD and ARND.

Astley and Claren (2000) at the University of Washington promoted a diagnostic protocol centered on descriptions of dysmorphology to define conditions with the continuum of FASD.

Their model results in a 4-digit coding that reflects growth parameters, facial characteristics, brain effects, and fetal exposure to alcohol. For each characteristic, a score of 1 through 4 is assigned, indicating 'normal' or 'no exposure' as '1', and 'unknown' or 'untested' as '2'. '3' and '4' rankings reflect lower and higher departure from the norm or significant fetal exposure. The codes that are generated are connected to clinical diagnoses such as "Fetal Alcohol Syndrome" at '4444'. When growth or face characteristics do not support a diagnosis of the complete syndrome, the term "neurobehavioral disorder" is applied for a 'brain' ranking of '3', while "static encephalopathy" is assigned when the 'brain' rank is '4'.

While facial characteristics may be helpful in confirming an impression of FASD, a face rank of '4' does not in itself diagnose FASD, and a rank of '1' does not exclude one of those conditions. Similarly, growth data indicating differences significantly below the norm can support a diagnosis of FAS if the other criteria are met, but in isolation are of limited clinical value.

The dysmorphology categories in the UW protocol do not address specific presenting problems, and offer limited clinical utility to assist the design of therapy or long term management. "Neurobehavioral Disorder" can be distinguished from "Static Encephalopathy" as a matter of degree of brain deficits, but the distinction does not direct clinical decision making.

As Hoyme etal. point out (2005), both Institute of Medicine and UW diagnostic protocols suffer from ambiguities in clinical application, especially regarding identification of FASD in those with evidence of brain injury, but without physical findings supporting an FASD diagnosis. The protocol described by Hoyme etal attempts to minimize false positive identification by directly exploring potential genetic and/or environmental influences that could explain the observed symptoms. They also discuss the categories of FAS and partial FAS 'without confirmed maternal alcohol exposure', which can be very useful in cases where pathology is clear but historic details lacking.

STATE MENTAL HEALTH SERVICES

Mental health resources in Alaska are disproportionately distributed, with the majority restricted to urban and suburban settings. Regional mental health systems have been developed across the state, but have frequently depended on urban centers for evaluation and treatment plans. Like most of the US, these systems have not differentiated FASD or other causes of brain injury as important issues in mental health pathology. Problems are characterized as Axis 1 diagnostic conditions in the 5-axis model of the DSM IV, and are assigned specific therapy targeting the condition, often without regard to underlying or related medical etiology.

Recent policy changes at Alaska's Behavioral Health Division have attempted to influence this clinical reality. Substance abuse and mental health agencies and programs are now required to screen new and existing clients for history of brain injury (including FASD), and treatment planning must reflect this new information. As a consequence, many providers around Alaska are gaining awareness of the high incidence and prevalence of this group within the larger mental health and substance abuse client populations. Understanding of the need to adjust treatment strategies is growing, but at a slower pace, and with limited state resources ready to provide those alternatives.

FASD CLINICAL RESOURCES

Fetal Alcohol Spectrum Disorders have been gaining attention and resources in Alaska, especially over the past 5 years, via state distributed federal funds in several programs. Most of the effort has focused on increasing diagnostic capacity, using the University of Washington diagnostic "4-digit coding" model. Presenting problems and other historic detail are secondary issues in this diagnosis-centered approach, with treatment deferred via referral to appropriate resources.

Local communities in Alaska have been supported by state funding to develop FASD diagnostic teams. Local teams from across the state have been trained in the UW diagnostic model. The operations of these teams have varied, depending upon the continued involvement of the team members and availability of support funding.

A few of the participating communities have active diagnostic teams with regular clinics; the population seen is usually limited to those with a certainty of fetal exposure to alcohol. Assignment of a 4-digit FASD code with related diagnostic condition defines the clinic product. Most of the community teams have held few or no clinic evaluations, focusing instead on improving local perceptions and resources. The primary impact of this clinical effort has been to dramatically increase awareness of FASD as a reality in Alaska, followed by growing recognition of the need for effective prevention, as well as the need for treatment of those who have the condition.

ALASKA'S TELE-BEHAVIORAL HEALTH (TBH) PROJECT

The Alaska Psychiatric Institute (API) is located in Alaska's largest city of Anchorage, and serves as the state's inpatient treatment facility for residents with severe mental health problems. The TBH project was conceived as a model of mental health service delivery to remote locations around the state, using videoconference technology to support telemedicine clinics. A growing number of sites in Alaska have gained connection to the system, with variable levels of use of the clinical resources.

Professional services available via this program include Developmental/Behavioral Pediatrics, Child and Adolescent Psychiatry, Psychology (clinical testing and support of local treatment), as well as support of local social work, case management resources, and billing procedures.

While telemedicine is a central component of the project, the diagnostic process always includes direct, onsite examination by the pediatrician, at some point prior to determination assignment of final diagnosis. Initial contacts are often by videoconference to triage the cases and discuss available information, which helps to guide referrals for needed assessments. Contact via telemedicine also is well suited to clinical management of identified problems, such as assistance with medical management, ongoing review of treatment plans, participation in IEP or case conference meetings, etc.

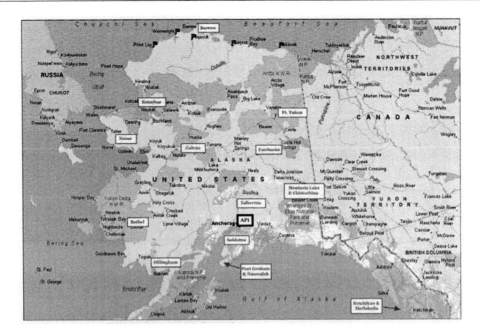

Figure 1. Alaska TBH clinic sites in operation or planning.

When an FASD condition is suspected, the diagnostic procedures used is a combination of IOM and UW models. One site (Soldotna) includes an active state-sponsored FASD diagnostic team; reported diagnostic results include a 4-digit code. However, the narrative diagnoses and overall diagnostic protocol used in this and the remaining sites is an adaptation of the revised Institute of Medicine criteria described by Hoyme etal. Problem solving and long term management are defining elements of the clinical interactions, with design and ongoing facilitation of an adaptive and adjusting treatment plan as the goal of each contact.

CLINICAL ASSESSMENT

Clinical contact begins with a referral to the local clinic site, from a variety of sources. Many of our clients have spent their lives within their biologic family in the local community, and an extended family member may initiate the request for help with a specific problem. Others may be in the foster system, with the request for evaluation coming from a child protection provider to help support the placement. Schools initiate some contacts, while others come to us with history of corrections placement, or with other legal complications. A significant and growing number of referrals is made up of adults with long histories of functional problems, who are hoping for better definition of and explanations for their troubles.

Assessment Protocol:

1. Definition of presenting problems
2. Inventory of available information
   a. Medical records and other data about pregnancy, delivery, infancy, etc
   b. School performance information

      c. Child Protection Service records

      d. Psychiatric and other mental health service records

      e. Psychologic test results

3. Clinical interview and examination by physician

4. Assessment by other related disciplines (OT, PT, SLP, psychology), as indicated

5. Assignment of diagnoses

6. Treatment Plan design and adjustment

The list above is not a sequential ranking, since the severity of presenting problems often dictates beginning treatment prior to resolution of diagnoses, especially when FASD or related conditions are being considered. For children of school age, ADHD is a very common presenting problem prompting the referral (often including an extended period of unsuccessful treatment).

Definition of the presenting problems is an essential first step, and assists in assigning clinical priority. An imminent change of placement takes precedence over a more chronic learning problem; screening for potential issues in a young child with history of fetal exposure to alcohol is often the lowest priority. Clarification of the source of the referral is also essential. Not only does this information determine the recipients of the clinic report, it also helps to determine the community resources which may be available to assist with the treatment planning. The need for releases of information is also directed by the referral source, and at times may slow the process as appropriate signatures are sought.

The presenting problems of our clinical population reflect their complicated lives, as discussed above. Comorbidity is the rule, and problems usually cross several domains of setting and discipline. ADHD may be the named concern on a referral from a teacher, parent, or daycare setting, but in most cases the diagnosis and treatment includes other elements. Child protection services constitute the largest referral source for these clinics. While ADHD is often on the list of presenting concerns for patients referred by this route, the need for child protection service intervention is an absolute marker for family disfunction and emotional trauma. Assessment for RAD, PTSD, other anxiety disorders, and other mental health conditions is often an essential component in such cases.

Decisions about the timing and setting of the first clinical contact with the client are often dictated by the severity of the presenting problem. Depending upon access and logistics, this may be via videoconference or in person. In that visit, the child is seen with one or more care providers who can describe the circumstances prompting the referral. Presumptive diagnoses may be assigned, and an initial treatment plan designed and put into action. The treatment plan often includes referral for additional assessment as indicated (OT, Speech/Language, psychologic testing,...). A return visit would be scheduled to evaluate responses to the initial therapy, and to allow review and discussion of any new information. Often, diagnoses can be assigned at this point, with adjustments to the treatment plan as necessary.

In other cases where the presenting problems are less emergent, the initial client-physician contact may be postponed until all necessary information is gathered. If diagnosis of FASD is a primary goal of the consultation, additional assessment by other professionals may be scheduled prospectively, so that reports and test results can be reviewed at the time of the physical exam and interview.

For cases of possible FASD and related conditions, a completed diagnosis often depends upon the accuracy of information available about the pregnancy. Both the intake paperwork and the clinic interview can address the question of alcohol exposure, but the respondents may not have first hand knowledge. It may be necessary to explore alternate routes to the information. Child protection service records and other law enforcement may include episodes that occurred during the pregnancy. Members of the extended family or the local community may be willing to provide information, especially if the potential for helping the client is emphasized. Medical records of the pregnancy and early infancy may include clues, but often access to the maternal chart is restricted by lack of release.

When a biologic parent is available, how the question is asked may impact the answer received. Most women will respond in the negative when asked if they drank during pregnancy, in spite of a history of early drinking. We have found better success by asking how far along the pregnancy was when the woman became aware of her new status. Next comes questions about the need for medical treatment or special testing, etc, during prenatal medical care. Then we ask if she smoked cigarettes in the pregnancy, used medications or street drugs, or drank alcohol. Regardless of the answer, we ask if she smoked or drank in that period of time before she became aware of the pregnancy. Very often, there is a pause, a reconsideration, and a change in response. It is essential to minimize stigma and to avoid any sense of blame in the clinical interviews and exam. Again, an emphasis on problem solving, linked with improving access to support services and therapies helps to keep attention on the child, and away from blame for caretakers.

Family history may reveal other individuals with learning or behavior problems, in a familial pattern such as uncomplicated ADHD, dyslexia, or an autistic spectrum disorder. Review may also reveal mental health pathology in the extended family, with disrupted parenting and individuals affected by an array of mental health diagnoses. The context of chronic substance abuse in individuals, or generational abuse within families may further complicate the interpretation of this information. Since FASD is a recent diagnostic construct, it was seldom mentioned or considered much beyond the past 15-20 years. Brain injury by any cause, including FASD and head trauma, has recently gained clinical recognition and new appreciation of the significance, which may justify a reassessment of diagnoses and treatment plans of affected individuals. Bipolar disorder is a good example of a diagnosis very frequently assigned to brain injured individuals with extreme emotional reactivity, often without supportive family history, and without attention to significance of that underlying etiology.

Review of family history may also provide suggestions of FASD in parents, grandparents and others, which could certainly affect the need for services, as well as direct some discussion toward the competence of affected caretakers. Parents with FASD may have exposed and/or unexposed children; their ability to provide appropriate childcare may be a significant factor in the child's presenting problems. Careful consideration of sources needs to accompany review of family history. The information may often be third party hearsay, presented without supporting detail. Mental health diagnoses are particularly problematic, given the high frequency of missed diagnoses regarding FASD, RAD, PTSD, etc. Bipolar disorder is an extremely common diagnosis assigned to children in Alaska, in numbers far beyond the low incidence described in diagnostic series elsewhere. Many of those diagnosed with bipolar disorder have histories including fetal exposure to neurotoxins as well as other causes of brain injury which may not have been appreciated. Similarly, diagnosis of ADHD is a very common historical detail in both family and personal histories, but often details to support the accuracy of the diagnoses is not available.

In our clinical experience, evaluation of an affected child often leads to review of siblings; assessment of one or more parents may follow (especially the mother, since she is most likely to be the children's care provider). Long term management of children with FASD may include treatment and support for an affected custodial parent(s) as a primary focus.

Imaging studies of the brain, particularly by MRI, have been used to support diagnosis of FASD, and abnormalities (particularly of midline structures) have been described (Swayze et al 1997), but clinical use is limited by expense and risk of sedation, as well as logistical issues of access to the technology. Several MRI studies have linked corpus callosum differences in FASD to neuropsychology deficits, but the clinical utility has not been established (Streissguth et al. 2002, Sowell et al 2001). Functional imaging studies by MRI and other modalities remain research tools at this time, although clinical availability is approaching quickly. As these techniques become more available, the balance of risk to benefit should be reevaluated, especially if the results can help to direct therapy. At this time, we do not routinely use imaging in our clinical protocols.

Onsite Clinical Assessment

The physical examination is often dominated by observation of the client during the interview of accompanying providers. When the client is a young child, their interactions with both familiar and new contacts often provide helpful information about their ability to communicate and form relationships with others, as well as their ability to explore the environment, process information and to solve problems. Interactions with the parent/provider may reveal problematic discipline or dysfunctional patterns of interaction. Attention to developmental milestones is always important with younger clients, especially in relation to reported concerns of providers.

Measurements of height, weight and head circumference are taken at each exam, and may support diagnosis of growth delay or microcephaly. Some children, especially those with histories of abuse, neglect, or multiple complicated changes in placements, are extremely resistant to close or extended physical contact by an unknown adult. Measurement of head circumference often supersede the limits of such a child. Placement of a small plastic ruler next to the eyes for measurement of palpebral openings can be far too intrusive and effectively destroy earlier rapport. The relative value of dysmorphology should be weighed carefully in such cases. When a resistant child has a complicated family history, PTSD or RAD may be suggested by their behavior. Sensory integration problems should also be considered, with referral for further assessment when appropriate.

Digital photographic imaging can be an invaluable tool in these evaluations. Young children who are resistant to contact may warm to the examiner when shown a picture of themselves or a parent on the camera. Most become closely engaged in the process, and are excited to view the pictures. Sequential images, taken over a series of clinical visits, can also be helpful, often by reminding the child of a past pleasant contact and reestablishing rapport. Discussion of the images is often an easy way to generate language and communication samples to aid assessment. A child who is unwilling to allow close physical examination often will tolerate photography, which may permit assessment and recording of facial stigmata supportive of FASD.

"Clumsiness" or frequent accidents while running or handling objects can be common presenting concerns in young children with FASD, especially those with attention problems. It can be important to distinguish easy distractibility and risk-taking behavior from more physiologic causes such as poor motor coordination or central nervous system deficits or delays.

A variety of neurologic abnormalities may be found in the population of individuals with FASD. Findings suggestive of cerebral palsy may be present in infants and young children; milder symptoms often fade as childhood progresses. Hyper reflexia or minimal asymmetry may be detected in a child with delayed motor milestone achievement or discoordination. Early or late emergence of laterality, or mixed dominance may be soft signs of neuromuscular difference. Assessment by a occupational or physical therapist skilled at assessment of children with neuromuscular differences may be helpful, especially if accompanied by recommendations for effective therapy.

DIAGNOSTIC ASSIGNMENTS AND CHARACTERIZATIONS

One 'product' of this clinic process is the diagnostic statement. Our diagnostic assignments for individuals with FASD conditions use Institute of Medicine categories as a starting point, but with the emphasis on presenting problems rather than on etiology. Evidence for brain injury is the key clinical component; confirmation of fetal alcohol exposure supports an FASD determination. Typically, the diagnostic statement for a clinic evaluation would include "FASD" to support and explain a diagnosis of brain injury, qualified by clinical descriptors that define the related problems (e.g., "Static encephalopathy related to a Fetal Alcohol Spectrum Disorder, with severe deficits in language-based learning, attention, and social judgment"). Other diagnoses are given appropriate weight when present, including environmentally derived mental health conditions such as Post Traumatic Stress Disorder or Reactive Attachment Disorder. When mental health problems derive from that brain injury of FASD, a diagnosis is used to reflect that origin (e.g., Mood Disorder secondary to brain injury caused by FASD).

The relevant Institute of Medicine categories are often not added to the narrative statement, in the interest of clarity for the patient, family, and others. While many or most patients belong to Partial FAS and ARND groups, use of the terms in clinic would often be unnecessarily confusing.

Many patients seen in this clinic fit criteria for ADHD, but seldom as an isolated problem. As mentioned above, RAD and PTSD are very common comorbidities in populations at risk for FASD. The TBH clinic provides access to resources experienced at identification and treatment of these conditions. Often a primary contribution of the clinic assessment is to bring focus to the primary role these conditions may be playing in the life of the patient. This re-casting of the diagnosis may involve significant changes in treatment, especially regarding medication regimens. Polypharmacy is a very frequent component of pre-clinic treatment models for our presenting patients, often with significant adverse effects to daily function. These affects may include sleep disorders, medical problems (e.g., tardive dyskinesia, thyroid disfunction), exacerbation of cognitive deficits, and disruptions of attention. Not infrequently, the outcome of clinic for such patients is the reduction of the existing drug regimen to monotherapy or no medications at all, while emphasizing environmental accommodations and community support.

In each case, the organizing focus of the evaluation is on defining the presenting clinical problem and providing recommendations for therapy. If the problem is related to a chronic condition such as brain injury with permanent sequelae, development of a long term management plan will be emphasized. Follow up clinical visits will always be offered to assist with adjustments to the plan for the existing problems, and to allow assessment of new issues that will emerge later in life. The initial clinic evaluation is often followed by a shift in emphasis to the permanence of the underlying condition as an explanation for recurrent acute episodes of behavior or functional problems. Changing the perceptions of care providers and family members may be the most effective intervention in gaining real control of the problem at hand.

Case Example

Multiple siblings commonly present together in a clinic setting. One of the group may have a more immediate problem prompting the referral, but often there are additional issues of concern for each of the other family members. Keeping the details straight for the individuals within the family can be a challenge, since environment and genetic variables are often similar, but not identical for the group. The individuals discussed here are composites derived from our clinical experience. The pattern of history and descriptive information does not represent actual clients or a specific family, although most of the details are drawn from real situations.

A family of 4 siblings presented in late September with their primary caretaker, a maternal aunt who is also adoptive mother to the two oldest children. The younger two have recently joined their older siblings after removal from the home of their common biologic mother and her partner (father of the youngest child). Concerns about school function for several of the children were raised by teachers, and added to family concerns about the others to prompt this visit. A statement of the clinical question by their aunt was "We know their mother drank. Do they have FASD, and how can we help them in school?"

(Time constraints, clinic logistics, and realities of family child care in such cases usually result in a combined examination of the family as a group. Family history gathering is non repetitive and more efficient, although it can be difficult to keep the details straight where they differ. Physical examination benefits from observation of the children as they interact with each other and their care providers.)

The children include: Alexi at 14 years, Martin at 11 years, Henry at 8 years, and Karen at 4 years of age. When Alexi was born, their mother was 16 years old and living with her parents. She remained in that home through the birth and infancy of Martin, with maternal grandmother providing most of the childcare. Near the end of her third pregnancy with Henry, the father of the children was killed in a car accident. She quickly became involved with another man, and substance abuse by both escalated. She used alcohol in each of her pregnancies, but tended to decrease her use as the gestation proceeded. Prior to Henry's birth, she and her partner left the community for Anchorage, but the older children remained with their grandmother, who shared their care with a maternal aunt. Eventually, the aunt and her husband adopted Alexi and Martin.

Alcohol use in the fourth pregnancy continued through the full term, in a recurrent bingeing pattern. Child protective workers became involved with the family shortly after that birth due to concerns about neglect of basic child care. Henry and Karen were removed on several occasion due to neglect, and placed in a sequence of foster homes alternating with returns to their mother's care. In the last year prior to this clinic visit, they accompanied their mother to a residential treatment program for substance abuse that allowed children to accompany their mother into the treatment setting. Her partner did not participate in treatment, but lived nearby. He occasionally provided care for Henry, and continued to actively use alcohol in his lifestyle. On discharge from the treatment program, the children's mother rejoined her partner, and quickly returned to her previous pattern of heavy alcohol use and neglect of her children's care. With this latest removal, the child protection service workers indicated their intention to seek termination of parental rights. The tribe of enrollment indicated interest in becoming involved, and the maternal aunt's petition for custody was granted, with the children joining their siblings in that family's home during late August just as school started.

Maternal family history includes extensive substance abuse by multiple family members, including the maternal grandmother during several of her own pregnancies. The biologic mother was her last child, with the highest fetal exposure to alcohol. Her childhood and school history was marked by high activity and short attention span, with many episodes indicating poor judgment or risk taking behavior. She received special education support through her school years, but details are not available, since most school files were not kept long after graduation. While she did graduate from high school, she has retained limited functional reading skills. She is unable to manage money on her own, and has no effective job skills. Several older siblings share fetal alcohol exposure and similar stories of developmental and academic problems. The grandmother denied use of alcohol in her first pregnancies, and those oldest children (including the adopting aunt) had more normal childhood and school histories. No other individuals in the extended family were reported to have histories of learning problems, although others were noted to have had problems related to substance abuse. There is also no clear history of mental health problems distinct from the pattern of chronic substance abuse.

The father of the older three children had a similar pattern to that of the mother, including the extended family pattern of substance abuse. Again (to the degree history was available), chronic substance abuse was common. Learning, behavior, and school problems were described for those with drinking mothers, but not in other individuals. Multiple partners in a sequence of frequent family disruption was also common. While he also had a pattern of chronic alcohol abuse, he was able to maintain extended periods of sobriety. During those periods, he was a positive influence for the mother and their children, and contributed to their care.

Pregnancies for the older children were uncomplicated except for certainty of alcohol exposure, as witnessed by the maternal aunt and confirmed by medical and legal records. Deliveries were normal, and developmental milestones were met in the normal range, although Martin's language skills always lagged behind his sister's earlier pattern. He also was viewed as "clumsy", and could not ride a bicycle independently until the age of 8 years. He is right handed, but that preference did not clearly establish until the age of 5, after a long period of ambidexterity of relatively poor coordination. His athletic abilities are below the norm, and he shows some mixed dominance (preferring to kick balls with his left foot and using knives with his left hand).

Both children began school without major difficulties or differences from their peers. Their academic performance has been in the low to middle range. There have been no concerns regarding behavior problems for either child. Both have been well behaved in the home, and have engaged willingly in the family's very consistent daily routine of chores and activities. That routine includes regular, repetitive reminders from the parents so ingrained in their family patterns that they have become invisible to the participants. School teachers have reported a similar level of compliance in the children, but which has required a similar level of structure and regular verbal reminders, assisted by visual cues of charts and observed peer behavior.

The father of the fourth child comes into the story with the death of the other man, and during an extended drinking binge begun by the (pregnant) mother during the funeral ceremonies. His own pattern of alcohol use was a more persistent daily use that enabled her to continue her binge behavior on a nearly continuous basis. Allegations of domestic violence toward the mother have been made, but never substantiated. No information is available regarding his childhood, school history, or extended family.

The third child, Henry, was born several weeks premature, with growth delays and facial features that supported a diagnosis of Fetal Alcohol Syndrome. Developmental motor milestones were normal or advanced, and he was described as "a very active child." His fine and gross motor function was not impaired, and coordination was normal to advanced. However, he has had a low threshold for distraction, and prominent impulsivity that has at times resulted in injury through shifts in attention, sudden changes in direction, etc. Athletic skills have typically been advanced compared to same age peers. Speech production was delayed, and marked by persistent disarticulation and slow emergence of word combinations and complex concepts. He often has required frequent reminders to stay on task, but without suggestion that opposition contributed to his lack of compliance. His behavior toward peers at times has been aggressive in the past, but this behavior has not been observed in the current setting. He has remained small for age, with persistence of facial features suggestive of FAS.

The fourth pregnancy was marked by the heaviest maternal alcohol use and the addition of frequent street drug use (cocaine and methamphetamine), which continued through to the full term uncomplicated delivery. Infancy and early childhood were complicated primarily by the recurrent allegations of neglect and possible domestic violence, disruptions of placement. Developmental milestones were met on a normal to advanced schedule.

This year, teachers for both older children have expressed concerns about their ability to meet expectations. Alexi has been having trouble keeping up with science and math activities. Martin, the 11 year old, has moved to a larger and more urban middle school setting from a village elementary school. In the smaller setting, he was one of the higher functioning children among a group with high incidence of developmental problems (most related to FASD). Teachers in the current school have noted problems with both behavior and attention, and have expressed concern about his cognitive capacity to do grade level work.

Meanwhile, the third child, Henry, joined a mixed 2nd and 3rd grade classroom, where he rapidly became the most challenging student in that group. His attention span was short and easily distracted, and his reading ability (in 3rd grade placement) lagged at late first grade levels. The classroom teacher and special education support teacher both raised questions about possible ADHD, which prompted this referral. The additional concerns about the older children resulted in a full review of the entire family, with the youngest (Karen) included due to her high level of fetal exposure to alcohol and the related worries about possible later problems.

Physical examination of the group was largely normal. Henry continues to be small in stature and weight for age (about 7th percentile, with a proportional head circumference (10%). Growth parameters for the others were within normal limits. Palpebral fissures for Henry were more than 2 standard deviations below the norm, while Martin's eye openings were between one and two SD below the mean; measurements for Alexi and Karen with within one standard deviation of the mean. Likert scale assessment of philtrum/upper lips for the group were 2/2 for the oldest and youngest, with scores for Martin at 4/3, and 5/4 for Henry. Using UW criteria, these latter scores are consistent with early fetal alcohol exposure. Overall, Henry's physical presentation is consistent with the full Fetal Alcohol Syndrome. Martin's fine motor coordination was not stuttering, with an intention tremor that emerged with challenge and was worse on the right. He preferred his right hand, but writing skills are poorly developed. Speech production was limited in the older children, who preferred to let their adoptive mother speak for them. They often waited for her to respond to questions directed at them, and at times required repetition to answer. The remainder of the exams were normal.

Clinical observations of social interactions with family and others showed Henry to have the most problems in this brief controlled encounter. He needed frequent reminders to return to task, and tended to push limits at every opportunity. He remained in good humor, and easily complied when reminded or redirected. His language was less mature for age than for his siblings, with frequent fragmented sentence structure and occasional garbled speech that was difficult to interpret. Karen appeared to play a role of favor as the youngest in the group, expecting and receiving special treatment and extra consideration in her own exploration of those social limits. She seemed to be very sensitive to the tolerance levels of each of her siblings, but was able to play to that edge without quite offending. The older two contributed to the interview and exam somewhat independent of their younger siblings, but did at times fall into rolls as older sibling/ part time providers in manners that suggested healthy adjustment.

Psychologic assessment of IQ and academic achievement was done for each of the three older children, and included Vineland Adaptive Behavior Scales for Alexi and Martin. Connor's behavior scoring was done for Henry at first contact, and repeated after 3 months, prior to a return clinic visit. Karen was included in clinic due to her known high level of fetal exposure; however, her normal level of function in multiple settings made psychologic testing for her a low priority. Local speech/language assessment resources were relatively unavailable, and again a low apparent priority.

Alexi's IQ scores were: full scale 81, verbal 75 and performance 89. Word recognition and reading comprehension were delayed by one grade level on oral reading, but dropped to a two grade deficit on silent reading. Remedial reading support was encouraged, with oral input for academic information (books on tape and oral reading support), as well as alternative oral testing with extended time in a low distraction environment. Vineland Adaptive scores were lower than expected in each area, consistent with a passive young lady with adequate superficial verbal skills, but limited depth to communication capacity, who may often find herself in situations beyond her capacity. Daily living performance also lagged, supporting need for regular structured supervision to attain a semi-independent lifestyle. Her low scores on interpersonal relationships, combined with her attractive appearance and a passive personality that is easily overwhelmed by stress, suggest an individual at high risk of victimization. The school counselor was encouraged to develop a curriculum of "Sexuality and appropriate touching" for presentation to Alexi and her classmates.

Martin's Full Scale IQ was 86, with a verbal/performance split of 15 points. In 7th grade, his academic achievement scored in high 3rd to low 4th grade. On the Vineland, communication lagged by a year, social skills by 2 years, and daily living skills by three years. Attention varied by the context, with academically challenging situations making for high distractibility. In social settings of active play he was well controlled, but his capacity to interact successfully dropped off rapidly as verbal skills came into play. His social success was highest among preferred younger playmates. Accommodations to the curriculum and classroom that minimize distractions while providing alternative sources of information (oral reading and more demonstration, with the assistance of peer tutors) has resulted in improved attention and reduced distractibility.

Henry had a full scale IQ of 81, with verbal scoring at 70 and performance at 89. Distractibility was significant, and easily elicited, especially as the cognitive challenge increased. His overall activity level was high. A behavior scale ranking for home showed moderately high activity and easy distractibility, but not to the point of significance. School ranking on the same scale at the beginning of the year was highly significant for activity, distractibility and impulsivity. After 4 months in the stability of the new placement, the parental behavior ranking had moderated slightly, but initial scoring from school showed no change. Discussion with the teacher, with the suggestion that she consider only the past week's performance resulted in considerable gains in moderation, and she acknowledged that her first effort had included memories of earlier behavior. His reading ability was at early second grade level at the start of the 3rd grade school year, and had shown no progress in that first month. Since then, after 3 months of close attention and support by the classroom and special education teachers, his performance had advanced by 6 months, though he still lagged behind expected grade level. A medication trial has been discussed, but deferred at this time due to strong resistance from the foster family and custodial case worker. His steady progress via classroom and curricular modifications has supported this conservative approach, although we may need to reconsider the issue at future clinic visits. It seems highly likely that he will continue to have problems with attention and distractibility, and likely that he will benefit from a stimulant trial as academic challenges increase. We will follow his progress with regular contact, and address this issue in the future. As his function levels out, a Vineland Adaptive Behavior Scale will be added to the assessments.

Diagnoses for the children have been assigned, with recommendations for therapeutic intervention: 1. Alexi: mild static encephalopathy associated with fetal alcohol exposure as a Fetal Alcohol Spectrum Disorder, presenting as deficits in higher level learning, communication, and executive function, impacting organization, memory and interpersonal relationships. Using UW criteria, her 4- digit code is 1144, and IoM category is ARND. Recommendations for therapy are as above, with accommodations to classroom and curriculum that stress oral reading and other sources of information input, as well as attention to her immature or maladaptive social skills.

2. Martin has a similar diagnosis: mild static encephalopathy associated with fetal alcohol exposure as a Fetal Alcohol Spectrum Disorder, presenting as deficits in higher level learning, communication, and executive function, impacting organization, memory and interpersonal

relationships. His facial stigmata combine with soft neurologic signs and cognitive deficits to support a diagnosis of Partial FAS (UW code 1344). His problems of attention and distractibility fit a pattern of Attention Deficit Disorder without hyperactivity, and currently seem controlled without medication after curriculum adjustment. Again, regular clinical monitoring will be maintained to assure that he is able to meet the growing academic challenges. Medication for attention problems does not seem necessary at this time, but could be reconsidered in the future.

3.Henry had the most problematic behavior and impaired cognitive performance of the group, some of which reflects adjustment reactions to the new living setting. A diagnosis reflecting the fetal alcohol exposure seems clearly justified, especially in the context of physical features and growth abnormalities, but the absolute level of cognitive impairment is unclear as he makes improvement in the new residential stability. In his case, we assigned: "Static encephalopathy related to FASD, with problems in learning, attention and social function." UW code: 3444, with IoM category of Fetal Alcohol Syndrome. It is possible that he may have elements of PTSD reflecting his extremely disruptive early family life, but his steady progress in the current environment leaves that as a potential issue for later review. Continued monitoring and future psychological reassessment will allow us to revisit the diagnoses and to make adjustments as indicated. ADHD is a likely additional diagnosis, now reserved until his social and academic progress has leveled out. While stimulant medication may indeed be very helpful in moderating his classroom behavior and focusing his academic performance, the issue will need to be approached carefully to gain acceptance by a reluctant family.

4.Karen is an interesting child, given her high level of fetal exposure to alcohol and street drugs. She has the most normal developmental progress of the group, which suggests that her father's genetic contribution may have had some positive influence. She remains at risk of subtle cognitive problems as she grows older and faces increasingly sophisticated cognitive and social challenges. Her early disrupted life history represents a substantial risk of poor functional outcome, as noted by Streissguth, etal (2004). We will continue to monitor her progress as we follow her siblings, but have deferred any diagnoses at this time, beyond a statement of the risks inherent in her exposure. (UW code is 1124).

MEDICATION MANAGEMENT

The issue of medication management in rural and remote regions deserves further discussion, with Henry as a useful example. While it is very likely that this case would show clear benefits from use a daily low dose stimulant, the social and logistic realities intrude quickly. Henry's story represents a composite of numerous current and past cases, with a variety of medication success and failures. Henry's home region is like much of rural and remote Alaska, with only one fulltime general physician to serve a widely distributed small population, who has little experience or interest in managing psychotropic medications of any kind. Many residents choose to get their medical care in Anchorage, which is at least 4 hours away by a single highway through winding mountain roads. Use of a Schedule 2 medication requires monthly contact with the prescriber, which strains the capacity of our consulting physician in his monthly contacts (as well as the ability of case managers to successfully schedule contacts with that broadly spread clientele). There is widespread distrust or misunderstanding of medication use, especially as treatment for mental health conditions. Clients frequently choose to discontinue one or more medications, usually without notifying the case manager or prescriber.

In addition, many of the mental health and school function problems are primarily impacted by environmental variables such as family stability and substance abuse, and the impact of medication is often secondary or adjunctive to more primary family support and treatment for parental problems. On the positive side, since hyperactivity and distractibility are high frequency conditions in our population, affected individuals are less likely to stand out in a classroom setting as major disrupters of the process. Teachers in these regions often become expert at dealing with disproportionately affected classroom populations. The associated high frequency of learning problems also make curricular accommodations a more important first intervention than consideration of stimulants. Having said that, when the teachers have achieved appropriate accommodations and still see attention problems in a student, they become the most effective advocates to convince the family of the need to consider a medication trial. Often, successful compliance with a drug regimen is driven by a motivated teacher who ensures that the family follows through with clinic visits, prescriptions and other recommendations.

REFERENCES

Anderson, Thayne I., *Alaska Hooch, The history of alcohol in early Alaska*, Hoo-Che-Noo, Fairbanks, AK, 1988)

Astley SJ, Clarren SK. Diagnosing the full spectrum of fetal alcoholexposed individuals: introducing the 4-digit diagnostic code. *Alcohol Alcohol.* 2000;35 :400 –41

Furman, L What is Attention-Deficit Hyperactivity Disorder (ADHD)? *J Child Neurology* 2005; 20(12):994-1003

Klassen AF, Miller A, and Fine S Health-Related Quality of Life in Children and Adolescents who have a diagnosis of Attention-Deficit Hyperactivity Disorder *Pediatrics* 2004 Nov; 114(5):541-547

Hoyme HE, May PA, Kalberg WO, Kodituwakku P, Gossage JP, Trujillo PM, Buckley DG, Miller JH, Aragon AS, Khaole N, Viljoen DL, Jones KL, and Robinson LK A Practical Clinical Approach to Diagnosis of Fetal Alcohol Spectrum Disorders: Clarification of the 1996 Institute of Medicine Criteria *Pediatrics* 2005; 115: 39-47

O'Malley KD, and Nanson J Clinical implications of a link between Fetal Alcohol Spectrum Disorder and Attention-Deficit Hyperactivity Disorder *Can J Psychiatry* 2002 May; 47(4):349-54

Perry, BD, Applying Principles of Neurodevelopment to Clinical Work with Maltreated and Traumatized Children *in* Webb NB, *Working with Traumatized Youth in Child Welfare* Guilford Press, NY, NY 2006

Sowell ER, Mattson SN, ThompsonPM, JerniganTL, Riley EP, Toga AW Mapping callosal morphology and cognitive correlates: effects of heavy prenatal alcohol exposure *Neurology*, 2001 Jul 24; 57(2):235-44

Stratton KR, Howe CJ, Battaglia FC, eds. *Fetal Alcohol Syndrome: Diagnosis, Epidemiology, Prevention, and Treatment.* Washington, DC: National Academy Press; 1996

Streissguth AP, Bookstein FL, Barr HM, Sampson PD, O'Malley K, Young JK. Risk factors for adverse life outcomes in fetal alcohol syndrome and fetal alcohol effects. *J Dev Behav Pediatr.* 2004 Aug;25(4):228-38.

Swayze VW, Johnson VP, Hanson JW, Piven J, Sato Y, Giedd JN, Mosnik D, Andreasen NC Magnetic resonance imaging of brain anomalies in fetal alcohol syndrome. *Pediatrics* 1997 Feb; 99(2):232-40

DEVELOPMENTAL HISTORY QUESTIONNAIRE

Client Name: Birth date: age:

Address:

name of person filling out form: phone #:

   relationship to client:

Client's primary physician/address:

What is the goal of this clinic visit?

Medical Risk factors:

   How far along was the pregnancy when the mother became aware?   Father:

   When was 1st OB prenatal visit?

   Were there any illnesses, or were medications used in pregnancy?:

   Were tobacco, drugs, or alcohol used during pregnancy?:

      mother: father:

Was the delivery premature?

Were there problems with the delivery?

Any illness or other problem before discharge home after birth?

Has s/he had any problems with eating or growing?

Have height, weight, or head circumference ever been abnormal?

Has s/he ever had a brain injury from an accident or an infection?

Developmental Risk factors:

Has anyone ever worried about this child's development?

Milestones: Age when s/he first sat alone:

Age when s/he first crawled:
Age when s/he first walked:
Age at first single words:
Age at first word combinations:
Age when toilet trained for urine: for stool:

Behavior: Any problems?
Any previous evaluation?:   age of child/result:

Sleep:
        Typical bedtime/waking time:
        Time to sleep onset:
        Any history of snoring or pauses in breathing?:
        Level of awareness in daytime (sleepy, wide awake, needs naps):
        Frequent nightmares, sleepwalking, other abnormalities:

Medications:
current drugs/reason/effect:
other drugs tried/results:

Allergies:
School Concerns:
        Education diagnoses (SED, etc) ?
        Was the child ever held back?   When/why?

Learning problems: Testing results: IQ Full Scale: Verbal: Performance:
Other testing done (please bring copies):

Behavior problems at school:
Special Education program?   Is there an IEP?   Date of last plan:
(if you have an IEP, please provide a copy)

Family History: (Inherited problems in family members)
                Mother's side   Father's side

Medical conditions:
Learning problems:
(reading, ADHD...)
Mental Health:
(bipolar d/o, depression, substance abuse...)

History of child abuse/neglect:
Age of child, who was responsible:
Has the child ever been removed from the home?   How many times?

Who has legal custody at this time?
Who does the child live with now?

Other information:
Any previous Developmental Disability diagnosis?:
Receiving State-funded DD services?

Any previous Mental Health diagnosis?:
Previous psychiatric admissions or outpatient visits:

Testing and other evaluations: Please bring or send copies of school report cards and any reports by physicians, psychologists, or others which may help to understand the problems we'll be looking at in clinic.

Please feel free to add any other information or comments on the back of this page.

In: ADHD and Fetal Alcohol Spectrum Disorders (FASD)   ISBN: 1-59454-573-1
Editor: Kieran D. O'Malley, pp. 199-216   © 2008 Nova Science Publishers, Inc.

Chapter 11

MUTI-MODAL MANAGEMENT STRATEGIES THROUGH THE LIFESPAN

Kieran D. O'Malley[*]

INTRODUCTION

The treatment of FASD needs a *multi-modal approach* postulated initially by O'Malley in 1997. This management approach needs to be flexible with the ability to incorporate new strategies being ever present. The multi-modal approach is predicated on the initial multi-dimensional assessment of the patient (Jones, et al 1973a, Jones, et al 1973b, Stratton, et al, 1996, Astley and Clarren 1997, Koren, et al 2003). Already this type of approach has been proposed and studied in child and adolescent psychiatry in the management of mental retardation, language and learning disorders and more recently ADHD. The dysmorphology examination only quantifies the developmental disability i.e. dysmorphic, FAS, or non-dysmorphic, ARND. It is the quantification of the neuropsychiatric disorder(s) that is the central guide to management (King, et al 1998, Kapp and O'Malley 2001, Lemay, 2003, O'Malley and Storoz , 2003, O'Malley, 2003).)

The multi-modal approaches to management can be divided into different components: Individual, Dyadic (parent/child or adolescent), Family, Group, Advocacy. The biggest challenge to management is a pervasive ' therapeutic nihilism' that exists in the medical community about FASD. I once worked in a large Canadian city where a good number of family physicians and pediatricians refused to diagnose FAS or ARND (especially if there were no facial features), as 'there was nothing to do'... Hopefully, the next generation of patients with FASD will not continue to be undiagnosed and untreated.

---

[*] Kieran D.O'Malley M.B., D.A.B.P.N.(P); Lecturer / Adjunct Faculty, Dept. of Psychiatry and Behavioral Sciences and Henry M. Jackson School of International Studies, University of Washington, Fetal Alcohol and Drug Unit, Suite 309, 180 Nickerson Street, Seattle, WA, 98109; Contact kieranom@u.washington.edu : August 24th 2004

1. INDIVIDUAL THERAPY

The best approach is an *indirect non-verbal* one using art, guided play or sand- tray therapy as modes of connecting with the patient. Art and drama therapy can enhance the patient's self awareness and increase their ability to express themselves. Patients with FASD often have problems expressing themselves, not because of a low IQ, but because of a specific deficit in language processing. The language deficit is called alexithymia, i.e. an inability to have words for emotions. This concept was first described in patients with psychosomatic disorders , and later in patients with temporal lobe epilepsy (post surgery). This deficit is often subtle, and in childhood it is not uncommon to find that the child with FAS or ARND has been labeled as Oppositional Defiant Disorder (ODD), because they do not give an appropriate explanation for a social situation or confrontation i.e. an episode of aggression to a peer is seen as deliberate rather than understood in the light of an inability to verbally express frustration over constant verbal teasing. The non-verbal therapy gives the patient an opportunity to express themselves in a different modality. So a child emotionally or physically abused at home or at school can show a picture into their world through their play i.e. a sand-tray picture evolves of a school classroom where children are shouting and hitting each other, or stealing books etc.

Cognitive Behavioral therapy does not always work as these patients do not link cause and effect consistently and have executive function problems (i.e. problems in planning band organization, working memory and a lack of understanding the gist of a complex situation). Nevertheless, it is possible with repeated sessions and tasks to help a patient begin to connect the consequences of their negative actions i.e. a child or teenager is repeatedly brought through a common situation where they are creating problems at home such as always placing dirty boots on the clean carpet in the winter-time. Operant conditioning plans can, and do, work. The secret is to persevere, and also to have the parents be consistent in their consequences. This is the time where positive re-enforcement for the child who shows the ability to escapee a negative behavior, is often more rewarding to the child (and also the adult!). This approach is also valuable as the parent or teacher frequently needs support to help them understand that the child or adolescent with FAS or ARND is not deliberately defiant, but often does not comprehend the negative consequences of a certain behavior. A common conceptualization of patients with FASD is that they 'live in the moment'.This is true but does not have to be an insoluble problem. Sometimes in fact, it is the adult who is' stuck in the moment' that hinders the child from connecting with the adult and their environment. It is always salutary to remember that children or adolescents with FAS or ARND are brain-damaged and impulsive, and thus their actions and reactions are not inevitably deliberate volitional acts set to harass the over-worked parent!

Reality–based psychotherapy can play an ongoing role in the management of adolescent or young adult patients with FASD navigating jobs or relationships. These patients are often impulsive, destructive, and intermittently suicidal and can benefit from.a relational approach described by Bleiberg, 2001 in severe personality disorders. The relational approach of Bleiberg coupled with a sensitivity to the frequently encountered transgenerational trauma issues, (Horowitz, 2003) is a good combination. Dialectical Behavior Therapy seems to be too sophisticated for the FASD population, as the language is often too complicated and the concepts underpinning this model assume intact working memory.Therefore, the person has consistent reference points for their behaviors This is not the situation in FASD, where memory of past events can be a floating piece of water , constantly changing and moving. The essence of the reality-based therapy is formed from the therapeutic alliance where the therapist offers consistent reference points for the patient, and in effect becomes , for a time, their 'auxiliary brain.' Chapter 7 written by Kathy Page offers many good examples of this type of approach.

Examples:

a. A teenage boy with ARND and a normal IQ was failing in school. He responded in psychotherapy to a regular CBT approach, which helped organize his work programme at the school, and changed his attitude from one of defeat to one of success, albeit in small increments.

b. MS a 8-year-old girl with FAS, mild MR and severe PTSD due to early trauma responded slowly to regular non-verbal therapy, which included the sandtray. This approach was still useful until she was in her early teens and her PTSD symptoms had disappeared.

2. SPECIAL EDUCATION

The FASD population benefit from understanding the concept of 'multiple intelligence', as they have strengths and weaknesses in different areas and do not conform to standard developmental disability/ low IQ global delays. Formal cognitive testing such as WISC IV or Stanford -Binet can show impairment in the patient's verbal or visual attention and memory, with specific mathematics disorder. Commonly, school special education programs are frozen in the mental retardation model of developmental disability. This school education model does not connect with FASD as 75% of these patients have a normal IQ. This is a specific of developmental neuropsychiatric population that needs, and merits, a more holistic understanding. These are the children and adolescents who have organically- driven impulse disorders(ADHD), affective instability or even pervasive developmental disorder features who do not conform to old classifications. They need to be seen for what they are, complex learning disorder individuals with major unseen language deficits in social cognition and social communication. However it is the marked discrepancy between cognitive ability and functional ability, as measured by Vineland Adaptive Behavioral Scales (VABS), in communication, socialization and daily living skills that becomes the essence of the developmental disability in FASD(Streissguth, et al 1996). A special education class, teacher's aide, speech and language therapist and an occupational therapist (if the patient has fine or gross motor problems or visual- motor co-ordination problems) are often needed. Their individual, and collective, work is enhanced by placing it in Gardner's world of multiple intelligence(Gardner, 1993). These children and adolescents need to have a school system that can seek, recognize, and celebrate their skills in non-traditional arenas i.e. figure skating, pow- wow dancing, art, culture. Only then can school start to become a place for growth and companionship, rather than a world of constant denigration and blame (Kapp and O'Malley 2001).

Examples:

a. A severely physically hyperactive and impulsive 10 year old girl with FAS was unable to be contained in a regular school or special education class in a regular school, but responded well to a small specialized DD (LD) class with 8 pupils and 1 teacher and a teacher's aide.

b. A 8-year-old boy with ARND and MRI evidence of heterotrophic gray matter in corpus callosum of the brain area failed in a regular school. However, he succeeded in a specialized DD (LD) school which used a multi-sensory teaching approach.

3. Speech and Language Assessment and Therapy

It is necessary to establish the patient's level of receptive/expressive language disorder, and can be very important in showing that the child or adolescent with FASD may have a good vocabulary, grammar and syntax, but those words are often disconnected from the patient's thoughts or feelings. Narrative discourse analysis is a useful assessment as it gives a picture of the patient's ability to comprehend and generalize social situations. Many patients with FASD have Alexithymia, or " no words for emotions".(Sifneos , 1974, Kapp and O'Malley, 2001). This impedes their ability to fully express emotional distress about a situation, so the patient often acts out their feelings with physical action i.e. hitting some-one or breaking a chair. Sometimes the child , adolescent or even adult expresses their emotional feelings, whether positive or negative, through somatic symptoms i.e. recurrent headache, abdominal pain. A Speech and language therapist can often become the eyes , ears and mouth of a child with FAS or ARND and ' translate' this world for the teachers or parents. Skills borrowed from work with autistic spectrum patients are an appropriate fit (Nowicki, et al , 1992, Coggins, et al 2003).

Examples:

a.   A 10-year-old Russian boy, with a normal IQ, was labeled as being a trouble –maker with ADHD and ODD. When a diagnosis of ARND was made a Speech and Language assessment showed his deficits in social cognition and social communication. The boy was subsequently given specialized language therapy, which helped him in his ability to communicate his needs and frustrations. In turn, his teachers also began to understand his impulsive and reactive behavior as a consequence of his previously undiagnosed language disorder.

This example repeats itself many times over and over. The key to helping the child with FAS or ARND, irrespective of IQ, appears to be doing a proper language assessment, including a discourse analysis (which analyses the social use of language). This allows the teachers to see the social cognition and social communication deficits. As well it opens the door for both the teachers and the parents to be able to see the autistic features sometimes embedded in the child or adolescent with FAS or ARND.

4. MEDICATION THERAPY

Although this is used quite extensively with children and adolescents with FASD, it is important to remember that there are no FDA approved medications for the condition. Thus, the use of medication in FASD has not been properly evaluated, and as O'Malley and Hagerman 1998, have commented, the brain of a prenatally brain-damaged infant or young child is especially vulnerable to atypical medication response and untoward side effects It is critical for the physician to remember that Patients with FASD constitute an acquired brain-injury population(Ikonomidou , et al, 2000, Bookstein, et al 2001). Generally, if medication is being considered, it is essential to have a recent complete medical by a family physician or pediatrician to rule out any alcohol related birth defects (ARBD) e.g. kidney or cardiac problems to name a few. The role of medication is one of symptom control in order to facilitate other modalities of treatment. There is considerable literature on psychopharmacotherapy of patients with mental retardation (MR) and/or brain injury, both of which are relevant to the FASD population. Some studies have been performed on children or adolescents with MR and co-morbid psychiatric disorder.

There have been only five studies on the use of psychostimulants in FASD and no clear algorithm has been established. *No other class of medications have been scientifically tested in FASD patients* Early evidence from animal and human studies suggests that dextro-amphetamine may be more efficacious for the ADHD symptoms of FASD children and adolescents than ,the universally prescribed first line ADHD medication, methylphenidate. Methylphenidate does relieve the ADHD symptoms of FASD patients but is also less effective if IQ is under 50. Other medications that are clinically useful for the ADHD symptoms include, Adderall XL and the second-generation bi-modal psychostimulants. Strattera is increasingly being used, but may have cardiotoxicity in FASD because of its nonadrenergic action, and prenatal alcohol's known effect on the developing heart.

The general principle in using medication in patients with FASD is to always start with low dose *mono-therapy.* This is important as the patient may show a paradoxical excitation effect or over-sedation effect in the first 48 hours due to the underlying organic brain damage. If only one medication has been used then it is easier to isolate the drug as the author of the changed mental status. As well medication may ' unmask' secondary psychiatric problems. This is especially true of SSRI's in children or adolescents with FASD. So unmonitored long term usage of SSRI in a FASD child/ adolescent used for depressive symptoms may unmask an affective instability syndrome (similar to rapid cycling Bipolar disorder) which is a product of the organic brain damage due to prenatal alcohol and maybe familial loading for Bipolar Disorder. SSRI's may also induce extrapyramidal side effects (EPS) because of the underlying organic brain damage (Sher 2003).

Polypharmacy is a very common problem in FASD patient management. It is almost impossible to begin to unravel the clinical presentation from delayed and /or immediate drug side effects when up to 5 or 6 drugs are being used. It is really much better to move one drug at a time, carefully evaluating subjective and objective clinical response. As well, the primary psychiatric presentation of the developmental disability is the key to understanding the good, bad or indifferent medication response in the FASD patient .It is also far to say that FASD patients with quantified structural brain abnormalities (identified on CAT Scan or MRI) will invariably be the most complex and unpredictable ones to manage. When two or more medications are being utilized it is important to only change the dosage of one medication at a time i.e. a SSRI is being used with a GABAergic agent for the management of Mood disorder with panic attacks in an adolescent with FASD then only change the dosage of either the SSRI or the GABA agent. This will help to clinically evaluate the positive or negative effect of increased drug dosage. A commonly forgotten point in treating FASD patients is to understand that their atypical drug response may not just be due to organic brain damage from prenatal alcohol , but also the toxic effect of the alcohol on the developing liver. This makes a drug such as Paroxetine especially problematic because it interferes with the cytochrome P450 2D6 liver isoenzyme pathway which is utilized by most of the psychotropic agents. So it increases the likelihood of drug toxicity of multiple drug therapy in FASD patients.

Intermittent Explosiveness Episodes (Rage attacks), respond to carbamazepine, valproic acid or GABA agents, such as gabapentin This Explosiveness can be related to a Complex Partial Seizure Disorder, or sometimes is seen in patients with "hyperactive" symptomatology who did not respond to the psychostimulant. It also may be precipitated by too long a treatment with a SSRI. Valproic acid usage in pre-pubertal girls or adolescents with FASD is not recommended as precocious puberty often develops this population, and valproic acid has been implicated in causing polycystic ovarian problems, so complicating endocrine/ hormonal balance. It is critical to evaluate if these episodes are truly explosive ones or are really panic attacks. These panic attacks can be precipitated by certain triggers such as misunderstanding a teacher's class instructions, or overwhelming social situation such as a party or shopping centre with too many sensory stimuli.

Psychotic Features (such as auditory or visual hallucinations) respond to mellaril (check EEG, for QT) suspension or neuleptil oral drops alone, or anti-convulsants such as carbamazepine or valproic acid if the patient has an epileptic focus in the temporal lobe, and clinical presentation of complex partial seizures. The newer atypical anti-psychotics may have a use here e.g. risperidone, olanazepine, seroquel or clozaril. Recent work on the atypical antipsychotics has shown that they can double the risk of abnormal glucose metabolism including diabetes, hyperprolactinaemia and pancreatitis all potential problems in the FASD population. This population is also more likely to need benztropine as they develop EPS easier. Parentral medication such as fluanxol has proven effective in once month regime, in the schizoaffective population of FASD patients.

Sleep Disorders are pervasive in FASD patients and can often underpin the psychiatric clinical presentation. They respond to melatonin, trazadone or l-tryptophan.

Medications that should be used with caution in FASD patients:

- -Lithium Carbonate causes cardiac, renal and thyroid problems. As prenatal alcohol already can cause cardiac and renal problems this medication really compounds the potential clinical morbidity of FASD.
- -Tricyclic Antidepessants (amitriptyline, imipramine, desipramine, clomipramine) cause cardiac toxicity, sudden death, lower the seizure threshold and are lethal in overdose All of these issues are especially relevant in FASD patients and the unpredictable liver aborption makes toxicity at therapeutic levels a definite risk (Bonthius , et al 2001).
- -New Antidepressants affecting seratonergic and nor-adrenergic systems. (Effexor), may cause cardiotoxicity in a vulnerable population because of prenatal effect on noradrenergic neurotransmitter system and also alcohol effect on developing heart.

- -First Generation Antipsychotics (chlorpromazine, stelazine, nozinan and haldol) cause excess sedation, increased risk of EPS and possible liver toxicity. These side effects are all potentially magnified in the FASD population due to organic brain damage and prenatal alcohol effect on developing organ systems such as heart , liver and kidney (Hannigan, et al 1996, O'Malley and Hagerman , 1998, Hagerman 1999).

Examples:

a.   An 11-year-old boy MC with above average IQ is diagnosed with ADHD and co-morbid Mood disorder and treated with Desipramine 25mgs BID. He lives with his professional parents, both of who work. His dosage is increased to 30 mgs BID and within 1 day he impulsively hits two boys at school with little provocation. An emergency assessment revealed that his mother drank alcohol throughout her pregnancy with MC. She did not report this in the initial clinical assessment as her husband was a functioning alcoholic and she drank far less than him so she felt that it was not relevant. The Desipramine was stopped and he was started on Dexedrine. He had no more explosive episodes. A follow-up tricyclic blood level showed his level on the borderline of toxicity despite the low dose, suggesting atypical liver metabolism consistent with the prenatal alcohol exposure history. (MC denied taking extra tablets and so was taking the prescribed dosage when the blood level was done).

b.   A teenager with ARND and ADHD was treated with Methylphenidate. Risperidone was added to his treatment regime by the family physician because of aggression. This precipitated a hypomanic switch, which stopped when the Risperidone was discontinued. This suggested sensitivity to the 5HT receptor action of Risperidone and is an example that has been repeated in at least 3 other cases.

c.   A 20 year old Native American with ARND was admitted to an acute care psychiatric ward with increased suicidality and panic, which came on shortly after Effexor had been prescribed by his adult psychiatrist. These symptoms abated when the Effexor was discontinued and the patient subsequently responded to Neurontin (gabapentin).

d.   A 7-year-old adopted Caucasian boy, JS, was diagnosed with Childhood Schizophrenia. He did not respond to a series of different antipsychotic medications. He was subsequently assessed in a FAS clinic and fulfilled criteria for ARND as his birth mother had a well-documented history of using alcohol in her pregnancy with JS. An EEG showed complex partial seizure disorder. His first rank psychotic symptoms of auditory and visual hallucinations disappeared a number of weeks after he was started on Carbamazepine.

5. SEX EDUCATION

Patients with FASD have pervasive problems with social boundaries and become a major issue in adolescence and young adulthood. These patients may crave touch, because of their tactile integration problems, and can then find themselves accused of being sexually inappropriate. The prevalence of physical or sexual abuse in the FASD population leads to a very vulnerable individual. The teaching of sexual boundaries in this developmentally delayed population requires a specialized trainer. These patients often do not learn from experience or consistently link cause and effect, thus a non-verbal approach using non-ambiguous art or role playing drama therapy techniques can be beneficial. A family physician/paediatrician can have an important role in discussing basic sexual development sexually transmitted diseases and birth control. Sex education is best done in individual counseling, but sometimes can be taught in a group setting with other developmental disability patients of the same gender to decrease misunderstandings and potential embarrassment (Brown, 1993, see Novock-Brown, Chapter 8).

Examples:

1. There seems to be an almost ' double standard' in basic sexual health education as many school child and teenage programmes are not sensitive to the cognitive learning needs of patients with DD, especially FASD. This effectively excludes them from fundamental, common sense education in the boundaries in social relationships.

2. In my limited clinical experience the most disturbed children and teenagers with FASD are those who have experienced sexual or physical abuse (especially same sex abuse) before 10 years of age. These patients have many sexually inappropriate behaviors (SIB) and their impulsivity and misreading of social cues makes them   particularly at risk for becoming involved with the legal system.

6. DENTAL CARE

Patients with FASD should have a regular dental assessment because of common orthodontic problems. These problems may lead to decreased self-esteem, especially if he or she is teased at school. Dental care needs to be organized as part of a general self-awareness of personal hygiene. The misunderstandings involved in dental care and the fear and pain sometimes involved in treatment require a dentist familiar with patients with a developmental disability, including the possible interaction between the patient's psychotropic medication and the dental medication or anesthetic.

Examples:

1. A dentist wanted to give a general anaesthetic to an 11-year-old girl with FAS and major orthodontic problems to do prolonged surgery. A pre-operation ECG showed sinus arrhythmia. In consultation with a paediatric cardiologist and child psychiatrist the dentist elected to do the operation with local anaesthetic over 3 sessions. This proved safer and also was successful.

2. Another dentist did not understand why his teenage patient BD (with ARND) was so anxious. The child/ adolescent   psychiatrist contacted him (at the parents' request) and informed him of the boy's ARND. The dentist had been previously unaware of this Developmental Disability. He then explained the simple dental surgery i.e. wisdom tooth extraction with visual drawings and this decreased BD's anxiety.

7. PARENT/CHILD DYAD

Therapy is needed in infancy and early childhood to address attachment and parenting issues with the birth or adoptive/ foster mother. Here, the therapist needs to actively balance the infant or young child's behaviors which reflect their brain damage i.e delayed suck reflex, poor feeding,or poor habituation to the parent's natural anxiety in the simple act of parenting. It is always important to remember that the infant or child is not the author of his or her behavior's, and so the parent's perceived rejection may really be a misunderstanding of the developmental neuropsychiatric disorder. Parents who are still under the influence of an addictive disorder or have FAS or ARND themselves may not respond consistently to an infant or young child's cues. However, a temperamentally difficult to settle or slow to warm infant does not necessarily herald an insecure attachment. It prefaces challenges, but does not preclude true bonding. In fact, it is the unpredictable disorganized attachment paradigm, a product of neurological sensory integration problems, that is the hallmark of FASD. Infant interventions such as swaddling, cradle-board, feeding strategies or sensory integration techniques are all very helpful.(O'Malley and Streissguth 2006).

In adolescence, individuation and identity issues arise and are especially important in adoptive children, especially in cross-culturally adopted children This type of dyadic therapy is more taxing for the therapist as they must be vigilant in their appreciation that the teenager who is speaking in monosyllables , expressing non-sequitors, is also suffering from organic brain damage and so needs an advocate to help them express their sense of self i.e. a teenager who wants to separate from their Caucasian adoptive parents and seek connection with their birth family may be unable to express this anxiety in words . Thus, the teenager acts out at home for no apparent reason, or suffers daily headaches and pain with no medical etiology discovered.

Example:

a.   A young mother with ARND binge drinks through her pregnancy with AN. She is involved with an advocate throughout the pregnancy and when AN is born she is involved in weekly parent/infant sessions which greatly help her bonding and her competence in basic parenting.

b.   Dyadic therapy is also useful with adults. KD, a 21-year-old adult woman, with ARND becomes involved in a relationship with a LE, a 22-year man with ARND. They both want to marry, but understand their disability so they enter into regular dyadic therapy with a counselor. This greatly helps their relationship and offers a neutral voice to clarify misunderstandings. The counselor is also able to do systemic work with both KD's and LE's adoptive parents and KD's social service support team to allay their anxieties about this relationship and so gain their support.

8. FAMILY THERAPY

Family Education approaches help reduce the family's fear by explaining the nature of FASD and giving realistic expectations for treatment response. Frequently families have been blamed by previous professionals as the cause of their child's psychiatric disorder. Local FASD support groups are a good source of reference material , and can help parents in families with newly placed FAS or ARND children as these parent groups offer the wealth of collective ' parent knowledge'.

Instrumental Family Therapy addressing basic family functioning such as the daily living routines of the child/ adolescent with FAS or ARND or even the parent with FAS or ARND. It is helpful to draw up daily timetables of chores and schedules, and to stick them on the door or fridge. Parents have also found it useful to have a list of these child expectations on a paper or board and have the child tick them off on a daily basis (with a pencil or felt pen).

Adoptive families commonly need time to grieve the loss of their "idealized" self, which is brought on by the child's FAS or ARND diagnosis. One clinical model that is useful in dealing with the family's grief is the model proposed by Kubler Ross in her definitive book, Death and Dying. Although the parallels may not be readily apparent, the stages of denial, anger, despair, bargaining and acceptance are a deceptively simple but respectful way of acknowledging the differing perceptions of parents, or even other sibs, to the arrival of a child with FAS or ARND. Traditionally it is the mother who reaches a level of acceptance long before the father. However, like all so called truisms, exceptions are not commonly the rule and the father and the father may prove be be more accepting of the FASD than the mother..

The *family burden* of managing a child or adolescent with FAS or ARND and the effect this disorder has on the other family members is a constant theme in therapy and is even more complicated when dealing with a guilty-feeling birth mother in recovery. This burden has generally four components: the medical needs , the mental health or psychiatric needs, the economic needs, and the emotional burden or compassion fatigue in the parents.(Grosch and Olsen , 1994, Figley, 1995, Cummings, et al , 2000,Gelo and O'Malley 2001). Planned Regular Respite Care is a most important component, as is proper , detailed post-adoption plan, with clear delineation of the state, or provincial, financial support. Mental health professionals have a key role in writing support letters to social service agencies to advocate for financial aid for birth, adoptive or foster parents who have children or adolescents with FASD.

Examples:
1.   A teenage boy with ARND is disruptive in school and home. His adoptive mother supports the teenager, but the adoptive father refuses to accept his disability. Although he responds to CBT and medication he has to be placed in a residential centre.

2.   A young couple has adopted a child and gradually they begin to see signs of prenatal alcohol, exposure. They pursue a nearly diagnosis of FAS (under 3 years) and start early interventions, including sensory integration. The both parents work together and the child remains in the home 4 years later with on going professional support, specialized school and respite care.

3.   A teenage boy with ARND impulsively tries to hang himself in response to other hangings in his local area. He dos not succeed, as he does not tie the knot properly. His birth mother (with ARND) is unable to support him because of her own mental health issues, which are consistent with a Mixed Personality Disorder. At one stage he is prescribed 1 cc of fluoxetine, but the mother dispense 5cc. He becomes quite hypo-manic but settles when the dose is reduced to 1cc. Again. He is admitted to a specialized Adolescent Psychiatric Day Hospital that provides support for his mother. The structure of the Day Hospital and the mother/ son support is beginning to achieve success and he is less depressed and impulsive and his mother is feeling more empowered in dealing with him.

4.   A Caucasian family adopts a 5-year Native American girl with FAS. They also have an older natural sib, a 9-year-old boy. The parents are very attentive to the care of their FAS

child and after a few years her brother becomes quite resentful, as he feels neglected. This type of story repeats itself in many families in which there is a mixture of special needs, (FAS or ARND) children and natural children. These blended families may be a challenge and it is always important for the parents to be vigilant to the needs of their non-special needs children, irrespective of their age.

9. GROUP THERAPY

A *support group for parents or caregivers* provides a way to exchange ideas about different methods that have succeeded in the management of their child with FASD (e.g. sensory integration, language therapy, medications), or a place to acknowledge their son or daughter's unique talent (art, sport, music).

The *therapeutic group approach* for young adults with FASD can offer an opportunity to discuss the effect of FASD on their lives and encourage better ways of functioning in social relationships and work situations (a forum for collective problem-solving) .This group has many of the classical curative features described by Yalom. It's universality and non-judgmental structure greatly enhances the group's cohesion and effectiveness (O'Malley 2005). Recent experience with a parallel group process, whereby the parents or guardians were seen at the same time as the patient with FAS or ARND (with a parent facilitator), proved an invaluable supportive forum for positive parent affirmation, and practical nuts and bolts guidance.

Examples:

1.   A young adult group of patients with ARND with 6 participants functions well as a group as the group deal with the every day problems of life by   ' joint problem – solving'. The group identity i.e. FAS or ARND forms an immediate bond with the group members as they engage in similar stories of life's foibles.

2.   A young woman's group with FAS and ARND is not as successful as the participants do not seem to be able to work together. and have too many individual emotional unmet needs. More careful screening may be help for future such groups.

10. ADVOCACY

Patients and caregivers need to have para-professional advocates who work one-on-one with alcoholic and substance-abusing women forming a therapeutic and protective alliance and helping them navigate through the mental health, addiction and social services. The University of Washington Parent-Child Assistance Program is a good example (Grant et al 1999). FASD children are born to women who commonly have co-morbid addictive and psychiatric problems, and thus sensitivity and knowledge of these two areas are important to help break the cycle of victimization that FASD children may inherit. The advocacy role exists from infancy to adulthood, and is a key part of the professional relationship that is formed with the teacher, or mental health professional. These patients are commonly called ' orphan' patients as they do not fit the expected mould of mental retardation, 75% not being mentally retarded, and 75 to 80% do not display the classical and 75 to 80% do not display the classical facial dysmorphology, and so are a hidden population of a complex developmental disability.

11. THERAPIST SUPPORT IN THERAPY

Patients with FASD are complex clinically, frequently come from chaotic family backgrounds and need a multi-modal treatment approach. All of these components can be overwhelming to the individual primary care provider, or the caregiver/parent. It is essential to provide respite care options and shared therapy for the clinician, as this type of patient truly needs a multidisciplinary approach occurring concurrently. A regular schedule of case management meetings, usually monthly or 2 monthly, is a method of anticipating problems and sharing their management. This approach commonly avoids the onset of Compassion Fatigue in the primary care provider or parent/ caregiver (Grosch, et al, 1994, Figley, 1995). Horowitz nicely describes a suitable therapeutic stance in his recent book (Horowitz 2003).

Example:
1. Regular parent and professional support groups are very helpful for parents of children with FASD, but they also serve as an essential regular grounding for the professionals involved with these children, adolescents and families.

12. HOUSING

Respite housing and care is worth organizing as part of an initial ' post-adoption agreement' A young hyperactive/ impulsive patient with FASD benefits most from a well-structured, predictable respite home environment. This is an essential ingredient in any long-term treatment plan as patients with FASD pose developmental and neuropsychiatric challenges throughout the lifespan. The provision of *appropriate independent housing* becomes a key part of management in the late teen and young adult years. They need to be in a protective home environment with some type of daily adult monitoring. The VABS gives a picture of the functional ability, and is a useful guide to the level of monitoring needed in an independent home environment (Streissguth, et al 1996). Also a suitable work placement ,and day to day financing may be done through the local Developmental Disability office in liaison with the patient's protective payee or guardian.

Examples:
1. GB is an 18-year Caucasian old with ARND who has just finished High school with a vocational diploma. She is receiving income support through the DD agency and has a social worker in the adult services that is instrumental in placing her with an adult couple in a first supported living placement.
2. AD is a 17-year Caucasian old with ARND who has left school and is working in a part time job with a vocational rehabilitation agency. He has a case manager who works in liaison with adult services to find him a placement with a 25-year male in a supported

independent living situation. His foster mother continues to manage his money in a public payee/ trustee role.

SUMMARY

The direction of treatment will come from the initial clinical evaluation. Thus, a child with ARND, mild variety, with some cognitive and language impairment but a history of abandonment by the birth parent and later physical/sexual abuse by a foster parent requires specific individual psychotherapy. On the other hand, a child or adolescent with Full FAS who is in a special education class and is markedly physically hyperactive and explosive needs a different approach, most likely with psychiatric involvement and medication. The initial dysmorphological screening assessment of FASD creates a platform for further clinical evaluation, the most important being a thorough psychiatric assessment, which will have create recommendations for child/ adolescent and family management. FASD is a transgenerational condition and screening tests for alcohol use in pregnancy by normally developing or FASD adolescents or young adults are an essential ingredient to holistic management. This chronic developmental and neuropsychiatric disorder ultimately needs a holistic 'developmental system of care' which incorporates the infant, but also includes the pregnant substance abusing mother who potentially is delivering the next generation of FASD patients (Streissguth, 1997, Streissguth and O'Malley, 2000, Streissguth, et al , 2004). This is becoming more important as researchers are recognizing the adult risk of alcohol addiction which is kindled by the effect of prenatal alcohol on the developing brain (Li, 2000, Baer, et al 2003). See Table 1. (Barr , et al 2001). (The age, gender and ethnicity of the patients in the clinical examples have been altered to protect their identity)

Table 1. Questions Used to elicit BARC Score

Estimate the following (write 0 if it never happened	Month or so before pregnancy	During this pregnancy
Number of times per month that you drank 5 or more drinks on one occasion		
Number of times per month that you consumed 3-4 drinks on an occasion		
Number of times per month that you consumed just 1-2 drinks on an occasion		
Did you drink alcohol almost every day, even if only a small quantity? (circle answer)	Yes No	Yes No

Note: The fourth question is redundant, but is suggested as a check on the first three questions, and seems to reflect the tone of many of the respondents.

REFERENCES

*Astley SJ and Clarren SK *Diagnostic Guide for Fetal Alcohol Syndrome and Related Conditions.* 1997,Seattle, WA: University of Washington.

Baer JS, Sampson PD, Barr HM, Connor PD and Streissguth AP A 21- year longitudinal analysis of the effects of prenatal alcohol exposure on young adult drinking. *Arch Gen Psychiatry,*2003, Vol. 60, April 377-385.

Barr HM and Streissguth AP Identifying maternal self- reported alcohol use associated with fetal alcohol spectrum disorders. *Alcohol Clin Exp Res*, 2001, Vol 25, No. 2, 283-287.

Bleiberg , E Treating personality disorders in children and adolescents. A relational approach. 2001, The Guilford Press, New York, London

Bonthius, DJ, Woodhouse, J, Bonthius, NE, Taggard, DA, and Lothman, EW Reduced seizure threshold and hippocampal cell loss in rats exposed to alcohol during the brain growth spurt. Alcohol Clin Exp Res,2001, Vol. 25, No. 1, 70-82

Bookstein FL, Sampson PD, Streissguth AP, Connor PL Geometric morphometrics of corpus callosum and subcortical structures in fetal alcohol effected brain. *Tetratology,* 2001,4, 4-32.

*Brown, Hilary J Sexuality and intellectual disability: The new realism. *Current Opinion in Psychiatry*, 1993, 6, 623-628.

Coggins TE, Olswang LB, Carmichael Olson H and Timler GR On becoming socially competent communicators: The challenge for children with fetal alcohol exposure, *International review of research in mental retardation*, 2003,Vol. 27, 121-150.

Cummings, EM, Davies, PT, Campbell, SB Developmental psychopathology and family process. 2000, The Guilford Press, New York, London

Figley, CR *Compassion Fatigue: Coping with secondary trauma stress disorder in those who treat the traumatized.* 1995, Publisher, Brunner/ Mazel, New York

*Gardner H *Multiple Intelligence. The Theory in Practice.* 1993, Harper Collins, New York.

*Grant TM, Ernst CC, and Streissguth AP Intervention with high-risk alcohol and drug abusing mothers: 1.Administrative strategies of the Seattle model of paraprofessional advocacy. *Journal of Community Psychology,*1999, 27, 1-18.

Grosch, WH and Olsen, DC *When helping starts to hurt. A new look at burnout among psychotherapists.* 1994, Publisher, WW Norton and Company Inc., New York/ London

Hagerman RJ *Neurodevelopmental Disorders. Diagnosis and Treatment. Fetal Alcohol Syndrome,* 1999, 3-59, Oxford University Press, New York, Oxford.

Hannigan, JH and Randall, S Chapter 9, Behavioral pharmacology in animals exposed prenatally to alcohol, 1996,191-213, *CRC Press, Inc.* USA

Horowitz,MJ Treatment of stress responsive syndromes, 2003, American Psychiatric Press, Washington DC

Ikonomidou, C, Bittigau, P, Ishimaru, MJ, Wozniak, DF, Koch, C, Genz, K, Price, MT, Stefovska, V, Horster, F, Tenkova, T, Dikranian, K, Olney, JW Ethanol- induced apoptotic neurodegeneration and fetal alcohol syndrome. *Science*, 2000,Vol. 287, 1056-1059

Jones KL and Smith DW Recognition of the fetal alcohol syndrome in early infancy. *Lancet*, 1973a, 2, 999-1101.

Jones KL, Smith DW, Ulleland CN and Streissguth A P Pattern of malformations in offspring of chronic alcoholic mothers *Lancet,* 1973b, 6, 1267-1270.

**Kapp FME and O'Malley KD *Watch for the Rainbows. True stories for educators and caregivers of children with fetal alcohol spectrum disorders*; 2001,64-83, Publisher Frances Kapp Education, Calgary, Canada.

King BH, State MW, Bhavik S, Davanzo P, Dykens Mental Retardation: A review of the past 10 years. 1998, Part I, in *Reviews in Child and Adolescent Psychiatry, AACAP*, 126-133.

Koren G, Nulman I, Chudley AE, Loocke C Fetal Alcohol Spectrum Disorder. *CMAJ*, 2003, 169 (11) 1181-1185.

Kubler-Ross On death and dying.

Lemay J-F, Herbert AR, Dewey DM, Innes AM A rational approach to the child with mental retardation for the paediatrician. *Paediat Child Health*,2003, Vol. 8, No. 6, 345-356.

Li TK Pharmacogenetics of response to alcohol and genes that influence alcohol drinking. *J Stud Alcohol*. 2000, 61, 5-12.

**Nowicki S and Duke MP *Helping the Child Who Doesn't Fit In*. 1992, Peachtree Publishers. Atlanta, Georgia.

O'Malley, KD, Multi-modal treatment approaches to children and adolescents with FASD (1997) Paper presentation. Part of the Indian Health Service National FAS training curriculum at the University of Washington, Seattle, 1997-2005

*O'Malley KD, Hagerman R.J Developing Clinical Practice Guidelines for Pharmacological Interventions with Alcohol-affected Children.1998, *Proceedings of a special focus session of the Interagency Co-ordinating Committee on Fetal Alcohol Syndrome.* Chevy Chase Ma, Sept 10TH and 11th, Centers for Disease Control and National Institute of Alcohol Abuse and Alcoholism (Eds.), USA, 145-177.

*O'Malley KD and Streissguth AP Clinical intervention and support for children aged zero to five years with fetal alcohol spectrum disorder and their parents / caregivers Revised. 2006, In: Tremblay RE, Barr RG, Peters RdeV, eds. *Encyclopedia on Early Childhood Development (online)*, Montreal, Quebec: Centre for Excellence for Early Childhood development: 1-9 Available at, http://www/excellence-earlychildhood.ca/documents /OMalley-StreissguthANGxp.pdf.

*O'Malley KD and Storoz L Fetal alcohol spectrum disorder and ADHD: diagnostic implications and therapeutic consequences. *Expert Review of Neurotherapeutics*,2003, July, Vol. 3. No. 4, 477-489.

O'Malley, KD Youth with Comorbid Disorders. Chapter 13, 276- 315, in *The Handbook of Child and Adolescent Systems of Care*, 2003, Pumariega AJ and Winters NC (eds.) Jossey- Bass, San Francisco.

Sher, L.Developmental alcohol exposure, circadian rhythms, and mood disorders. *Can J. Psychiatry,2003,* vol. 48, No. 6, 428

*Stratton KR, Rowe CJ and Battaglia FC *Fetal Alcohol Syndrome: Diagnosis, epidemiology, prevention and treatment in medicine* . 1996, National Academy Press, Washington DC.

*Streissguth, A.P., Barr, H.M., Kogan, J. and Bookstein, F.L. Understanding the occurrence of secondary disabilities in clients with fetal alcohol syndrome (FAS) and fetal alcohol effects (FAE). ,1996, *Final Report, August, C.D.C. Grant R04.*

**Streissguth AP *Fetal alcohol syndrome. A guide for families and communities 1997,*. Brookes Publishing, Baltimore.

*Streissguth AP and O'Malley KD Neuropsychiatric implications and long-term consequences of fetal alcohol spectrum disorders. *Seminars in Clinical Neuropsychiatry*, 2000,5, 177-190.

**Streissguth, AP, Bookstein, FL, Barr, HM, Sampson, PD, O'Malley KD, Kogan Young Risk factors for adverse risk outcomes in fetal alcohol syndrome and fetal alcohol effects. *Developmental and Behavioral Pediatrics*, 2004, Vol. 25. No. 4, 228-238

* Recommended for primary care physicians or psychologists
** Recommended for families

1. Fetal Alcohol Syndrome (FAS) (adapted from Stratton et al 1996, also see Tables 1&2 Chapter 1)

A. Confirmed maternal alcohol exposure

B. Evidence of a characteristic pattern of facial anomalies that includes features such as short palpebral fissures (2 SD or greater below mean), and abnormalities in the premaxillary zone (i.e. flat upper lip, flattened philtrum and flat midface)

C. Evidence of Growth retardation, as in at least one of the following:

- low birth weight
- decelerating weight over time not due to nutrition (less than 3rd percentile for height and weight),
- disproportional low weight to height.

D. Evidence of CNS neurodevelopmental abnormalities, such as:

- structural brain abnormalities, i.e.decreased cranial size at birth, microcephaly (head circumference less than 3 rd percentile), partial or complete agenesis of the corpus callosum, cerebellar hypoplasia,
- neurophysiological abnormalities, complex partial seizure disorder, absence seizure, other seizure,
- neurological hard or soft signs(as age appropriate):
    - motor:
        - gross motor function; poor tandem gait, positive romberg test, balance problems,
        - fine motor function, fine motor problems with evidence of constructional apraxia, poor hand-eye co-ordination motorically disorganized in the under 5 year age group,
    - sensory:
        - abnormal sensation upper or lower limbs,
        - neurosensory hearing loss,
        - abnormal visual, auditory, gustatatory, olfactory or tactile sensations, including hallucinations, includes craving touch

and can make the patient a victim of false accusation of
sexually inappropriate behavior
- Regulatory disorder, type 1, 11 or 111, in under 5 year age

2. Alcohol Related Neurodevelopmental Disorder (ARND)
A. Confirmed maternal alcohol exposure
B. No characteristic pattern of facial anomalies
C. No or little growth retardation
D. Evidence of CNS neurodevelopmental abnormalities, such as:
- structural brain abnormalities i.e. decreased cranial size at birth
- microcephaly, partial or complete agenesis of the corpus callosum, cerebellar hypoplasia, decreased hippocampal size
- neurophysiological abnormalities i.e complex partial seizure disorder, absence seizure, or other seizure
- neurological hard or soft signs (as age appropriate),
    - motor:
        - gross motor problems, poor tandem gait, positive romberg sign, balance problems
        - fine motor problems, poor eye-hand co-ordination, intentional tremor, motorically –disorganized in the under 5 year age group
    - sensory:
        - abnormal sensation upper or lower limbs,
        - neurosensory hearing loss,
        - Abnormal auditory, visual, gustatatory, olfactory, or tactile sensations,(including hallucinations), including craving touch and can make the patient a victim of false accusation of sexually inappropriate behavior
        - Regulatory Disorder, Hypersensitive or Hyposensitive, in the under 5-year age group
- and/or evidence of complex pattern of behavior, cognitive or language abnormalities that are inconsistent with developmental level and cannot be explained by familial backround or environment alone:
    - Behavioral:
        - attentional problems, visual and auditory
        - poor impulse control
        - working memory problems
        - poor adaptive functioning
    - Cognitive:
        - complex learning disorder with inability to link cause and effect
        - specific deficits in mathematical skills
        - marked split between verbal and performance IQ, over 12-15 points

- poor capacity for abstraction and metacognition
- deficits in school performance
- poor insight
- impaired judgment
  - Language:
    - deficits in higher level receptive and expressive language i.e.the patient does not fully comprehend the "gist" of a social situation
    - -impairment in social interaction
    - -problems in social perception, cognition and communication
    - -problems in expressing emotions, Alexithymia, where the patient does not have the words to express feelings and acts them out ,or expresses them, physically

In: ADHD and Fetal Alcohol Spectrum Disorders (FASD)
Editor: Kieran D. O'Malley, pp. 217-247

ISBN: 1-59454-573-1
© 2008 Nova Science Publishers, Inc.

Chapter 12

FETAL ALCOHOL SPECTRUM DISORDERS (FASD) IN THE ADULT: VULNERABILITY, DISABILITY, OR DIAGNOSIS - A PSYCHODYNAMIC PERSPECTIVE

Arthur K. Sullivan[*]

ABSTRACT

An adult with FASD presents a multitude of diagnostic and therapeutic challenges. Because the diagnosis still rests upon retrospective information, and often is not made until the life trajectory is firmly set, these patients may be referred for psychiatric evaluation from a wide range of settings. Associated with significant Axis I comorbidities, including depression, anxiety, and stress-related disorders, characterologic issues often take the forefront of practical management. From this point of view, an understanding of how the associated neurological lesions interact with developmental difficulties are relevant to management of the patient who has greater than 50% chance of requiring psychiatric intervention during his/her lifetime. Many factors work against the individual's attaining an adaptive repertoire of mature ego defenses, mature object relations, or a cohesive self. This paper reviews some of the major characteristics of FASD from a psychodynamic point of view, including the following: 1) potential impact of major neurological vulnerabilities on later psychological functioning; 2) early mother-child interactions that may lead to difficulties in the attachment process and their consequences; 3) deficits of cognitive and attentional processes that are recognized in later life by impulsivity and limitations in executive function; and 4) finally, a discussion of these findings in the context of alexithymia as a unifying construct around which to organize clinical thinking and further research.

---

[*] Present address: Dr. A.K. Sullivan; Department of Psychosocial Oncology and Palliative Care; Princess Margaret Hospital/ University Hospital Network; 610 University Avenue; Toronto, Ontario; Canada; Tel: 416-946-4525; e-mail: arthur.sullivan@uhn.on.ca

I. INTRODUCTION

John was a navy vet who had served his two years on dry land with a maintenance crew, and now at age 39 found himself in a veteran's hospital recovering from septic shock. Various diagnoses appeared on the record including depression, alcoholism, heroin addiction, and antisocial personality disorder. Many times he had held a gun to his head but had never managed to pull the trigger. His entry into the world was on a table in a tavern where the owner, his aunt, had hired a waitress, his mother, and remunerated her with one hot meal a day and free beer to keep her going the rest of the time. He recalled few personal details before junior high school when he began to enjoy fast cars and booze, resulting in frequent arrests for public mischief and brawling. However, there was minimal evidence otherwise for a conduct disorder during adolescence. While in the military he was introduced to heroin, and for the first time in his life found relief, though transient, from abiding anxiety and low self-esteem. After discharge he went through withdrawal and began to work in construction, only to develop back pain for which he was prescribed opiate analgesics. With irregular attendance on the job he was fired and assumed the life of a vagrant stowaway on freight trains, finding enough odd jobs to maintain a heroin addiction for himself and a female friend to whom he exhibited affection, loyalty, and devotion. The two shared custody of a small dog that accompanied them on their travels back and forth across the country. During the recent hospital admission, he expressed a firm desire to enroll once again in a methadone replacement program; because he could not organize himself to come on time for his doses, he had been discharged from another two years before.

Jane was an engaging woman of 45, referred for psychiatric evaluation by a radiation oncologist who was treating her for a malignant brain tumor; he felt that she was atypically "slow" and seemed not to grasp his explanations. She was one of eight children, and her mother had consumed alcohol heavily throughout all of her pregnancies. During high school she had managed to pass the basic courses by "my personality and charm" until she dropped out after grade 10. She herself drank heavily through three pregnancies, each the product of a different "abusive relationship". She had never been hospitalized except for her deliveries, and had lived independently working at various service jobs. Although neuropsychological testing measured a full scale IQ of 83, she was not able to follow through any of the Wisconsin card sort routines or Trails B tests of executive function, impulsively chasing the cues to wrong conclusions. Her opening words of the interview were, "I have fetal alcohol syndrome"; when asked how she knew that, she replied, "I'm not sure, but I think that's what they told me last year at AA."

A recently pregnant young woman sat in a restaurant sipping Perrier water and lemon while the family circle around her shared a bottle of expensive wine. From across the table, her uncle (a physician) delivered his lecture on the dangers of fetal alcohol effects and junior's outlook for loss of IQ points should she waver from abstinence. Another young woman nearby, overhearing the conversation, came to ask if she could join the discussion. She related how she was the youngest child of a single mother who had been severely depressed during pregnancy, had abused alcohol throughout, and died two years later. After passing through several foster homes and institutions, at age 13 she was placed with a teacher couple who had mentored her intensely through high school graduation and a year of junior college. During the next seven years she tried to live independently, starting and failing various academic and technical programs, living in perpetual financial disarray even though she had inherited comfortable means; she already had entered and left several "poor choice" relationships. For the past two years she had found stable employment as a clerk in an office that provided clear guidelines, structure, routine, and expectations. She had never heard of the fetal alcohol syndrome, and now wondered if she might have been so afflicted. One could imagine her upper lip as being a bit more thinned and flattened than usual – however, a picture of her older half-brother, a successful cardiologist now in his third marriage, showed similar features.

These illustrations from real life,[1] extending what once was a challenge for only the pediatrician, demonstrate some of the complexities and ambiguities of FASD, and draw our attention to issues that confront medical practitioners across the range of disciplines. Some individuals who have made it into adulthood bearing the consequences of maternal alcohol over-ingestion are aware of it while others are not, but all of them navigate life guided by the state of mind and body they have internalized through their accumulated experiences and relationships. Deviations from a healthy adaptive progression through developmental milestones can begin very early under the influence of genetic aberration or exposure to a neurotoxin. A near infinite number of influences impact on biological substrates, and in the cases described above, a small turn in the prism of fate could have changed the story of one into the other. As exemplified by more than thirty years of research into the fetal alcohol syndrome (FAS), many of these influences are set in motion even before birth. Thus, from a psychodynamic perspective the question arises as to whether the anatomic lesion(s) associated with FASD, assumed to be a reflection of altered neuronal connections and pathways within the brain, define a particular vulnerability to later expression of the character traits repeatedly observed in the syndrome. If so, can this condition be used as a model to explore how an individual forms his[2] internal representational world and how it can go awry?

Although a wealth of animal data exists on behavioral consequences of prenatal alcohol exposure, this review is limited to human studies. It aims to offer a framework around which to organize thoughts when performing a psychiatric assessment of an adult patient with a clinical history of prenatal alcohol exposure: 1) first, summarizing underlying functional disabilities in the cognitive, linguistic, and behavioral domains by which the clinical syndrome of FASD is recognized; 2) then, considering psychiatric comorbidities in the context of possible relational antecedents and consequences; and 3) finally, exploring how these patterns might be viewed in a psychodynamic context. For a summary of the fetal alcohol syndrome, a review by Olson (Olson, Morse, and Huffine, 1998), and the monograph of Streissguth and Kanter (Streissguth and Kanter, 1997) offer background details.

---

[1] To maintain confidentiality, identifying details of these individuals have been modified.
[2] Throughout this paper, "his" or "he" is used for convenience in a gender-neutral manner.

II. UNDERLYING VULNERABILITIES

A. Biological

1. "There is no Such Thing as a Baby"

In the decade following its original description, the fetal alcohol syndrome of the newborn, came to be characterized by growth inhibition, craniofacial abnormalities, and severe mental retardation (Jones, Smith, Ulleland, and Streissguth, 1973; Jones, Smith, Streissguth, and Myrianthopoulos, 1974). Subsequent publications (reviewed in Abel, 1981) reported further behavioral consequences in the newborn, infant, and toddler periods, including irritability, sleep disorders, and hyperactivity. In the first three days after full term birth, exposed infants showed increased tonicity of reflexes and level of activity, even when the mothers had abstained from alcohol after the second trimester, excluding an explanation of alcohol withdrawal alone (Coles, Smith, Fernhoff, and Falek, 1985). Acoustical analysis of crying on postnatal day three showed that emissions from infants of drinking mothers were more turbulent (dysphonation) and of a different frequency (formant frequency) than those of non-drinking mothers (Nugent, Lester, Green, Wieczorek-Deering, and O'Mahony, 1996). During the early months, some babies showed ineffective sucking to the extent that they required tube feedings for most of the first year (Van Dyke, Mackay, and Ziaylek, 1982). Beyond such extreme examples, however, more subtle disruption of the mother-infant feeding unit might occur. Considering the high comorbidity of alcohol abuse and eating disorders in women, the latter condition could add another contributing influence (Fischer, Anderson, and Smith, 2004; Keel, Dorer, Eddy, Franko, Charatan, and Herzog, 2003; Loxton, and Dawe, 2001; Sinha, and O'Malley, 2000; Dansky, Brewerton, and Kilpatrick, 2000). Indeed, a prospective study monitoring the sucking patterns of infants of mothers with eating disorders found that their daughters sucked faster and were weaned later, and at age 5 demonstrated more negative affect (Agras, Hammer, and McNicholas, 1999). Thus, even the earliest channels of communication and attachment that will enable optimal affect regulation in later life could be disrupted from the beginning. This situation well illustrates Winnicott's oft quoted observation (cited in the heading above) that an infant cannot be understood in isolation, but only as a mother-child in a nursing couple (Winnicott cited in Greenberg and Mitchell, 1983). Such considerations potentially could apply even to babies who would be adopted in the early days and weeks of life.

2. Evolving Disabilities During Childhood

As these babies become toddlers and preschoolers, further difficulties arise in domains of performance that intensify with increasing demands of socialization and education.

Inattention/Hyperactivity

The capacity to focus and sustain attention at will is a basic necessity upon which representation of a continuous self, others, and world will develop. Hyperactivity, distractibility, and short attention span was a recurrent observation in early descriptions of FAS (Aronson, Kyllerman, Sabel, Sandin, and Olegard, 1985), and studies outside of the laboratory confirmed that by age 3-5, children of mothers who drank more than occasionally throughout pregnancy exhibited shorter periods of focused attention and more fidgeting during mealtime (Landesman-Dwyer, and Ragozin, 1981). At the same time, multiple lifestyle variables related to social class also appeared to impact on the incidence and expression of the primary characteristics of FASD, including attention deficit hyperactivity disorder/ADHD (Landesman-Dwyer, and Ragozin, 1981). Note that prior observations had pointed out that early school age children, even from economically comfortable homes, whose intelligence lay within the normal range of IQ, still encountered difficulties related to hyperactivity, short attention span, and incapacity to apply self to learning, suggesting problems of a complexity greater than a mere learning disability (Shaywitz, Cohen, and Shaywitz, 1980). In various target populations the diagnosis of ADHD is made in as many as 70% of children with FASD (Burd, Klug, Martsolf, and Kerbeshian, 2003), and discussion continues as to whether the disease process differs from those without a history of alcohol exposure. Hyperactivity has been reported often in children exposed to alcohol during prenatal life, and the clinical manifestations and treatment issues appear to be more complex than in those without such a history (O'Malley, and Nanson, 2002; O'Malley, and Storoz, 2003).On the one hand, parental ratings of hyperactivity among 5-12 year olds with a diagnosis of ADD were similar in children with or without a history of prenatal alcohol exposure. Likewise, the two groups demonstrated identical profiles on laboratory indices of maintenance of attention, modulation of arousal, and inhibition of impulsive responses (Nanson, and Hiscock, 1990). However, these authors also called attention to the difficulty in dissecting which elements resulted from the neurological lesion(s), in contrast to those acquired as a result of past environmental disruption. On the other hand, interpretation of their difficulties with tests measuring attention was compounded by deficits in visual/spacial comprehension, encoding of information, and flexibility in problem solving, whereas children with "simple" ADHD alone were identified by problems more restricted to their ability to focus and sustain attention (Coles, Platzman, Raskin-Hood, Brown, Falek, and Smith, 1997; Coles, 2001).Relatively simple measures of attention (e.g., Freedom from Distractibility index from the Wechsler Intelligence scale) and caregiver observation (Achenbach Child Behavior checklist) were able to differentiate children with histories of heavy prenatal alcohol exposure from controls matched for social status and ethnicity (Lee, Mattson, and Riley, 2004). The capacity to control attention has been linked to the successful development of social competence, and deficits appear to predict aggressive behaviors in elementary school children (reviewed in Wilson, 2003). Within this model, a child who can adeptly shift attention and not become fixated upon a negative bias can broaden the inflow of information, and thus modulate emotional activation. A shift from input laden with hostility or rejection to a more positive focus will lead to the more adaptive behavioral regulation that is essential to develop healthy social interactions (and by implication, more developed object relations). Wilson (2003) has presented experimental evidence that kindergarten children who were considered aggressive and rejected by their peers took a longer time to shift attention from an angry to a happy stimulus (human face), showed less cooperative interactions, and more negative behaviors in the test situation.

In his classic work on patterns underlying character disorders, Shapiro has defined the "Impulsive" as one of four fundamental "neurotic styles" (Shapiro, 1965), and the DSM-IV lists impulsive traits as one of the cardinal descriptors of both borderline and antisocial personality disorders. While expressed in a wide range, from individual trend to pervasive pattern of cognition, affective experience and behavior, the severely impulsive do not grasp the normal feeling of deliberateness and intention, and can even defensively disavow it.

Integration and organization of mental function into a sustained intentionality that enables further construction of internal working models of the world fall behind. A concrete immediacy guides action and the future takes care of itself. From a classic psychodynamic point of view, in the highly impulsive individual, primitive drives/impulses ("id") and their derivatives are not as well modulated by "ego" executive function (see executive function below), and the influences of external prohibition and authority are not internalized into a mode of thought and subjective emotional experience conceptualized as "superego". Current research efforts are attempting to define and operationalize the construct of impulsivity, and elucidate how it relates to executive function (Moeller, Barratt, Dougherty, Schmitz, and Swann, 2001).

Standardized Intelligence Quotient and Memory

Neuropsychological testing of preschoolers demonstrated subnormal scores on several verbal, motor, and perceptual performance scales (Janzen, Nanson, and Block, 1995). By school age, children in most studies showed an intelligence level below the norm as measured by standardized IQ tests, generally in proportion to the extent of physical malformation (reviewed by Mattson and Riley, 1998; Streissguth and O'Malley, 2000). However, prenatal alcohol exposure at an undetermined threshold, even when subsequent abnormalities of facial morphology or growth retardation are not evident, can result in lowering of both verbal and performance IQ (Mattson, Riley, Gramling, Delis, and Jones, 1997). Further examination of children in kindergarten through grade 7 showed that while short-term object recall did not differ from controls, delayed recall was less, as was ability to recreate a spatial arrangement, plan a solution to a maze, and draw an accurate representation of a clock face(Uecker, and Nadel, 1996; Uecker, and Nadel, 1998). This raised suspicion of a diffuse pathological process involving at least hippocampal, parietal, frontal, and cerebellar areas. Further refinements of experimental protocols allowed dissection of memory and attentional process into subcomponents in a group of higher functioning adolescents of age 9-18 (Kodituwakku, Handmaker, Cutler, Weathersby, and Handmaker, 1995). Although in this study the subjects did not differ from controls in story or design memory, those with a diagnosis of FAS performed less well on tasks of increasing complexity involving manipulation of information in working memory, as well as in planning, sequencing and changing strategies to attain a goal. Contrary to expectation, they did not find any impairment on tests of self-regulatory ability (e.g., inhibition of dominant responses), leading the authors to propose that prenatal alcohol exposure may involve disruption of memory circuits in the central executive system. Exclusion criteria of the experimental protocol, however, may have led to removal of the more severely affected children with concurrent ADHD. As long-term studies extended into secondary school, it became evident that IQ alone was not the best predictor of disability (extensively reviewed by Streissguth, Barr, Kogan, and Bookstein, 1996, and references therein). A specially selected subgroup of 8 young adults (age 16-27) from the Seattle follow-up study diagnosed with FAS, but a full scale IQ >90 and within the average range for academic achievement, was assessed with a battery of tests to probe integrity of frontal lobe functions. Results showed that as a group, their scores were below the norm on tests requiring sustained attention and capacity to override distraction during a learning task (Kerns, Don, Mateer, and Streissguth, 1997).

Language and Communication

Associated with IQ is the capacity to transform consciousness into symbols, and use them to manipulate ideas, reflect upon the self, and communicate the results. Early case reports of children with FAS documented a decreased capacity to comprehend prepositions, follow 2-stage commands, and appreciate prosody of speech, along with failure to engage at school (Shaywitz, Caparulo, and Hodgson, 1981). In a small series (8 subjects, age 4.5-9.5) designed to dissect components of speech and carefully control for cultural variables, researchers found that children with full FAS had not developed a normal capacity for language in multiple domains. These included impaired production of sounds, storage of words in short-term memory, production of accurate sentences in spontaneous conversation, and comprehension of single words, syntax, and verbal commands (Becker, Warr-Leeper, and Leeper, 1990). However, prospective studies examining children yearly for the first three years of life suggested that alcohol exposure alone without expression of dysmorphic features (e.g., FAE) was not as strong a predictor of expressive or receptive language deficits as was the home environment (Streissguth, Barr, Sampson, Darby, and Martin, 1989; Greene, Ernhart, Martier, Sokol, and Ager, 1990). Others showed that exposure even after the first trimester of organogenesis, at an apparent threshold of a mother's one drink/day during the second trimester, was associated with poorer reading and spelling performance at age six while difficulties with arithmetic appeared to be more related to the alcohol dose (Goldschmidt, Richardson, Stoffer, Geva, Day, 1996). A potential confound in this was the observation that 23 of 29 FAS children between ages 4-12 with retarded speech development had untreated recurrent serous otitis media associated with conductive hearing deficit verified by analysis of auditory evoked potentials (Rössig, Wässer, and Opperman, 1994). Whether this is a result of dysmorphic features and aberrant auditory canals, caregiver neglect, or some other cause(s) is not known.

Mattson and coworkers have published a series of papers aimed to characterize the learning deficits particular to children and adolescents exposed to alcohol *in utero*.

They found that when compared to control samples matched for age, gender, and ethnicity, children with FAS showed less ability to learn and recall words and did not show the same degree of improvement from repeated exposure as the controls. Since recall of previously learned words was like the norm, they concluded that the neurological defect was one of encoding (Mattson, Riley, Delis, Stern, and Jones, 1996). This pattern was consistent in both children with facial dysmorphology (i.e., FAS) and those similarly exposed to alcohol but without the characteristic constellation of bony defects (i.e., FAE) (Mattson, Riley, Gramling, and Delis, 1998). Using refinements of the test paradigm to distinguish patterns of memory retrieval, they found that while both FAS and Down's children showed defects in explicit memory (with FAS approximately halfway between Down's and controls), in FAS implicit (primed) memory remained intact (Mattson, and Riley, 1998). Other findings that recognition memory was better preserved than speed of information processing was consistent with this (Jacobson, 1998). Controversy continues as to whether this is related more to lesions in the basal ganglia, tempolimbic connections, or both.

Another component of language that is used in social interactions to communicate emotional content is the capacity to comprehend affective prosody. This was tested in eleven right-handed adult males (age 34-56) with a history of prenatal alcohol exposure, with demonstration of a clear deficit pattern similar to comparison subjects who had suffered right or left hemispheric damage (Monnot, Lovallo, Nixon, and Ross, 2002). The authors point out that this function is primarily located in the right parietal area, which must communicate through the corpus callosum to coordinate with other parts of the brain (e.g., Broca's and Wernicke's areas on the left) in the production of speech. This may be especially relevant to recent findings on structural defects in the corpus callosum in individuals with FAS described below.

Finally, extreme deficit in communication and language is one of the major characteristics of autism, the incidence of which was increased in case series of children with severe FAS (Nanson, 1992) or FAE (Harris, MacKay, and Osborn, 1995). Also, family studies have documented a high incidence of maternal alcoholism associated with probands presenting with the regressive form of autism (Miles, Takahashi, Haber, and Hadden, 2003).

Executive Function

After storage and retrieval of information, the brain must evaluate it adaptively when called upon to mediate between an internal call for action and external prohibitions. Experimental psychology approaches this task through the construct of "executive function" (EF) (Royall, Lauterbach, Cummings, Reeve, Rummans, Kaufer, LaFrance, and Coffey, 2002). Four domains of this include planning, cognitive flexibility, selective inhibition, and concept formation/reasoning. Giancola (2004), based upon experiments designed to measure interaction between EF and aggression, has concluded that "EF is more than the sum of its parts...is related to, and even predicts, the expression of aggressive and violent behavior." This is highly reminiscent of Freud's description of the phenomenology of the ego.

Again, in a manner not related to IQ, alcohol exposed children performed less well in both verbal and nonverbal based tasks of EF, consistent with damage to the frontal lobes (Mattson, Goodman, Caine, Delis, and Riley, 1999; Schonfeld, Mattson, Lang, and Delis, 2001). The tapping inhibition test, which reflects function of the frontal-subcortical circuit, given to 4 year old children of mothers who abused multiple substances during pregnancy, revealed lower scores related to alcohol intake but not to cocaine or marijuana use (Noland, Singer, Arendt, Minnes, Short, and Bearer, 2003). Examining mutual influence between IQ and executive function with an expanded battery of tests, Connor *et al* found that some apparent deficits were fully explained on the basis of IQ alone, while others (Wisconsin card sort, Stroop, trail making, and figure fluency generation) were more specific to alcohol damage (Connor, Sampson, Bookstein, Barr, and Streissguth, 2000). This is consistent with what had been reported previously by the same group on younger children's disproportionately lower performance using the Vineland instrument. Furthermore, the presence of typical facial dysmorphology was not associated with a more severe deficit in EF than were those similarly exposed to alcohol but lacking those features.

The tests most affected by chronic prenatal alcohol exposure reflect an individual who is disabled in the capacity to shift tasks when rules are not certain, maintain complex attention, and work with information in the presence of distraction. This pattern is similar to patients with damage to the orbitofrontal cortex due to other causes who show deficits in certain motivation-based executive tasks (reviewed by Kodituwakku, Kalberg, and May, 2001). Such deficits translate into a range of behavioral problems that correlate with lower scores on measures of executive function (e.g., perseverative errors on the Wisconsin card sort), and reversal of learned response-reward associations to changing conditions (e.g., visual discrimination reversal test, an "emotion" related measure) (Kodituwakku, May, Clericuzio, and Weers, 2001). Laboratory studies on non-clinical populations have shown that men testing in the lower range of EF also displayed a more aggressive response to provocation, as well as increased aggression after a test dose of alcohol (Giancola, 2004). The first clear evidence linking neurophysiological abnormalities to potential brain damage came with reports of complex partial seizures and abnormal EEG rhythms in the non-dominant or both temporal lobes (O'Malley, 1998). Further precision came with clear demonstration on MRI imaging of morphological abnormalities in the corpus callosum (Bookstein, Sampson, Streissguth, and Connor, 2001). The Seattle group further documented two patterns - callosal thickening associated more often with a deficit in EF, and callosal thinning associated with motor dysfunction (Bookstein, Streissguth, Sampson, Connor, and Barr, 2002). Thus, evidence exists for a clinically significant diffuse process involving at least the frontal, parietal, and temporal areas, as well as the corpus callosum, that can predict behavioral consequences.

B. Psychological

With physical malformations and related neurological deficits documented, investigators in Germany reported several studies on the psychological sequellae of FAS/FAE, based primarily on caregiver reports of children followed in a large clinic for developmental disabilities. By age 4-10, children with physical stigmata of alcohol embryopathy had exhibited stereotyped habits, difficulty with peers, dependency, and temper tantrums in association with decreased performance in measures of visual perception (e.g., figure-ground relationships) and verbal expression (Steinhausen, Nestler, and Huth, 1982). Observations on the whole group (both FAS and FAE) confirmed hyperkinetic behaviors and "social problems" most frequently (Steinhausen, and Spohr, 1998). Longitudinal studies found that along with these problems, as well as difficulties with speech and sleep, states of depression and anxiety became manifest (Steinhausen, Willms, and Spohr, 1993). They also noted that some children with less severe cognitive deficits improved over the course of 36 months (Steinhausen, Göbel, and Nestler, 1984), and drew attention to a trend that children with alcoholic fathers manifested more problems with conduct, while those with alcoholic mothers exhibited more "disturbance of emotions". Other longitudinal studies in Seattle, documented a wide range of maladaptive social behaviors compatible with a generalized skills deficit (reviewed by Kelly, Day , and Streissguth, 2000). However, the degree of severity of behavioral difficulties is multifactorial. Although results based on caregiver observation (e.g., Child Behavior Checklist) consistently pointed to problems in the "social, attention, and aggressive" domains, socioeconomic status of parents tended to be associated with internalizing problems (e.g., depression/anxiety), and deficit in verbal IQ with externalizing behaviors (e.g., acting out) (Mattson, and Riley, 2000). Using further screening tools based on caregiver observation (Personality Inventory for Children), other laboratories confirmed that as a group children with both FAS and FAE were outside of the norm on most indices of behavioral functioning, indicating a high incidence of potential psychopathology, including psychosis (Roebuck, Mattson, and Riley, 1999). Such conclusions, however, demand caution, as "psychosis" subscales so defined are neither sufficient for nor necessarily supportive of a psychiatric diagnosis of a psychotic disorder and its prognostic implications. Interpretation of diagnostic inferences from such instruments relies upon selection of an appropriate comparison group. Thus, when compared to a clinical sample of children (age 1.5 to 10.5) referred for a variety of behavioral problems, those who had been exposed to alcohol in the prenatal period did not differ from those who had not on measures of communication, daily living skills, or socialization (Vineland Adaptive Behavior Scales) (Whaley, O'Connor, and Gunderson, 2001). Over the period from infancy through latency, however, their rate of decline was significantly faster than the others, even after controlling for factors such as multiple home placements. In a recent update of the Seattle cohort, time spent in a stable nurturing home was reported to be the most influential protective factor for the five major secondary disabilities (inappropriate sexual behavior, disrupted school experience, trouble with the law, confinement to a mental health facility or correctional institution, and drug/alcohol problems) (Streissguth, Bookstein, Barr, Sampson, O'Malley, and Young, 2004). Furthermore, in a population of inner city adolescents identified as part of a follow-up study based in a prenatal clinic (i.e., not referred for evaluation of behavior problems), those who had been exposed to alcohol *in utero* did not self report any more delinquent behaviors than the non-exposed group. The investigators found that life stress, substance use, and low level of parental supervision were more predictive of a wide range of aberrant behaviors (Lynch, Coles, Corley, and Falek, 2003). Thus, it still is not fully resolved the extent to which prenatal alcohol exposure contributes to the behavioral phenotype of the evolving adult with FASD, independent of exposure to the consequences of an alcoholic mother, father, and their living environments (Weinberg, 1997).

III. ADAPTATION TO LIFE: INHIBITIONS

A. Attachment

At some point in the first weeks and months of life, an infant emerges from the world of somatosensory impression into one of causes, effects, and formed memories (Phillips JL, 1975). During this time his biological and psychological endowments activate behavioral patterns necessary to attract the caregiving on which survival depends. This inclination to attachment, or object seeking, is a fundamental life process that sets the template for how an individual will form a representation of his inner and outer world, and acquire the capability to regulate his affects in the years to come (Schore, 1994). Attachment theory and its experimental basis are described in recent expositions (Goldberg, Muir, and Kerr, 2000; Fonagy, 2001). Empirical studies often approach the study of attachment using the experimental paradigm of the "strange situation", in which a child (usually around 12 months of age) and caregiver are exposed to brief encounters of separation and reunification in order to activate the process. The resulting patterns form the basis of a broad classification into secure, insecure, and disorganized types, which can be transmitted across generations and correlate with certain psychopathologies in later life. In a study of children with a history of prenatal alcohol exposure, >50% of the one-year olds exhibited "insecure" attachment behaviors. Mothers of insecure infants reported drinking more than twice the alcohol during their pregnancy than did mothers of secure children. The difference was most marked for the disorganized/disoriented pattern that has been identified as a risk factor for development of more severe character disorders in adulthood (O'Conner, Sigman, and Brill, 1987). Again, toxin/alcohol exposure itself may not be the only factor of consequence. In assessing the stability of attachment pattern from 12-18 months in relation to various parental characteristics, investigators found that it tended to be stable for the most part; of note, this group was selected to exclude the more heavily exposed children (> 0.5 oz/day). The mothers of children whose attachment pattern remained "insecure" from 12 to 18 months, more often were depressed, endorsed more symptoms of alcohol-related difficulties, and expressed more negative affect during play with the child. These children expressed more negative affect in other experimental situations. In addition, examination of paternal interaction patterns showed that more alcohol abuse was associated with lower levels of paternal positive affect and decreased sensitivity during a standardized play situation. Marital aggression and adjustment alone were not related to the attachment pattern toward either parent (Edwards, Eiden, and Leonard, 2004). Recent studies examined the behaviors through which a mother's own disorganized/unresolved attachment style may convey an insecure or disorganized pattern toward her child. They found that in a community derived sample, the children of mothers with unresolved attachment patterns had a greater tendency to behave in a disorganized manner in the strange situation procedure. Accordingly, infants in the disorganized/insecure group had mothers who displayed more disrupted affective communication in the Atypical Maternal Behavior Instrument. However, statistical analyses applied by the authors inferred that factors other than the atypical behaviors of the mother mediated between unresolved maternal attachment and infant disorganization. They suggested further studies to clarify if maternal physical handicap, mental health, or family relationships may supply the missing links (Goldberg, Benoit, Blokland, and Madigan, 2003). Thus, much research remains to be done to precisely define if/where alcohol exposure itself, and the subsequent neuropathological lesions borne by the child, lead to impairment of the attachment-seeking mechanisms early in life.

B. Parent Distress

In Western societies at least, disorganized and insecurely attached toddlers tend to coexist in environments with insecurely attached mothers. This raises questions about the internal state of a mother whose alcohol dependency so overrides "primary maternal preoccupation" (Winnicott, 1975) that she continues to drink at critical stages of her pregnancy: what is her background, what does she bring to the mother-child relationship, and what of her own accumulated trauma does she transmit? What are the consequences of a child's exposure to alcohol – the teratogen – apart from and in synergy with the behavioral manifestations and projections onto/into the child of a mother whose personality and defensive structure had led her to an alcohol dependent or addictive lifestyle? The psychoanalytic literature has begun to acknowledge the transgenerational transmission of trauma. (Share, 1994; Share, personal communication, 2001;[3] Volkan, Ast, and Greer, 2002) At the investigational level, the study has yet to be done comparing the outcome of children of drinking mothers stratified for equivalent attachment and trauma history.

Mother/caregiver-child bonding can unfold in many ways that would influence subsequent personality development, and the consequences of being born into a family in

---

[3] Share L. The psychoanalytic theory and method of Bernard Bail: an overview. Paper presented at the meeting of the American Psychoanalytic Association, December 20, 2001, New York.

which one or both parents are alcoholic can be profound (reviewed by Murray, 1989). Difficulties include those of poor parental role modeling, disturbed development of trust and identity, patterns of avoidant coping behavior, dysfunctional adolescent and adult relationships, and economic disadvantage. In a sample of all birthmothers in the state of Minnesota who had received prenatal care during the year 2000 and agreed to complete a survey on alcohol use, 20% of responders reported continued alcohol use by the time of their first prenatal visit. The drinkers tended to report more depressed mood than the abstainers, to initiate prenatal care later, and perceive more problems related to alcohol ((Meschke, Holl, and Messelt, 2003). In an unselected population of women presenting for prenatal care to an inner London hospital in the 1980's, investigators found that about half of the women drank some alcohol as late as 36 weeks. Perhaps surprisingly, the prototypic pattern of the drinking mother was a woman who was married, employed, older, and of higher educational and social attainment. The heaviest consumers (> 70 gm/wk of absolute ethanol or > 1 drink/day), however, segregated into three patterns: (1) smoking, unmarried, minimally educated, unhappy to be pregnant, and having received psychiatric treatment; (2) non-smoking, married, more education, not unhappy to be pregnant, and unlikely to have been treated for any psychiatric condition; (3) smokers, intermediate in other categories. Thus, at least in this population, mothers who continued to drink most heavily during pregnancy appeared to inhabit a wide social spectrum (Heller, Anderson, Bland, Brooke, Peacock, and Stewart, 1988). Unfortunately, data were not presented on the relative incidence of FASD in the subgroups. Mothers of preadolescent children, living in a residential facility for treatment of drug or alcohol dependence, completed self-report questionnaires on their own childhood experiences in relation to their later parenting styles. The majority of these women reported growing up under adverse family circumstances, and the more neglectful and negative the home environment, the more difficulty they reported with parenting distress and problematic parenting behaviors. These authors reviewed evidence that parenting stress can lead to over-reactive and inconsistent styles, that in turn can escalate the child's problematic behaviors, perpetuating the cycle. Furthermore, in keeping with the psychodynamic processes of anger displacement, maternal depression was found to be associated with inconsistent discipline, and use of guilt and anxiety as a means of exerting control over an unruly child (Harmer, Sanderson, and Mertin, 1999). In an urban substance abuse clinic, MMPI-2 scores of a multiracial population of pregnant women who continued to abuse alcohol in addition to other substances were compared with those who did not. The former showed a trend toward more endorsement of depression in addition to psychopathy, but the difference was found only in the white subpopulation (Miles, Svikis, Kulstad, and Haug, 2001). Another study of women incarcerated for repeated convictions for driving while intoxicated showed that most had begun drinking by age 15, were not living with a partner, abused multiple substances, gave birth to her first child by age 20, and often had cared for the child while under the influence of a substance (Goldberg, Lex, Mello, Mendelson, and Bower, 1996). Sixty percent had drunk throughout pregnancy, 28% already had delivered a low-birth weight infant, and in two thirds the child had not lived with her for significant periods of time; attempts at reunification generally were not successful. In an extremely economically disadvantaged group (a high risk Native American population), retrospective review of medical records found that the mothers of children born with FAS were much more likely to have problems with substance abuse, more mental health interventions, frequent suicide attempts, unintentional injuries, and sexual abuse. At least one third of the case mothers themselves had cognitive dysfunction suggestive of FAS (Kvigne, Leonardson, Borzelleca, Brock, Neff-Smith, and Welty, 2003).

Parenting seen from the child's point of view also can be instructive. A survey of elementary school age children from predominantly white upper and middle class homes whose mothers had sought treatment for alcoholism perceived (Children's Report of Parental Behavior Inventory) more control through guilt, leading authors to suggest that the mother's conflicts over her own alcohol abuse were being projected onto the child (Marcus, and Tisne, 1987). A longitudinal study with two multiethnic cohorts of junior high school students in Los Angeles confirmed previous studies that had proposed that selection of peers and disruptive behaviors (e.g., fighting, dangerous activities, destruction of property) were major determinants of alcohol use before high school. They went on to show that parental monitoring and a positive parental relationship (e.g., praise of child, communication of pride, fun time together, and expression of affection) was protective against disruptive behaviors and vulnerability to peer pressures to drink. Time spent with and communication with the child in grade 7 was a predictor of a perceived positive relationship in later grades (Cohen, Richardson, and LaBree, 1994). These findings could be interpreted in the context of a developing individual's notion of self-worth, with adolescent alcohol use a symptom of dysfunctional coping in the face of insecure attachment. Among residents of a home for boys (age 13-19) with recurrent drug and alcohol problems, only 21% had been living in two parent households, the mothers tended to have had more marriages, divorces, and children with multiple partners, and both parents generally were of lower socioeconomic status than controls matched for ethnicity and location of residence. In the situations where fathers were absent, maternal alcohol abuse and antisocial characteristics correlated with greater severity of substance related problems in the youth. Although other family process variables were elicited, none predicted severity (Gabel, Stallings, Young, Schmitz, Crowley, and Fulker, 1998). Frank *et al* have drawn attention to the possibility that adjustment problems can be related to paternal alcohol consumption as well. They found that for 22% of mothers with a history of cocaine abuse, the father of the child also had a drug and/or alcohol problem. These mothers tended to experience significantly more mental and physical abuse and deliver babies weighing 97 gm less than the others; however, head circumference (a severity marker for FAS) was not different (Frank, Brown, Johnson, and Cabral, 2002). By the teen years, children of alcoholic parents, especially when both were affected, had a higher incidence of oppositional defiant disorder and conduct disorder diagnosable by structured interviews (Reich, Earls, Frankel, and Shayka, 1993). Thus, from the point of view of "secondary disabilities" and psychopathology in later life, perhaps the more accurate descriptor of the condition could be the "parental alcohol abuse syndrome". The many currents leading to inclusion of a misnamed (according to those authors) "fetal alcohol syndrome" into the medical diagnostic vocabulary, with subsequent creation of an academic industry around it, have received attention from the sociological perspective (Armstrong, 1998).

IV. ADAPTATION TO LIFE: PSYCHOPATHOLOGY

Whatever the nature and origin of the disabilities, the social consequences of FASD is not trivial. In a prospective study of all youths remanded to a British Columbia detention center for evaluation over the course of one year, the diagnosis of FAS or FAE was made in 23%, and *in only 3 of the 67 had it been made prior to incarceration* (Fast, Conry, and Loock, 1999). This implies, in a manner similar to the case illustrations at the beginning of this chapter, that as late as the mid-1990's the diagnosis of FASD still went undetected most of the time. As these children enter adulthood, in many of them patterns of mental illness have already begun to unfold. Several investigations focusing on the neurological consequences of FAS also probed its psychological manifestations. The German prospective study that had followed a cohort of >150 children found that by pre-school age, a global psychopathology rating obtained from structured assessments increased in relation to the severity of the morphological damage and with institutionalization. Most notable were trends to enuresis, eating, speech, hyperkinetic disorders, stereotypies, and depression (Steinhausen, Willms, and Spohr, 1994). An attempt to describe a behavioral phenotype, again based on the results of parental report using the Developmental Behavioral Checklist, identified subscales ("disruptive, self-absorbed, anxiety, antisocial behavior, and communication disturbance") that seemed to distinguish individuals with FAS/FAE from the control population (Steinhausen, Willms, Metzke, and Spohr, 2003). However, such correlation between prenatal alcohol exposure and subsequent psychopathology has been called into question by investigators using statistical methods designed to control for highly interrelated variables. In their sample, Hill *et al* found that the apparent association between retrospectively estimated maternal alcohol consumption and child/adolescent externalizing disorders, depression, and ADHD did not remain when *family* history of alcoholism was considered. They concluded that the familial predisposition to alcohol dependence led to other behaviors such as smoking and drinking during pregnancy, and to associated psychopathology (Hill, Lowers, Locke-Wellman, and Shen, 2000). The first study to report combined use of parental report and psychiatric interviews with the children themselves (both full FAS and alcohol related neurodevelopmental disorder with IQ>70, age 5-13) found that 61% had symptoms consistent with a mood disorder (major depression, adjustment disorder with depression, and bipolar disorder). In none of them was a diagnosis of psychotic disorder made, indicating either a major difference between the study population of the previously cited reports, or perhaps, underscoring that in these days of "operationalization" and standardized instruments, talking with your patients is still important (O'Connor, Shah, Whaley, Cronin, and Gunderson, 2002). By early adulthood, structured clinical interviews (SCID) of 25 subjects with FAS/FAE and IQ >70 indicated the presence of a DSM-IV/Axis I disorder in 92%, with substance abuse disorders (60%), major depressive disorder (44%), brief psychotic disorder (28%), and bipolar disorder (20%) being the most frequent designations (Famy, Streissguth, and Unis, 1998). However, only 18/25 had received any psychiatric treatment. Considering that this group tended to be derived from an environment relatively rich in medical resources, this figure may be an overestimate of the psychiatric care generally available to persons living with FASD. To date there have not been any studies reported investigating the adult personality structure of individuals with FASD viewed from any of the major psychoanalytic models, including ego psychology, object relations, or self psychology.

V. ALEXITHYMIA AS A UNIFYING MECHANISM

The capacity to process experience into emotions, and then attend to them, regulate them, and find words to communicate them in a reciprocal manner to another is a defining achievement for the human species and a developmental aspiration for each human being. Within the spectrum of individual potential is a wide range of attainment with many points of vulnerability along the way. As a broad measure of psychological functioning, the capacity (or lack thereof) to identify and communicate feelings has been operationalized in the construct of alexithymia – literally, no words for emotions. Although first used by Sifneos (1973) to describe patients who seemed unable to make progress during psychoanalytic therapy, and who tended to focus unexpressed emotion onto somatic components of arousal, alexithymia has become a unifying concept in efforts to understand and dissect mechanisms in many areas of psychopathology. Hundreds of research reports on the subject have relied upon a standardized instrument, the Toronto Alexithymia Scale (TAS-20) (Parker, Taylor, and Bagby, 2003). Many key elements of childhood FASD relevant to adult psychiatry (e.g., primary deficits in attention, memory, language, executive function, and affect regulation, along with adaptive response to environmental adversities) might foreshadow alexithymic traits or defenses. In earlier reviews Krystal (1988), McDougall (1982), and Taylor, Bagby, and Parker (2000) described psychoanalytic thinking, and more recently Taylor has summarized current research (Taylor, 2000; Taylor and Bagby, 2004) on the topic. Larsen, Brand, Bermond, and Hijman (2003) have reviewed some of the applications of neurobiological studies to alexithymia research. In the following, we present selected aspects of the alexithymia construct that may provide insight into understanding patients with FASD.

Alexithymics Processes Emotion Differently and May Reflect a Lateralized Function within the Brain

Clinical observations had suggested that patients with congenital absence of the corpus callosum or disruption following surgical transection for epilepsy appeared to be alexithymic. Thus, full appreciation of emotional awareness may depend upon communication between lateralized functions within the brain (Gazzaniga, 2000). Taylor (2000; 2004) further proposed that in individuals testing "high" on measures of alexithymia, interhemispheric cooperation might be insufficient to enable the usual emotional processing on the right side. Further evidence arising from indirect measurement of transcallosal conduction using a technique of ipsilateral motor inhibition after transcranial magnetic stimulation of the motor cortex showed that in non-clinical samples of alexithymic males, but not females, left to right hemispheric transfer was facilitated. (Apparently, faster does not necessarily mean better.) The significance of this in relation to possible neuroanatomic correlates is not yet defined (Grabe, Möller, Willert, Spitzer, Rizos, and Freyberger, 2004). However, imaging and electrophysiological studies have added further strength to support a neurological basis for alexithymic traits. Magnetic resonance imaging of healthy college students found that the size of the right anterior cingulate gyrus correlated with the total score on the TAS-20 in both men and women, but most markedly for men. The authors proposed that this association could represent a dysfunctional organization of the neuronal inhibitory mechanism that directs attention toward emotional cues, and functions to down regulate emotional processing (Gündel, López-Sala, Ceballos-Baumann, Deus, Cardoner, Marten-Mittag, Soriano-Mas, and Pujol, 2004). Functional imaging studies have enabled further anatomic correlations in individuals with high and low alexithymia.[4] Selected subjects were shown images of faces displaying happy, sad, or angry emotions in increasing intensity. Ax-h individuals had less blood flow in several loci in the right frontal and parietal areas with compensatory increase on the left. Furthermore, the anterior cingulate and insula were less activated in response to angry faces. A negative correlation with right cerebral blood flow and the TAS was found after presentation of angry and sad faces, but not for happy or neutral probes. These results were interpreted as suggesting a deficit in cognitive comprehension of emotion in the Ax-h subjects, consistent with other evidence that the right parietal area is essential for emotional processing, and right frontal for comprehension of facial and vocal expression. Differences were not found in the limbic areas, compatible with the view that this area may be specialized more for the perceptual aspects of emotion (Kano, Fukudo, Gyoba, Kamachi, Takawa, Mochizuki, Itoh, Hongo, and Yanai, 2003. Further confirmation of active processes within the brain has come from a study of the EEG response to emotionally charged visual stimuli (visual event related potentials following presentation of violent pictures). Ax-h subjects perceived and processed the emotional information of the probe, but did not report positively to questioning as to whether they had noticed it. The authors interpreted this to imply that such individuals use incomplete or inconsistent cognitive schemas to appraise and attach meaning to emotional information. They further speculated that this apparent dissociation between perception and meaning might be an adaptive process whereby adverse childhood experience resulted in developing preventive avoidance. The consequences of this, perhaps recognized as maladaptive interpersonal behaviors, could impede relationships and lead to psychiatric symptoms of anxiety and depression (Franz, Schaefer, Schneider, Sitte, and Bachor, 2004). Similarly, examination of theta frequency event-related synchronization of subjects viewing pleasant and unpleasant pictures detected differences between Ax-h and Ax-l individuals, with lateralized differences – decreased left hemispheric and increased right synchronization (Aftanas, Varlamov, Reva, and Pavlov, 2003).

Since important steps in the production and comprehension of speech and emotion are lateralized, and finding words for emotions are inherent in the definition of alexithymia, the two phenomena might be associated. Data from a large birth cohort followed longitudinally in Finland, showed a statistical trend for adult Ax-h subjects to have learned to speak late (i.e., no words at age 1), and for late speakers to have slightly higher TAS-20 scores (Kokkonen, Veijola, Karvonen, Läksy, Jokelainen, Järvelin, and Joukamaa, 2003). Other studies from the same cohort demonstrated a greater tendency for Ax-h individuals to be the product of an unwanted pregnancy and originate from a family of more than 4 children (Joukamaa, Kokkonen, Veijola, Läksy, Karvonen, Jokelainen, and Järvelin, 2003).

---

[4] Unless otherwise stated, conditions described as "alexithymic" or "high alexithymia" refer to scores attained in the designated range on the TAS-20 instrument. Abbreviations: Ax-h = high alexithymia; Ax-l = low alexithymia.

Alexithymia Can Predict Psychopathology in Non-Clinical Populations

A survey of Swiss medical and nursing students using the TAS-20 showed a close correlation between alexithymia (> 60 on TAS-20), especially the factor reflecting "difficulty identifying feelings" (Factor 1 "DIF" of the TAS-20), and higher scores on measures of depression and borderline pathology, as well as a general perception of poor physical and mental health. On multivariate analysis, the correlation with depression appeared to be dependent on the presence of borderline characteristics (Modestin, Furrer, and Malti, 2004). In view of known associations between early emotional trauma, borderline pathology, and self-mutilation, Paivio et al hypothesized alexithymia to be a mediator between childhood trauma and later self-injurious behavior, suggesting that abusive and neglectful environments provide limited opportunities for children to learn how to effectively express and cope with painful emotions (Paivio, and McCulloch, 2004). They surveyed female undergraduate students with questionnaires about childhood trauma, self-injurious behaviors of non-suicidal intent, and the TAS-20, and found evidence for interaction between alexithymia, childhood abuse/neglect, later affect dysregulation, and self-injurious behaviors. Thus, difficulty in identifying and communicating feelings may lead to the externalizing behavior of deliberate self-injury. In a group of female university students assessed for attachment pattern by the Adult Attachment Scale (a self-report instrument of 18 items), secure attachment and alexithymia correlated inversely. Measures of negative affectivity and alexithymia were associated with each other and with both types of insecure attachment, suggesting that the experience of rejecting or inconsistent parenting may have impaired their formation of good attachment objects (Wearden, Cook, and Vaughan-Jones, 2003). These trends continue in patient populations. Exploring the notion of alexithymia as a mode of affect regulation in which inner experience is denied and focus turns to external conditions in response to difficulty identifying and describing feelings, investigators looked for common risk factors in a series of patients (non-psychotic) admitted to an inpatient unit. Using self report instruments to assess past sexual trauma, perception of their parental relationships, and the TAS-20, the occurrence of recalled sexual abuse alone (which included a wide range of severity) did not correlate with the degree of alexithymia, whereas the less caring or more overprotective the parents were perceived to be, the higher the alexithymia rating. Of note, both the highest and lowest scores were among the sexually abused, the lowest (mean of 44) was found in those who considered that they had received "optimal" parenting, whereas the highest (mean of 58) was among those who recalled inadequate parental care (Kooiman, Vellinga, Spinhoven, Draijer, Trijsburg, and Rooijmand, 2004). It would appear that an appropriate "holding environment" in which to process traumatic stress is relevant to the emotional capabilities of later life.

Evidence for the Somatization-Alexithymia Link

The notion of somatization refers to production of bodily symptoms, as if background somatosensory stimuli were amplified by mediators of anxiety and depression, or unnamed emotions were released through intense bodily sensations. Thus, other factors that organize emotional processing could influence these pathways, and (alexithymic) individuals who do not identify emotions normally may interpret the intensity of their emotional arousal through somatic sensations, which in exaggerated form can be communicated *non*-symbolically as physical symptoms. In recent years much research has attempted to provide empirical verification for these clinical observations, and for the most part followed prediction when healthy controls were the basis of comparison (reviewed by De Gucht, and Heiser, 2003). Ongoing large population studies in Finland have explored relationships among various psychiatric symptoms in the "non-clinical" population, and confirmed that trends toward depression, somatization, dissociation, and alexithymia were closely linked and partly overlapping, but on multivariate analysis remained distinct constructs (Lipsanen, Saarijärvi, and Lauerma, 2004). In another series of patients with a diagnosis of major depressive episode, the "somatization" subscale of the symptom survey (SCL-90) was correlated with female gender, high anxiety, somatosensory amplification, and alexithymia (both Factors 1 and 2 of the TAS-20), and in multivariate comparisons the contribution of alexithymia was independent of anxiety and depression (Sayar, Kirmayer, and Taillefer, 2003). The idea of somatization more recently has been operationalized as "medically unexplained symptoms", symptoms that cannot be adequately explained after a reasonable search for organic causes. Viewed in this manner, the association with alexithymia is less clear. For example, in a setting of primary medical practice, the persistence of symptoms (mostly fatigue, headache, backache, and abdominal complaints) over a six month period correlated strongly with negative affect, and reports of a higher number of symptoms with difficulty identifying feelings (Factor 1 of the TAS-20) (De Gucht, Fischler, and Heiser, 2004). However, other similar studies did not confirm this association (Kooiman, Bolk, Rooijmans, and Trijsburg, 2004).

Alexithymia Predicts Psychopathology

Viewing alexithymia as a personality dimension in relation to other measures of temperament and character among psychiatric inpatients and outpatients, high scores on the difficulty identifying feelings cluster (Factor 1 of TAS-20) predicted higher levels on *all* nine subcomponents of the symptom checklist instrument (SCL-90-R) (Grabe, Spitzer, and Freyberger, 2004). The Finnish population study cited above also found that the majority of alexithymic individuals were depressed, confirming past reports of the association between depression and alexithymic traits (Honkalampi, Koivumaa-Hankanen, Hintikka, Antikainen, Haatainen, Tanskanen, and Viinamäki, 2004). The severity of hopelessness, often viewed with dissatisfaction in life as a predictor of suicidal ideation in patients with depression, correlated with alexithymia (Haatainen, Tanskanen, Kylmä, Honkalampi, Koivumaa-Hankanen, Hintikka, and Viinamäki, 2004). In spite of debates as to whether alexithymia is a reflection of the anhedonia of depression, studies examining the factor structure of the TAS-20 and the Zung depression scale among patients admitted to an inpatient unit for psychosomatic disorders indicated that the two constructs are separate. Although 75% of those patients classified as Ax-h fulfilled criteria for depression, only 25% of Ax-l were depressed (Müller, Bühner, and Ellgring, 2003). Among outpatients treated for major depressive disorder with antidepressant medication, the general trend was for scores on both the Beck depression inventory and the TAS-20 to decline over a period of one year, suggesting that there may be a "secondary" form of alexithymia in reaction to the other elements of depression. Thus, the subpopulation of patients who were alexithymic at baseline, and remained so after two years, tended to recall more harsh parental discipline during childhood and unhappiness in the home than did those who became less alexithymic over time (Honkalampi, Koivumaa-Hankanen, Antikainen, Haatainen, Hintikka, and Viinamäki, 2004). Similarly, in a 10 week study of patients with major depressive disorder treated with paroxetine, reduction of >50% on the Hamilton inventory occurred in 54% of the non-alexithymic group but in only 22% of the alexithymics. Of the patients whose TAS-20 score dropped below the high alexithymia cutoff value, 50% had responded to medication, but only 9% of those that did not responded (Özsahin, Uzun, Cansever, and Gulcat, 2003). In a refugee population the degree of elevation of the TAS-20 Factor 1 score (difficulty identifying feelings) correlated with a diagnosis of post-traumatic stress disorder and endorsement of dysphoric affects, as well as a decreased serum prolactin level (a dopamine regulated endpoint). This is consistent with the anhedonia or "psychic numbing" aspects of PTSD (Söndergaard, and Theorell, 2003). Similarly, in a group of combat veterans, measures of PTSD symptoms and combat exposure correlated closely with the alexithymia measure, supporting the notion of alexithymia as a possible defense to an overwhelming emotional response to trauma (Badura A, 2003).

Alexithymia in Adults with FASD

In a preliminary survey of patients followed in the Seattle cohort (Sullivan, unpublished), ten adults with FAS or FAE were selected for IQ measuring in the near normal range (>84), and were assessed for alexithymic traits by the TAS-20. Compared to the established population norms, 6/10 of these subjects obtained scores in the range of "increased alexithymia"; of these, 3/6 measured in the "severe" range. This raises a question as to what directs an individual's repertoire of psychological defenses that enable the ego to shift attention and regulate anxiety when release through internal and interpersonal dialogue is not sufficient. Further studies are in progress to extend this observation in the context of individual defensive structure and self-concept in these persons.

VII. IMPLICATIONS FOR PSYCHOTHERAPY

A MEDLINE search on the topic did not identify any research publications on psychotherapeutic approaches directed to the particular needs of adult patients with FASD. In discussing neuropsychiatric disorders from a psychoanalytic point of view, Salomonsson (2004) focused on ADHD as a model, but much of his perspective could apply also to problems of FASD. Seen as having a disorder of behavioral inhibition, the individual would tend to act impulsively without reflecting on possible negative consequences. Such a malfunctioning "behavioral inhibition system" could limit normal development of the executive functions essential to establish psychologically mature relationships in modern society. Structural lesions involving the prefrontal cortex and connections with other regions provide the physical substrate for many of the problems of adaptation observed in FASD, and in this sense, the pattern of impaired ego function would fit a "deficit" model. Extending this to object relational terms, the problem lies with early deprivation in the experience of a good object that can be internalized and used to effectively contain and transform anxiety-provoking elements. Under stress, the part objects, split apart and in conflict, might find fleeting reprieve through projection in an effort to displace anxiety and prevent the self from further fragmentation. Under threat of attack, either impulse to flight or discharge of affect through action ("externalizing behaviors"), or both, often result. Children who have not experienced a sufficient source of safe containment for their emotional arousal would grow with an abiding sense of being misunderstood and invalidated, and come to expect rejection in the course of attempts to form relationships. In FASD, with further impairment of linguistic function, expression of anxiety through verbalization also would be impaired. On this background, working with and through the complex transference and countertransference phenomena that inevitably would come into play, modern psychodynamic approaches to psychotherapy may help the individual better comprehend and live with his inner world. However, the limitations and dangers inherent in any form of psychotherapy in regard to issues of dependency, regression, and acting out of conflictual aggressive impulses toward self and others could become especially challenging.

The initial description of the alexithymia phenomenon was based in part on the poor response of such individuals to insight oriented psychotherapy. Attempting to explore this empirically, recent studies have hypothesized alexithymia to be the opposite pole of a spectrum of emotional functioning from "psychological mindedness" (PM). For example, monitoring the response to psychotherapy (supportive vs interpretive) for complicated grief and another for assorted disorders (mostly depression spectrum), after matching for quality of object relations, investigators in the psychotherapy research unit at the University of British Columbia found that PM did not correlate with alexithymia - psychologically minded people may or may not be alexithymic. Yet, while PM predicted symptomatic improvement, the second factor of the TAS-20 (difficulty describing feelings) contributed only to symptom improvement in the supportive therapy group (McCallum, Piper, Ogrodniczuk, and Joyce, 2003). A follow-up study, focusing on residual symptoms in patients who had responded to the psychotherapy intervention, found that Factor 1 (difficulty identifying feelings) predicted severity of residual symptoms (Ogrodniczuk, Piper, and Joyce, 2004), leading to the speculation that individuals with this kind of impairment in recognition of emotion stimuli may not be able to communicate their internal states effectively to a therapist or be able to understand the therapists interventions. The authors suggested that a strategy focused early in the course of therapy on facilitating the process of verbal representation "by providing new labels for past emotional experiences and identifying previously unrecognized triggers of emotion" would be an important first step. As is the cornerstone of psychotherapy, early efforts to affirm the therapeutic alliance has received empirical support in studies on women with fibromyalgia showing greater satisfaction, and perhaps more effective engagement, in the alexithymic group when the clinical encounter generated a larger number of empathic responses (Graugaard, Holgersen, and Finset, 2004).

One of the "secondary disabilities" found in 49% of the subjects described by Streissguth et al in the Seattle follow-up study, irrespective of IQ, was inappropriate sexual behaviors (Streissguth et al., 2004). In fact, it was the most frequent of any of the "adverse life outcomes" they recorded, and of the females in the study who had reported this, 94% also had been victims of sexual and/or physical abuse and violence. Baumbach has reviewed treatment implications for adolescents with FAS/FAE who have become sexual offenders (Baumbach, 2002). Considering that deficits in response inhibition could lead to diminished capacity for contemplating action in response to strong internal (drive) and external stimuli, he advised that conventional behavioral measures aiming to instill self-control might prove ineffective. Compounded by limitations in working memory, with learned patterns of compensatory suggestibility and confabulation, these individuals may not be able to use exploratory or insight oriented psychotherapies as designed for other conditions. With deficits in executive functioning, on which is based the capacity to plan, sequence, and flexibly envision changing patterns, innovative therapies may need to assume a long-term view and focus on helping the individual find a sense of constancy in their self and object representations. Modifications of psychodynamic therapies such as "accelerated experiential-dynamic psychotherapy" (Fosha, 2000), which focuses on the experiencing of core affects in a safe holding environment – perhaps for the first time in the life of some individuals with FASD - may interrupt the alexithymic process and enable a new self-experience. Such speculations, however, await testing in the laboratory of systematic clinical investigation.

VIII. SUMMARY, CONCLUSIONS, AND QUESTIONS

Whether referred through a medical provider, a drug and alcohol rehabilitation clinic, a court/school/employer/clergy, a distraught spouse, or the person himself facing breakdown, someone with a history of sustained prenatal alcohol exposure often presents a complex past and a difficult present to unravel and understand. From the moment of his entry into the world, the dynamics of mother-infant reciprocity may have gone so amiss that he never attained the state of object constancy necessary for a secure and continuous self to emerge (Tyson, 1996). Failure to internalize a sound mental representation of a reliable caregiver that enfolds both the good and the bad (the Kleinian "depressive position,") would impede further maturation of the structures needed to sustain a stable sense of self into adulthood. Such adverse trends form not only the core phenomena that characterize a borderline personality disorder, but also create the soil in which a wider range of psychopathologies can take root. Studies on how the mother-baby unit forms in the context of FASD could shed light on how the attachment system develops and how it is derailed. For example, might a delayed or dampened social smile further attenuate the affective reciprocity already limited by insensitivity to the subtleties of maternal vocal communications (Tyson, 1990)? Such early biological vulnerabilities could then impose a state of "bad fit" upon even the most well-intentioned caregiver, increasing the risk for later physical and emotional neglect. Retrospective studies to identify patterns of resilience might be instructive, and perhaps provide insight into how to better train mothers to compensate while the child's brain still is in a period of relative plasticity.

As a pattern of slowed response inhibition of the infant turns into inattention of the toddler, and finally impulsive character traits of the adult, with all the inherent consequences of impaired regulation of sexual and aggressive impulses, acquisition of life skills that society demands may fall farther and farther behind that of the peer group. Compounding other cognitive deficits, impairment in verbal capacity may filter the normal flow of emotions from entry into consciousness where ego function could then manipulate them in a symbolic manner. Evidence exists that such alexithymia can be a risk factor for subsequent infirmities, including depression, post traumatic stress disorder, somatization disorders, and the externalizing behaviors that define "secondary disabilities". This leads to the thorny problem of moral and legal responsibility, and the extent to which sanctions might be mitigated because of them. (For current information on this issue see the website of the Fetal Alcohol and Drug Unit of the University of Washington, http://depts.washington.edu/fadu under heading of "Legal Issues".) Furthermore, the extent to which prenatal alcohol exposure contributes to the behavioral phenotype of the evolving adult with FASD, independent of exposure to the consequences of an alcoholic mother, father, and their living environments, is still not clear.

With maturation into late adolescence and the expectation of autonomy, ego/executive function assumes increasing importance. The intriguing observation that motivation (emotion) based executive function is impaired in youths with FASD, around the time problems with substance abuse begin to mount, suggests further loci of biological vulnerability. As experimental evidence has shown that alcohol increases aggression in males in the lower, but not higher, range of executive function among "healthy social drinkers", the question arises as to how this might be exaggerated in conditions of brain damage like FASD. If studies showing diminished sensitivity to emotional reward/reinforcement were to be confirmed, then inborn vulnerability of the dopaminergic reward pathway into the nucleus acumbens might also exist.

Which of the myriad neurophysiological measurements summarized in the preceding pages and elsewhere are relevant to a practical understanding of subsequent behavior and functioning of someone with FASD? No doubt the answer will require extensive research to determine which of the difficulties results from a decompensated neuropsychological process, and which is imposed by a deprived environment, independent of maternal consumption of alcohol over the safe threshold (if such exists). On the other hand, effective psychotherapeutic approaches for adult individuals with FASD may require exploration of broader indices of psychological function. From a psychodynamic perspective, a better grasp of ego defenses, object relations, and self-structure at a phenomenological and experiential level would paint a picture of what it is like to be a person living with this particular neuropsychological endowment, and how he has developed his individual style and reflects upon himself. Increasingly, such concepts are testable and can form a basis for evidence based treatment strategies. A challenge is to know what parts of the distinctiveness of FASD rest upon restrictions and limitations within the brain consequent to an unfortunate experiment of nature, which of its manifestations are products of a unique representational world of that individual's developing self, and how might relationships between the two lead to new understanding of the human mind.

ACKNOWLEDGEMENT

The author thanks Dr. Ann Streissguth for making the resources of the Fetal Alcohol and Drug Unit available, Dr. Deb Cowley (director of the psychiatry residency program) for her guidance and flexibility, and Dr. Andrew Saxon (director of the fellowship program in addiction psychiatry) for his abiding support. The author was supported by a fellowship in Addiction Psychiatry through the Seattle Veteran's Administration Medical Center and the

Department of Psychiatry and Behavioral Sciences of the University of Washington College of Medicine.

REFERENCES

Abel, E. (1981). Behavioral teratology of alcohol. *Psychological Bulletin, 90,* 564-581.

Aftanas, L., Varlamov, A., Reva, N., and Pavlov, S. (2003). Disruption of early event-related theta synchronization of human EEG in alexithymics viewing affective pictures. *Neuroscience Letters, 340,* 57-60.

Agras, S., Hammer, L., and McNicholas, F. (1999). A prospective study of the influence of eating-disordered mothers on their children. *International Journal of Eating Disorders, 25,* 253-262.

Armstrong, E. (1998). Diagnosing moral disorder: The discovery and evolution of fetal alcohol syndrome. *Social Sciences in Medicine, 47,* 2025-2042.

Aronson, M., Kyllerman, M., Sabel, K., Sandin, B., and Olegard, R. (1985). Children of alcoholic mothers. Developmental, perceptual, and behavioral characteristics as compared to matched controls. *Acta Paediatrica Scandanavica, 74,* 27-35.

Badura, A. (2003). Theoretical and empirical exploration of the similarities between emotional numbing in posttraumatic stress disorder and alexithymia. *Journal of Anxiety Disorders, 17,* 349-360.

Baumbach, J. (2002). Some implications of prenatal alcohol exposure for the treatment of adolescents with sexual offending behaviors. *Sexual Abuse, 14,* 313-327.

Becker, M., Warr-Leeper, G., and Leeper, H. (1990). Fetal alcohol syndrome: a description of oral, articulatory, short-term memory, grammatical, and semantic abilities. *Journal of Communications Disorders, 23,* 97-124.

Bingol, N., Schuster, C., Fuchs, M., Iosub, S., Turner, G., Stone, R, and Gromisch, D. (1987). The influence of socioeconomic factors on the occurrence of fetal alcohol syndrome. *Advances in Alcohol and Substance Abuse, 6,* 105-118.

Bookstein, F., Sampson, P., Streissguth, A., and Connor, P. (2001). Geometric morphometrics of corpus callosum and subcortical structures in the fetal-alcohol-affected brain. *Teratology, 64,* 4-32.

Bookstein, F., Streissguth, A., Sampson, P., Connor, P., and Bar, H. (2002). Corpus callosum shape and neuropsychological deficits in adult males with heavy fetal alcohol exposure. *NeuroImage, 15,* 233-251.

Burd, L., Klug, M., Martsolf, J., and Kerbeshian, J. (2003). Fetal alcohol syndrome: neuropsychiatric phenomics. *Neurotoxicology and Teratology, 25,* 697-705.

Cohen, D., Richardson, J., and LaBree, L. (1994). Parenting behaviors and the onset of smoking and alcohol use: a longitudinal study. *Pediatrics, 94,* 368-375.

Coles, C. (2001). Fetal alcohol exposure and attention: moving beyond ADHD. *Alcohol Research and Health, 25,* 199-203.

Coles, C., Smith, I., Fernhoff, P., and Falek, A. (1985). Neonatal neurobehavioral characteristics as correlates of maternal alcohol use during gestation. *Alcoholism: Clinical and Experimental Research, 9,* 454-460.

Coles, C., Platzman, K., Raskin-Hood, C., Brown, R., Falek, A., and Smith, I. (1997). A comparison of children affected by prenatal alcohol exposure and attention deficit, hyperactivity disorder. *Alcoholism Clinical and Experimental Research, 21,* 150-161.

Connor, P., Sampson, P., Bookstein, F., and Barr, H., and Streissguth, A. (2000). Direct and indirect effects of prenatal alcohol damage on executive function. *Developmental Neuropsychology,* 18, 331-354.

Dansky, B., Brewerton, T., and Kilpatrick, D. (2000). Comorbidity of bulimia nervosa and alcohol use disorders: results from the National Women's Study. *International Journal of Eating Disorders, 27,*180-90.

De Gucht, V., and Heiser, W. (2003). Alexithymia and somatization. A quantitative review of the literature. *Journal of Psychosomatic Research, 54,* 425-434.

De Gucht, V., Fischler, B., and Heiser, W. (2004). Personality and affect determinants of medically unexplained symptoms in primary care. A follow-up study. *Journal of Psychosomatic Research, 56,* 279-285.

Edwards, E., Eiden, R., and Leonard, K. (1998). Impact of fathers' alcoholism and associated risk factors on parent-infant attachment stability from 12 to 18 months. *Infant Mental Health Journal, 25,* 556-579.

Famy, C., Streissguth, A., and Unis, A. (1998). Mental illness in adults with fetal alcohol syndrome or fetal alcohol effects. *American Journal of Psychiatry, 155,* 552-554.

Fast, D., Conry, J., and Loock, C. (1999). Identifying fetal alcohol syndrome among youth in the criminal justice system. *Journal of Developmental and Behavioral Pediatrics 20,* 370-372.

Fischer, S., Anderson, K., and Smith, G. (2004). Coping with distress by eating or drinking: role of trait urgency and expectancies. *Psychology of Addictive Behavior 18,* 269-274.

Fonagy, P. (2001). *Attachment Theory and Psychoanalysis.* New York: Other Press.

Fosha, D. (2000). *The transforming power of affect. A model for accelerated change.* New York: Basic Books.

Frank, D., Brown, J., Johnson, S., and Cabral, H. (2002). Forgotten fathers An exploratory study of mothers' report of drug and alcohol problems among fathers of newborn infants. *Neurotoxicology and Teratolology, 24,* 339-347.

Franz, M., Schaefer, R., Schneider, C., Sitte, W., and Bachor, J. (2004). Visual event-related potentials in subjects with alexithymia: modified processing of emotional aversive information? *American Journal of Psychiatry, 161,* 728-735.

Gabel, S., Stallings, M., Young, S., Schmitz, S., Crowley, T., and Fulker, D. (1998). Family variables in substance-misusing male adolescents: The importance of maternal disorder. *American Journal of Drug and Alcohol Abuse, 24,* 61-84.

Gazzaniga, M. (2000). Cerebral localization and interhemispheric communication. Does the corpus callosum enable the human condition? *Brain, 123,* 1293-1326.

Giancola, P. (2004). Executive functioning and alcohol-related aggression. *Journal of Abnormal Psychology, 113,* 541-555.

Goldberg, M., Lex, B., Mello, N., Mendelson, J., and Bower, T. (1996). Impact of maternal alcoholism on separation of children from their mothers: findings from a sample of incarcerated mothers. *American Journal of Orthopsychiatry, 66,* 228-238.

Goldberg, S., Muir, R., and Kerr, J. (2000). *Attachment Theory. Social, developmental, and clinical perspectives.* Hillsdale, NJ: The Analytic Press, Inc.

Goldberg, S., Benoit, D., Blokland, K., and Madigan, S. (2003). Atypical maternal behavior, maternal representations, and infant disorganized attachment. *Developmental Psychopathology, 15,* 239-257.

Goldschmidt, L., Richardson, G., Stoffer, D., Geva, D., and Day, N. (1996). Prenatal alcohol exposure and academic achievement at age six: a nonlinear fit. *Alcoholism: Clinical and Experimental Research, 20,* 763-770.

Grabe, H., Möller, B., Willer, C., Spitzer C., Rizos, T., and Freyberger, H. (2004). Interhemispheric transfer in alexithymia: a transcallosal inhibition study. *Psychotherapy and Psychosomatics, 73,* 117-123.

Grabe, H., Spitzer, C., and Freyberger, H. (2004). Alexithymia and personality in relation to dimensions of psychopathology. *American Journal of Psychiatry, 161,* 1299-1301.

Graugaard, P., Holgersen, K., and Finset, A. (2004). Communicating with alexithymic and non-alexithymic patients: an experimental study of the effect of psychosocial communication and empathy on patient satisfaction. *Psychotherapy and Psychosomatics, 73,* 73-92.

Greene, T., Ernhart, C., Martier, S., Sokol, R., and Ager, J. (1990). Prenatal alcohol exposure and language development. *Alcoholism: Clinical and Experimental Research, 14,* 937-945.

Gündel, H., López-Sala, A., Ceballos-Baumann, A., Deus, J., Cardoner, N., Marten-Mittag, B., Soriano-Mas, C., and Pujol, J. (2004). Alexithymia correlates with the size of the right anterior cingulate. *Psychosomatic Medicine 66,* 132-140.

Haatainen, K., Tanskanen, A., Kylmä, J., Honkalampi, K., Koivumaa-Hankanen, H., Hintikka, J., and Viinamäki, H. (2004). Factors associated with hopelessness: a population study. *International Journal of Social Psychiatry, 50,* 142-152.

Harmer, A., Sanderson, J., and Mertin, P. (1999). Influence of negative childhood experiences on psychological functioning, social support, and parenting for mothers recovering from addiction. *Child Abuse and Neglect, 23,* 421-433.

Harris, S., MacKay, L., and Osborn, J. (1995). Autistic behaviors in offspring of mother abusing alcohol and other drugs: a series of case reports. *Alcoholism: Clinical and Experimental Research, 19,* 660-665.

Heller, J., Anderson, H., Bland, J., Brooke, O., Peacock, J., and Stewart, C. (1988). Alcohol in pregnancy: patterns and association with socio-economic, psychological and behavioural factors. *British Journal of Addiction, 83,* 541-551.

Hill, S., Lowers, L., Locke-Wellman, J., and Shen, S. (2000). Maternal smoking and drinking during pregnancy and the risk for child and adolescent psychiatric disorders. *Journal of Studies on Alcohol, 61,* 661-668.

Honkalampi, K., Koivumaa-Hankanen, H., Hintikka, J., Antikainen, R., Haatainen, K., Tanskanen, A., and Viinamäki, H. (2004). Do stressful life-events or sociodemographic variables associate with depression and alexithymia among a general population? – A 3-year follow-up study. *Comprehensive Psychiatry, 45,* 254-260.

Honkalampi, K., Koivumaa-Hankanen, H., Antikainen, R., Haatainen, K., Hintikka, J., and Viinamäki, H. (2004). Relationships among alexithymia, adverse childhood experiences, sociodemographic variables, and actual mood disorder: A 2-year clinical follow-up study of patients with major depressive disorder. *Psychosomatics, 45,* 197-204.

Jacobson, S. (1998). Specificity of neurobehavioral outcomes associated with prenatal alcohol exposure. *Alcoholism: Clinical and Experimental Research, 22,* 313-320.

Janzen, L., Nanson, J., and Block, G. (1995). Neuropsychological evaluation of preschoolers with fetal alcohol syndrome. *Neurotoxicology and Teratology, 17*, 273-279.

Jones, K., Smith, D., Ulleland, C., and Streissguth, A. (1973). Pattern of malformation in offspring of chronic alcoholic mothers. *Lancet, 1,* 1267-1271.

Jones, K., Smith, D., Streissguth, A., and Myrianthopoulos, N. (1974). Outcome of offspring of chronic alcoholic women. *Lancet, 1,* 1076-1078.

Joukamaa, M., Kokkonen, P., Veijola, J., Läksy, K., Karvonen, J., Jokelainen, J., and Järvelin, M-R. (2003). Social situation of expectant mothers and alexithymia 31 years later in their offspring: a prospective study. *Psychosomatic Medicine, 65,* 307-312.

Kano, M., Fukudo, S., Gyoba, J., Kamachi, M., Takawa, M., Mochizuki, H., Itoh, M., Hongo, M., and Yanai, K. (2003). Specific brain processing of facial expressions in people with alexithymia: an H215O-PET study. *Brain, 126,* 1474-1484.

Keel, P., Dorer, D., Eddy, K., Franko, D., Charatan, D., and Herzog, D. (2003). Predictors of mortality in eating disorders. *Archives of General Psychiatry, 60,* 179-83.

Kelly, S., Day, N., and Streissguth, A. (2000). Effects of prenatal exposure on social behavior in humans and other species. *Neurotoxicology and Teratology, 22,* 143-149.

Kerns, K., Don, A., Mateer, C., and Streissguth, A. (1997). Cognitive deficits in nonretarded adults with fetal alcohol syndrome. *Journal of Learning Disabilities, 30,* 685-693.

Kodituwakku, P., Handmaker, N., Cutler, S., Weathersby, E., and Handmaker, S. (1995). Specific impairments in self-regulation in children exposed to alcohol prenatally. *Alcoholism: Clinical and Experimental Research, 19,* 1558-1564.

Kodituwakku, P., May, P., Clericuzio, C., and Weers, D. (2001). Emotion-related learning in individuals prenatally exposed to alcohol: an investigation of the relation between set shifting, extinction of responses, and behavior. *Neuropsychologia, 39,* 699-708.

Kodituwakku, P., Kalberg, W., and May, P. (2001). The effect of prenatal alcohol exposure on executive functioning. *Alcohol Research and Health, 25,* 192-198.

Kokkonen, P., Veijola, J., Karvonen, J., Läksy, K., Jokelainen, J., Järvelin, M-R., and Joukamaa, M. (2003). Ability to speak at the age of 1 year and alexithymia 30 years later. *Journal of Psychosomatic Research, 54,* 491-495.

Kooiman, C., Bolk, J., Rooijmans, H., and Trijsburg, R. (2004). Alexithymia does not predict the persistence of medically unexplained physical symptoms. *Psychosomatic Medicine, 66,* 224-232.

Kooiman, C., Vellinga, S., Spinhoven, P., Draijer, N., Trijsburg, R., and Rooijmand, H. (2004). Childhood adversities as risk factors for alexithymia and other aspects of affect dysregulation in adulthood. *Psychotherapy and Psychosomatics, 73,* 107-116.

Krystal H. *Integration and Self-Healing. Affect, trauma, alexithymia.* (1988). Hillsdale, NJ: The Analytic Press, Inc..

Kvigne, V., Leonardson, G., Borzelleca, J., Brock, E., Neff-Smith, M., and Welty, T. (2003). Characteristics of mothers who have children with fetal alcohol syndrome or some characteristics of fetal alcohol syndrome. *Journal of the American Board of Family Practice, 16,* 296-303.

Landesman-Dwyer, S., and Ragozin, A. (1981). Behavioral correlates of prenatal alcohol exposure: a four year follow-up study. *Neurobehavioral Toxicology and Teratology, 3,* 187-193.

Larsen, J., Brand, N., Bermond, B., and Hijman, R. (2003). Cognitive and emotional characteristics of alexthymia. A review of neurobiological studies. *Journal of Psychosomatic Research, 54,* 533-541.

Lee, K., Mattson, S., and Riley, E. (2004). Classifying children with heavy prenatal alcohol exposure using measures of attention. *Journal of the International Neuropsychological Society, 10,* 271-277.

Lipsanen, T., Saarijärvi, S., and Lauerma, H. (2004). Exploring the relations between depression, somatization, dissociation and alexithymia – overlapping or independent constructs? *Psychopathology, 37,* 200-206.

Loxton, N., and Dawe, S. (2001). Alcohol abuse and dysfunctional eating in adolescent girls: the influence of individual differences in sensitivity to reward and punishment. *International Journal of Eating Disorders, 29,* 455-62.

Lynch, M., Coles, C., Corley, T., and Falek, A. (2003). Examining delinquency in adolescents differentially exposed to alcohol: The role of proximal and distal factors. *Journal of Studies on Alcohol, 64,* 678-686.

Marcus, A., and Tisne, S. (1987). Perception of maternal behavior by elementary school children of alcoholic mothers. *International Journal of Addiction, 22,* 543-555.

Mattson, S., Riley, E., Delis, D., Stern, C., and Jones, K. (1996). Verbal learning and memory in children with fetal alcohol syndrome. *Alcoholism: Clinical and Experimental Research, 20,* 810-816.

Mattson, S., Riley, E., Gramling, L., Delis, D., and Jones K. (1997). Heavy prenatal alcohol exposure with or without physical features of fetal alcohol syndrome leads to IQ deficits. *Journal of Pediatrics, 131,* 718-721.

Mattson, S., and Riley, E. (1998). A review of the neurobehavioral deficits in children with fetal alcohol syndrome or prenatal exposure to alcohol. *Alcoholism: Clinical and Experimental Research, 22,* 279-294.

Mattson, S., Riley, E., Gramling, L., and Delis, D. (1998). Neuropsychological comparison of alcohol-exposed children with or without physical features of fetal alcohol syndrome. *Neuropsychology, 12,* 146-153.

Mattson, S., and Riley, E. (1999). Inplicit and explicit memory functioning in children with prenatal alcohol exposure. *Journal of the International Neuropsychological Society, 5,* 462-471.

Mattson, S., Goodman, A., Caine, C., Delis, D., and Riley, E. (1999). Executive functioning in children with heavy prenatal alcohol exposure. *Alcoholism: Clinical and Experimental Research, 23,* 1808-1815.

Mattson, S., and Riley, E. (2000). Parent ratings of behavior in children with heavy prenatal alcohol exposure and IQ matched controls. *Alcoholism: Clinical and Experimental Research, 24,* 226-231.

McCallum, M., Pipe, W., Ogrodniczuk, J., and Joyce, A. (2003). Relationships among psychological mindedness, alexithymia and outcome in four forms of short-term psychotherapy. *Psychology and Psychotherapy: Theory, Research and Practice, 76,* 133-144.

McDougall, J. (1982). Alexithymia, psychosomatosis, and psychosis. *International Journal of Psychoanalysis and Psychotherapy, 9,* 379-388.

Meschke, L., Holl, J., and Messelt, S. (2003). Assessing the risk of fetal alcohol syndrome: understanding substance use among pregnant women. *Neurotoxicology and Teratology, 25,* 667-674.

Miles, D., Svikis, D., Kulstad, J., and Haug, N. (2001). Psychopathology in pregnant drug-dependent women with and without alcohol dependence. *Alcoholism: Clinical and Experimental Research, 25,* 1012-1017.

Miles, J., Takahashi, T., Haber, A., and Hadden L. (2003). Autism in families with a high incidence of autism. *Journal of Autism and Developmental Disorders, 33,* 403-415.

Modestin, J., Furrer, R., and Malti T. (2004). Study on alexithymia in adult non-patients. *Journal of Psychosomatic Research, 56,* 707-709.

Moeller, F., Barratt, E., Dougherty, D., Schmitz, J., and Swann A. (2001). Psychiatric aspects of impulsivity. *American Journal of Psychiatry, 158,* 1783-1793.

Monnot, M., Lovallo, W., Nixon, S., and Ross, E. (2002). Neurological basis of deficits in affective prosody comprehension among alcoholics and fetal alcohol-exposed adults. *Journal of Neuropsychiatry and Clinical Neuroscience, 14,* 321-328.

Müller, J., Bühner, M., and Ellgring, H. (2003). Relationship and differential validity of alexithymia and depression: a comparison of the Toronto alexithymia and self-rating depression scales. *Psychopathology, 36,* 71-77.

Murray, J. (1989). Psychologists and children of alcoholic parents. *Psychological Reports, 64,* 859-879.

Nanson, J., and Hiscock, M. (1990). Attention deficits in children exposed to alcohol prenatally. *Alcoholism: Clinical and Experimental Research, 14,* 656-661.

Nanson, J. (1992). Autism in fetal alcohol syndrome: a report of six cases. *Alcoholism: Clinical and Experimental Research, 16,* 558-565.

Noland, J., Singer, L., Arendt, R., Minnes, S., Short, E., and Bearer, C. (2003). Executive functioning in preschool-age children prenatally exposed to alcohol, cocaine, and marijuana. *Alcoholism: Clinical and Experimental Research, 27,* 647-656.

Nugent, J., Lester, B., Green, S., Wieczorek-Deering, D., and O'Mahony, P. (1996). The effects of maternal alcohol consumption and cigarette smoking during pregnancy on acoustic cry analysis. *Child Development, 67,* 1806-1815.

O'Conner, M., Sigman, M., and Brill, N. (1987). Disorganization of attachment in relation to maternal alcohol consumption. *Journal of Consulting and Clinical Psychology, 55,* 831-836.

O'Connor, M., Shah, B., Whaley, S., Cronin, P., Gunderson, B., and Graham, J. (2002). Psychiatric illness in a clinical sample of children with prenatal alcohol exposure. *American Journal of Drug and Alcohol Abuse, 28,* 743-754.

O'Malley, K. (1998). Fetal alcohol syndrome and seizure disorder. *Canadian Journal of Psychiatry, 43,* 1051.

O'Malley, K., and Nanson J. (2002). Clinical implications of a link between fetal alcohol spectrum disorder and attention-deficit hyperactivity disorder. *Canadian Journal of Psychiatry, 47,* 349-354.

O'Malley, K., and Storoz, L. (2003). Fetal alcohol spectrum disorder and ADHD: diagnostic implications and therapeutic consequences. *Expert Reviews in Neurotherapeutics, 3,* 477-489.

Ogrodniczuk, J., Piper, W., and Joyce, A. (2004). Alexithymia as a predictor of residual symptoms in depressed patients who respond to short-term psychotherapy. *American Journal of Psychotherapy, 58,* 150-161.

Olson, H., Morse, B., and Huffine, C. (1998). Development and Psychopathology: Fetal alcohol syndrome and related conditions. *Seminars in Clinical Neuropsychiatry, 3,* 262-284.

Özsahin, A., Uzun, Ö., Cansever, A., and Gulcat, Z. (2003). The effect of alexithymic features on response to antidepressant medication in patients with major depression. *Depression and Anxiety, 18,* 62-66.

Paivio, S., and McCulloch, C. (2004). Alexithymia as a mediator between childhood trauma and self-injurious behaviors. *Child Abuse and Neglect, 28,* 339-354.

Parker, J., Taylor, G., and Bagby, R. (2003). The 20-item Toronto alexithymia scale. III. Reliability and factorial validity in a community population. *Journal of Psychosomatic Research, 55,* 269-275.

Phillips, J. (1975). *The origins of intellect: Piaget's Theory. 2nd Edition.* San Francisco: WH Freeman and Company.

Reich, W., Earls, F., Frankel, O., and Shayka, J. (1993). Psychopathology in children of alcoholics. Journal of the American Academy of Child and Adolescent Psychiatry, 32, 995-1002.

Roebuck, T., Mattson, S., and Riley, E. (1999). Behavioral and psychosocial profiles of alcohol-exposed children. *Alcoholism: Clinical and Experimental Research, 23,* 1070-1076.

Rössig, C., Wässer, S., and Opperman P. (1994). Audiologic manifestations in fetal alcohol syndrome assessed by brainstem auditory-evoked potentials. *Neuropediatrics, 25,* 245-249.

Royall, D., Lauterbach, E., Cummings, J., Reeve, A., Rummans, T., Kaufer, D., LaFrance, W., and Coffey, C. (2002). Executive control function: A review of its promise and challenges for clinical research. *Journal of Neuropsychiatry and Clinical Neuroscience, 14,* 377-405.

Salomonsson, B. (2004). Some psychoanalytic viewpoints on neuropsychiatric disorders in children. *International Journal of Psychoanalysis, 85,*117-136.

Sayar, K., Kirmayer, L., and Taillefer, S. (2003). Predictors of somatic symptoms in depressive disorder. *General Hospital Psychiatry, 25,* 108-114.

Schonfeld, A., Mattson, S., Lang, A., and Delis, D. (2001). Verbal and nonverbal fluency in children with heavy prenatal alcohol exposure. *Journal of Studies on Alcohol, 62,* 239-246.

Schore, A. (1994). *Affect regulation and the origin of the self: The neurobiology of emotional development.* Hillsdale, NJ: Lawrence Erlbaum Associates, Inc.

Shapiro, D. (1965). *Neurotic Styles.* New York: Basic Books, Inc.

Share, L. (1994). *If Someone Speaks, it Gets Lighter: Dreams and the reconstruction of infant trauma.* Hillsdale, NJ: The Analytic Press. 1994

Shaywitz, S., Cohen, D., and Shaywitz, B. (1980). Behavior and learning difficulties in children of normal intelligence born to alcoholic mothers. *Journal of Pediatrics, 96,* 978-82.

Shaywitz, S., Caparulo, B., and Hodgson, E. (1981). Developmental language disability as a consequence of prenatal exposure to ethanol. *Pediatrics, 68,* 850-855.

Sifneos, P. (1973). The prevalence of 'alexithymic' characteristics in psychosomatic patients. *Psychotherapy and Psychosomatics, 22,* 225-262.

Sinha, R., and O'Malley, S. (2000). Alcohol and eating disorders: implications for alcohol treatment and health services research. *Alcoholism: Clinical and Experimental Research, 24,* 1312-1319.

Söndergaard, H., and Theorell, T. (2003). Alexithymia, emotions and PTSD; findings from a longitudinal study of refugees. *Nordic Journal of Psychiatry, 58,* 185-191.

Steinhausen, H-C., Nestler, V., and Huth, H. (1982). Psychopathology and mental function in the offspring of alcoholic and epileptic mothers. *Journal of the American Academy of Child Psychiatry, 21,* 268-273.

Steinhausen, H-C., Göbel, D., and Nestler, V. (1984). Psychopathology in the offspring of alcoholic parents. *Journal of the American Academy of Child Psychiatry,23,* 465-471.

Steinhausen, H-C., Willms, J., and Spohr, H-L. (1993). Long-term psychopathological and cognitive outcome of children with fetal alcohol syndrome. *Journal of the American Academy of Child Psychiatry, 32,* 990-994.

Steinhausen, H-C., Willms, J., and Spohr, H-L. (1994). Correlates of psychopathology and intelligence in children with fetal alcohol syndrome. *Journal of Child Psychology and Psychiatry, 35,* 323-331.

Steinhausen, H-C., and Spohr H-L. (1998). Long-term outcome of children with fetal alcohol syndrome: psychopathology, behavior, and intelligence. *Alcoholism: Clinical and Experimental Research, 22,* 334-338.

Steinhausen, H-C., Willms, J., Metzke, C., and Spohr H-L. (2003). Behavioral phenotype in fetal alcohol syndrome and fetal alcohol effects. *Developmental Medicine and Child Neurology, 45,* 179-182.

Streissguth, A., Barr, H., Sampson, P., Darby, B., and Martin D. (1989). IQ at age 4 in relation to maternal alcohol use and smoking during pregnancy. *Developmental Psychology, 25,* 3-11.

Streissguth, A., Barr, H., Kogan, J., and Bookstein, F. (1996). *Understanding the occurrence of secondary disabilities in clients with fetal alcohol syndrome (FAS) and fetal alcohol effects (FAE). Final Report to the Centers for Disease Control and Prevention (CDC).* Seattle: University of Washington, Fetal Alcohol and Drug Unit, Tech. Rep. No.96-06.

Streissguth, A., and Kanter, J. (1997). *The challenge of fetal alcohol syndrome: overcoming secondary disabilities.* Seattle: University of Washington Press.

Streissguth, A., and O'Malley, K. (2000). Neuropsychiatric implications and long-term consequences of fetal alcohol spectrum disorders. *Seminars in Clinical Neuropsychiatry, 5,* 177-190.

Streissguth, AP, Bookstein, F., Barr, H., Sampson, P., O'Malley, K., and Young, J. (2004). Risk Factors for Adverse Life Outcomes in Fetal Alcohol Syndrome and Fetal Alcohol Effects. *Journal of Developmental and Behavioral Pediatrics, 25,* 228-238.

Taylor, G. (2000). Recent developments in alexithymia theory and research. *Canadian Journal of Psychiatry, 45,* 134-142.

Taylor, G., Bagby, R., and Parker, J. (2000). The alexithymia construct. A potential paradign for psychosomatic medicine. *Psychosomatics, 32,* 153-164.

Taylor, G., and Bagby, R. (2004). New trends in alexithymia research. *Psychotherapy and Psychosomatics, 73,* 68-77, 2004.

Tyson, P. (1996). Object relations, affect management, and psychic structure formation. The concept of object constancy. *Psychoanalytic Study of the Child, 51,* 172-189.

Tyson P. (1990). The development of the ego. In: P. Tyson P and R. Tyson, *Psychoanalytic Theories of Development. An Integration.* New Haven: Yale University Press.

Uecker, A., and Nadel, L. (1996). Spatial locations gone awry: object and spatial memory deficits in children with fetal alcohol syndrome. *Neuropsychologia, 34,* 209-223.

Uecker, A., and Nadel, L. (1998). Spatial but not object memory impairments in children with fetal alcohol syndrome. *American Journal of Mental Retardation, 103,* 12-18.

Van Dyke, D., Mackay, L., and Ziaylek, E. (1982). Management of severe feeding dysfunction in children with fetal alcohol syndrome. *Clinical Pediatrics, 21,* 336-339.

Volkan, V., Ast, G., and Greer, W. (2002*). The Third Reich in the Unconscious. Transgenerational transmission and its consequences.* New York: Brunner-Routledge.

Wearden, A., Cook, L., and Vaughan-Jones, J. (2003). Adult attachment, alexithymia, symptom reporting, and health-related coping. *Journal of Psychosomatic Research, 55,* 341-347.

Weinberg, N. (1997). Cognitive and behavioral deficits associated with parental alcohol use. *Journal of the American Academy of Child and Adolescent Psychiatry, 36,* 1177-86.

Whaley, S., O'Connor, M., and Gunderson, B. (2001). Comparison of adaptive functioning of children prenatally exposed to alcohol to a non-exposed clinical sample. *Alcoholism: Clinical and Experimental Research, 25,* 1018-1024.

Wilson, B. (2003). The role of attentional processes in children's prosocial behavior with peers: Attention shifting and emotion. *Developmental Psychopathology, 15,* 313-329.

Winnicott, D. (1975). Primary Maternal Preoccupation. In: *Through Paediatrics to Psychoanalysis.* London: The Hogarth Press.

Winnecott D. (1983). In J. Greenberg, and S. Mitchell (Eds.), *Object relations in psychoanalytic theory.* (p. 197). Boston: Harvard University Press.

INDEX

A

academic performance, 191, 194
academic problems, 190
academic progress, 194
acceptance, 132, 142, 194, 205
access, 70, 73, 74, 77, 88, 136, 152, 162, 165, 180, 185, 186, 187, 188
accuracy, 174, 185, 186
acetylcholine, 60
achievement, 48, 58, 132, 158, 165, 169, 188, 192, 193, 220, 229, 239, 247
acid, 31, 34, 38, 60, 203
activation, 3, 59, 219
activity level, 43, 44, 46, 112, 193
adaptation, 43, 45, 87, 97, 184, 233
adaptive functioning, 9, 10, 19, 26, 58, 96, 132, 134, 137, 213, 245, 247
addiction, 33, 74, 84, 103, 118, 206, 207, 216, 236, 239, 247
ADHD, vii, viii, 3, 5, 8, 9, 11, 13, 15, 16, 17, 18, 22, 36, 40, 51, 52, 53, 54, 55, 56, 57, 58, 59, 60, 61, 62, 63, 64, 65, 67, 95, 96, 100, 123, 124, 125, 126, 129, 131, 132, 133, 134, 135, 136, 137, 139, 140, 141, 143, 150, 154, 155, 157, 159, 164, 167, 168, 177, 179, 180, 185, 186, 188, 191, 194, 195, 197, 199, 201, 202, 208, 209, 211, 219, 220, 228, 233, 237, 242, 247
adhesion, 4
adjustment, 155, 185, 192, 194, 225, 227, 228
administrators, 84, 151
adolescence, 97, 100, 125, 128, 129, 132, 137, 141, 142, 144, 154, 176, 177, 180, 204, 205, 216, 236
adolescent behavior, 62
adolescent sex offenders, 156, 158
adolescents, 5, 10, 11, 12, 13, 14, 16, 45, 51, 52, 53, 55, 56, 57, 58, 60, 62, 66, 96, 100, 117, 131, 134, 135, 139, 140, 143, 149, 150, 154, 155, 157, 176,

200, 201, 202, 203, 206, 207, 209, 210, 220, 221, 224, 234, 237, 238, 241, 247
adrenaline, 60
adulthood, vii, 8, 29, 53, 58, 60, 104, 110, 117, 118, 137, 141, 143, 156, 204, 206, 217, 224, 228, 235, 240, 247
adults, viii, 10, 11, 12, 14, 28, 45, 64, 91, 104, 105, 106, 109, 110, 112, 113, 122, 125, 128, 129, 131, 132, 134, 135, 138, 139, 140, 150, 152, 157, 184, 233, 238, 240, 242, 247
adverse event, 53
advocacy, 12, 16, 21, 30, 70, 72, 91, 119, 206, 210
aetiology, 11, 29
affect, 11, 16, 30, 46, 54, 86, 132, 139, 142, 143, 144, 145, 186, 218, 225, 229, 231, 232, 234, 238, 240, 245, 247
affective disorder, 72
affective experience, 219
afternoon, 125, 152
age, vii, 4, 9, 10, 15, 16, 17, 18, 19, 26, 29, 30, 31, 32, 33, 34, 54, 56, 58, 62, 64, 70, 83, 86, 96, 98, 109, 117, 125, 126, 135, 136, 137, 138, 139, 140, 141, 142, 143, 144, 152, 154, 156, 158, 161, 162, 163, 165, 166, 168, 169, 175, 176, 177, 178, 185, 189, 190, 191, 192, 196, 197, 208, 212, 213, 216, 218, 220, 221, 223, 224, 226, 227, 228, 230, 239, 240, 242, 244, 247
agent, 1, 31, 60, 122, 203
aggression, viii, 41, 42, 132, 160, 200, 222, 223, 225, 236
aggressive behavior, 219
aggressiveness, 57
alanine, 28
alanine aminotransferase, 28
alcohol abuse, 11, 36, 64, 82, 92, 97, 134, 181, 190, 218, 225, 227
alcohol consumption, 28, 30, 31, 62, 96, 98, 133, 227, 228, 242, 247

alcohol dependence, 2, 3, 22, 92, 226, 228, 242

alcohol problems, 20, 118, 224, 227, 238, 247

alcohol use, 20, 28, 31, 34, 37, 67, 89, 91, 95, 104, 137, 181, 190, 191, 196, 207, 209, 226, 227, 237, 238, 244, 245, 247

alcohol withdrawal, 26, 29, 218

alcoholics, viii, 1, 2, 91, 242, 243, 247

alcoholism, 1, 3, 11, 20, 97, 174, 216, 222, 227, 228, 238, 247

alcohol-related aggression, 238, 247

alertness, 42, 44, 46

alexithymia, viii, 200, 215, 229, 230, 231, 232, 233, 234, 235, 237, 238, 239, 240, 241, 242, 243, 244, 245, 247

algorithm, 202

alienation, 71

ALT, 28

alternative, 81, 116, 178, 192, 193

alternatives, 151, 182

alters, 3, 58, 60, 170

ambidexterity, 190

ambiguity, 165

ambivalence, 75, 86

ambivalent, 51

American Psychiatric Association, 132, 136, 137, 153

American Psychological Association, 156

amnesia, 31

anatomy, 85

androgen, 150

anger, 107, 112, 117, 119, 136, 151, 205, 226

animals, 27, 54, 55, 57, 63, 95, 135, 210

anoxia, 17, 208

antidepressant, 150, 232, 243, 247

antidepressant medication, 150, 232, 243, 247

antisocial behavior, 141, 159, 228

antisocial personality, 180, 216, 219

antisocial personality disorder, 180, 216, 219

anxiety, 7, 51, 53, 57, 61, 72, 91, 110, 116, 129, 185, 204, 205, 215, 216, 223, 226, 228, 230, 231, 233, 234

anxiety disorder, 51, 53, 57, 185

apgar score, 28, 32

aphasia, 52

apraxia, 9, 19, 52, 212

argument, 162

arithmetic, 221

arousal, 29, 43, 44, 54, 64, 132, 133, 140, 150, 219, 229, 231, 234

arrest, 132, 142, 145, 146, 151

arson, 146, 147

arteries, 12

articulation, 88

aspartate, 28, 60

aspiration, 229

assault, 120, 139, 140, 144, 157

assessment, 5, 13, 14, 15, 16, 17, 49, 52, 72, 78, 87, 97, 100, 127, 139, 145, 147, 148, 149, 156, 157, 158, 162, 176, 185, 187, 188, 189, 192, 199, 201, 204, 207, 208, 217

assessment techniques, 16

assignment, 75, 107, 108, 183

assimilation, 150

association, 1, 2, 52, 53, 63, 67, 96, 100, 133, 223, 228, 229, 232, 239, 247

assumptions, 139

asymmetry, 62, 157, 188

atrial septal defect, 27

attachment, 15, 33, 51, 118, 119, 204, 215, 218, 224, 225, 227, 231, 235, 238, 239, 242, 245, 247

attacks, 203

attention, 5, 11, 12, 15, 16, 26, 28, 29, 30, 39, 40, 43, 44, 46, 48, 52, 54, 56, 57, 61, 62, 63, 64, 65, 66, 67, 75, 76, 80, 81, 96, 99, 101, 108, 112, 122, 123, 126, 127, 130, 131, 133, 134, 137, 141, 142, 155, 156, 158, 159, 162, 164, 170, 171, 174, 176, 177, 178, 183, 186, 188, 190, 191, 193, 194, 195, 217, 218, 220, 222, 223, 227, 229, 230, 233, 237, 238, 241, 242, 247

Attention Deficit Hyperactivity Disorder, 96, 155, 158, 159, 178

attitudes, 82

auditory evoked potentials, 221

Australia, 22

authority, 79, 105, 220

autism, 40, 61, 177, 178, 222, 242, 247

autonomy, 121, 236

autopsy, 4

availability, 180, 183, 187

avoidance, 7, 230

awareness, 3, 10, 42, 80, 105, 111, 115, 116, 123, 145, 148, 182, 183, 197, 199, 229

axons, 60

B

back pain, 216

bad behavior, 105

baggage, 180

bargaining, 205

barriers, 76, 79, 87

basal ganglia, 21, 64, 101, 221

basic needs, 144

beer, 17, 137, 209, 216

behavior, 9, 14, 19, 34, 35, 36, 39, 40, 41, 43, 44, 45, 46, 47, 61, 63, 75, 77, 78, 79, 80, 81, 82, 88, 91,

92, 101, 104, 105, 106, 107, 110, 111, 113, 118,
119, 121, 122, 125, 127, 128, 129, 133, 134, 135,
137, 138, 139, 140, 141, 142, 145, 146, 147, 148,
150, 155, 158, 162, 169, 178, 179, 180, 186, 187,
188, 189, 190, 191, 192, 193, 194, 200, 212, 213,
219, 222, 224, 226, 231, 236, 239, 240, 241, 244,
247
behavior modification, 118
behavior of children, 61
behavioral change, 90
behavioral disorders, 28
behavioral inhibition system, 233
behavioral manifestations, 225
behavioral problems, 14, 16, 26, 33, 34, 40, 45, 53,
62, 71, 87, 131, 162, 222, 224
beverages, 181
bias, 219
binding, 3, 60
binge drinking, vii, viii, 3, 17, 28, 208
bingeing, 190
biological markers, 59
biomarkers, 28
bipolar disorder, 30, 58, 72, 83, 186, 228
birds, 114
birth, 7, 9, 11, 16, 17, 18, 19, 29, 30, 31, 32, 34, 36,
53, 58, 69, 70, 72, 73, 74, 82, 83, 84, 85, 86, 87,
89, 97, 101, 125, 157, 161, 174, 189, 190, 196,
202, 204, 205, 207, 208, 209, 211, 212, 217, 218,
226, 230
birth control, 30, 70, 85, 86, 204
birth rate, 73
birth weight, 9, 17, 18, 32, 208, 211, 226
births, 3, 70, 72, 73, 76, 85, 90, 91, 134
birthweight, 97
BIS, 62
blame, 112, 115, 119, 120, 186, 201
blood, 15, 28, 54, 60, 120, 230
blood flow, 230
body, 12, 17, 26, 36, 39, 40, 43, 54, 60, 86, 95, 100,
113, 115, 123, 128, 133, 142, 144, 161, 166, 170,
208, 217
body fluid, 54, 60
body weight, 100
bonding, 29, 77, 205, 225
bone age, 17, 208
borderline personality disorder, 235
boys, 4, 100, 142, 154, 155, 156, 157, 158, 159, 227
brain, vii, viii, 4, 9, 12, 16, 17, 18, 19, 20, 21, 23, 27,
28, 29, 31, 34, 37, 38, 39, 40, 41, 42, 46, 51, 53,
55, 56, 57, 60, 67, 88, 89, 90, 95, 97, 98, 100,
101, 104, 105, 106, 108, 109, 110, 111, 112, 113,
114, 115, 119, 120, 122, 123, 131, 133, 137, 155,
158, 159, 163, 170, 179, 180, 181, 182, 186, 187,
188, 189, 196, 200, 202, 204, 205, 208, 209, 212,
216, 217, 222, 223, 229, 235, 236, 237, 240, 247
brain damage, viii, 4, 12, 34, 53, 60, 88, 90, 100,
109, 114, 115, 120, 122, 123, 133, 137, 202, 203,
204, 205, 223, 236
brain functions, 97
brain growth, 20, 98, 209
brain size, 133
brain stem, 98
brain structure, 51, 55, 97, 98, 163
brain tumor, 216
brainstem, 12, 98, 243, 247
breakdown, 41, 166, 235
breathing, 28, 36, 197
brothers, 112
bulimia, 238, 247
bulimia nervosa, 238, 247
burnout, 210

C

caffeine, 34, 61
calcium, 60
California, 103, 124
Canada, vii, 8, 21, 30, 51, 56, 63, 70, 95, 123, 156,
160, 210, 215
canals, 221
cancer, 3
CAP, 82
capillary, 97
carbohydrate, 28
cardiologist, 217
caregivers, 21, 22, 36, 45, 46, 65, 105, 106, 112, 126,
128, 137, 139, 141, 143, 144, 151, 153, 206, 210,
211
caregiving, 129, 224
case study, 81, 87, 141, 143
cast, 108
category d, 130
cell, 4, 20, 22, 27, 60, 209
cell death, 4
cell membranes, 60
central executive, 220
central nervous system, viii, 1, 26, 27, 40, 53, 54, 87,
96, 97, 101, 105, 113, 117, 120, 122, 161, 188
cerebellum, 4, 16, 52, 106
cerebral blood flow, 230
cerebral palsy, 53, 63, 188
cerebrospinal fluid, 54
changing environment, 29, 166
channels, 218
charm, 216
child abuse, 30, 81, 197

Child Behavior Checklist, 223
child development, 41, 175
child maltreatment, 158
child molesters, 156
child protection, 82, 184, 185, 190
childcare, 79, 186, 189
childhood, vii, viii, 6, 8, 15, 21, 25, 29, 36, 44, 47, 52, 53, 58, 62, 65, 87, 96, 97, 98, 100, 117, 127, 128, 129, 131, 132, 137, 138, 139, 141, 142, 144, 145, 156, 177, 180, 188, 190, 191, 200, 204, 226, 229, 230, 231, 233, 239, 243, 247
childhood disorders, 131, 177
childhood sexual abuse, 127, 129
cigarette smoking, 242, 247
circadian rhythm, 22, 211
circadian rhythms, 22, 211
class size, 99
classes, 81, 89, 105, 111, 141, 149
classification, vii, 6, 8, 13, 21, 32, 38, 53, 62, 96, 140, 160, 181, 224
classroom, 44, 99, 138, 173, 191, 193, 194, 195, 200
classroom teacher, 191
cleft palate, 97
clients, 23, 37, 72, 73, 74, 75, 76, 77, 78, 79, 80, 81, 82, 84, 85, 86, 87, 88, 89, 90, 91, 111, 121, 124, 126, 127, 151, 153, 177, 182, 184, 187, 189, 211, 244, 247
clinical assessment, 14, 176
clinical depression, 90
clinical diagnosis, 2
clinical disorders, 25
clinical presentation, vii, 4, 6, 13, 16, 57, 202, 203
clinical syndrome, 217
clusters, 8
CNS, 1, 4, 6, 18, 19, 27, 29, 30, 41, 55, 56, 57, 59, 104, 105, 117, 119, 128, 130, 134, 135, 136, 137, 138, 140, 141, 145, 146, 148, 149, 150, 153, 212
coaches, 151
cocaine, 14, 69, 83, 91, 191, 222, 227, 242, 247
cocaine abuse, 227
coding, 5, 181, 183
coffee, 120
cognition, 4, 10, 20, 38, 99, 112, 119, 179, 180, 213, 219
cognitive abilities, 166, 168
cognitive ability, 18, 55, 201, 209
cognitive deficit, 37, 87, 96, 127, 135, 136, 137, 146, 147, 148, 149, 152, 170, 188, 194, 223, 235
cognitive development, 47, 53
cognitive dysfunction, 22, 227
cognitive flexibility, 222
cognitive function, 5, 37, 180

cognitive impairment, 55, 80, 103, 129, 143, 145, 147, 148, 149, 150, 151, 194
cognitive performance, 194
cognitive process, 109, 130, 165, 166, 174
cognitive processing, 174
cognitive research, 166
cohesion, 164, 169, 206
cohort, 73, 224, 228, 230, 233
collaboration, 87, 89, 150, 151
collateral, 14
college students, 229
commitment, 90, 146, 149
communication, 5, 10, 16, 20, 52, 77, 79, 105, 119, 123, 124, 132, 139, 161, 162, 163, 164, 165, 166, 167, 168, 169, 170, 171, 172, 173, 174, 175, 176, 177, 178, 187, 192, 193, 201, 213, 218, 222, 224, 225, 227, 228, 229, 238, 239, 247
communication competence, 162, 163, 173
communication skills, 178
community, 3, 32, 34, 36, 70, 71, 73, 75, 76, 79, 87, 88, 90, 91, 95, 104, 112, 114, 121, 122, 123, 126, 127, 132, 143, 145, 146, 147, 151, 152, 153, 179, 180, 183, 185, 189, 225, 243, 247
community service, 70, 73, 87, 88
community support, 36, 151, 189
comorbidity, 92, 127, 133, 136, 179, 218
compassion, 205
compensation, 148
competence, 53, 75, 105, 161, 164, 166, 167, 168, 170, 186
competency, 148
complex partial seizure, 5, 9, 18, 19, 57, 203, 212, 223
complexity, viii, 58, 80, 219, 220
compliance, 76, 82, 84, 106, 151, 191, 195
complications, 37, 56, 69, 109, 179, 180, 181, 184
components, 45, 60, 97, 112, 114, 115, 150, 164, 167, 170, 171, 199, 205, 206, 221, 229
composites, 189
composition, 38
compounds, 51, 203
comprehension, 88, 96, 100, 105, 180, 219, 221, 230, 242, 247
compulsion, 129, 140
computation, 132
computer use, 152
concentrates, 18, 209
concentration, 111, 125
conception, viii, 30
conceptual model, 47
conceptualization, 200
concrete, 74, 75, 78, 79, 86, 88, 220
conditioning, 200

conduct, 51, 53, 61, 96, 132, 138, 162, 216, 223, 227
conduct disorder, 51, 53, 162, 216, 227
conduction, 229
confabulation, 235
confidentiality, 217
confinement, 33, 134, 139, 224
conflict, 86, 107, 108, 168, 172, 234
confrontation, 200
confusion, 126, 137
conscious awareness, 180
consciousness, 221, 235
consensus, 2, 47, 48, 65
consent, 109, 138
construction, 165, 216, 220
consulting, 194
consumers, 226
consumption, 28, 31, 34, 98, 99, 133, 156, 236
control, 10, 19, 44, 98, 99, 105, 110, 113, 120, 125,
    127, 130, 131, 133, 134, 136, 137, 148, 150, 151,
    155, 167, 189, 202, 213, 219, 221, 226, 227, 228,
    243, 247
controlled studies, 56
conversion, 60
conviction, 146, 147
coping, 76, 82, 129, 145, 156, 226, 227, 245, 247
coping strategies, 76
corn, 32
corpus callosum, 4, 9, 16, 17, 18, 19, 20, 22, 28, 29,
    34, 51, 97, 98, 101, 102, 106, 133, 187, 208, 209,
    212, 222, 223, 229, 237, 238, 247
correlation, 228, 230, 231
cortex, 222, 229
cost saving, 73
costs, 92
counsel, 148
counseling, 12, 74, 92, 204
crack, 81
craving, 9, 11, 19, 212
creatinine, 15
credit, 115
crime, 83, 128, 135, 141, 147
criminal justice system, 145, 146, 148, 155, 159,
    238, 247
critical period, 65
crying, 6, 7, 134, 218
CSF, 60
cues, 7, 46, 103, 130, 134, 138, 165, 166, 168, 169,
    170, 171, 174, 191, 205, 216, 230
culture, 181, 201
curiosity, 142, 143
curriculum, 193, 194, 210
cycles, 77
cycling, 202

cytochrome, 58, 203

D

daily living, 5, 16, 88, 134, 193, 201, 205, 224
damage, viii, 28, 55, 57, 65, 66, 69, 82, 98, 100, 104,
    105, 106, 107, 108, 109, 110, 112, 113, 114, 117,
    119, 120, 122, 123, 131, 133, 137, 160, 161, 202,
    221, 222, 228, 238, 247
danger, 113, 145, 150
dangerousness, 147, 148
data collection, 148
dating, 128, 136, 138, 143, 144
death, 53, 191, 203, 210
deaths, 4
decision making, 182
decision-making process, 86, 174
decisions, 82, 86, 89, 110, 172
deductive reasoning, 180
defects, 12, 34, 36, 56, 95, 98, 131, 140, 157, 181,
    202, 221
defendants, 145, 146, 148, 155
defense, 145, 148, 233
defensiveness, 42, 48
deficiency, 41, 95, 97, 98, 130, 161
deficit, 2, 40, 48, 61, 62, 63, 64, 65, 66, 67, 101, 119,
    130, 131, 155, 156, 158, 159, 162, 175, 176, 178,
    180, 192, 200, 219, 221, 222, 223, 230, 233, 238,
    242, 247
definition, 74, 104, 184, 230
delinquency, 241, 247
delinquent behavior, 132, 224
delirium, 14
delivery, 14, 29, 53, 73, 87, 150, 180, 183, 184, 191,
    196
delusion, 112
demand, 120, 223
dementia, 14
denial, 139, 205
density, 133
dentist, 173, 204
Department of Health and Human Services, 93, 154,
    155
depression, 4, 29, 52, 54, 61, 69, 72, 91, 103, 107,
    108, 132, 197, 215, 216, 223, 226, 228, 230, 231,
    232, 234, 235, 239, 241, 242, 247
depressive symptoms, 72, 202
deprivation, 47, 72, 233
derivatives, 220
desire, 165, 216
destruction, 227
detection, 144
detention, 83, 147, 227

developing brain, 2, 4, 11, 14, 21, 40, 55, 98, 137, 207

developmental disorder, 2, 21, 30, 32, 33, 61, 62, 201

developmental milestones, 17, 187, 190, 208, 217

developmental process, 127, 164

developmental psychopathology, 177

deviation, 192

diabetes, 3, 14, 55, 203

diagnostic criteria, 1, 10

diet, 31, 45

differential diagnosis, 13

differential treatment, 113

differentiation, 27

dignity, 121, 123

direct observation, 176

disability, vii, viii, 2, 5, 14, 15, 16, 21, 30, 33, 53, 56, 62, 89, 103, 109, 142, 145, 155, 157, 162, 199, 201, 202, 204, 206, 209, 219, 220, 243, 247

disappointment, 105, 117

discipline, 112, 185, 187, 226, 233

discomfort, 113, 126

discourse, 52, 164, 165, 167, 169, 201

discrimination, 41, 43, 67, 222

discrimination learning, 67

disequilibrium, 67

dislocation, 97

disorder, 2, 3, 5, 8, 9, 11, 14, 15, 17, 18, 19, 20, 22, 25, 30, 33, 36, 48, 51, 52, 53, 55, 57, 58, 61, 62, 63, 64, 65, 66, 67, 72, 96, 101, 104, 108, 119, 124, 130, 131, 132, 155, 156, 158, 159, 162, 176, 178, 180, 182, 186, 199, 201, 202, 203, 204, 205, 207, 208, 210, 211, 212, 213, 219, 223, 227, 228, 233, 237, 238, 242, 243, 247

displacement, 97, 226

dissatisfaction, 232

dissociation, 230, 232, 241, 247

distress, 7, 226, 238, 247

diversity, 80

DNA, 2, 3

doctors, viii

domain, 40

domestic violence, 69, 70, 75, 191

dominance, 188, 191

dopamine, 5, 11, 52, 54, 57, 62, 67, 133, 156, 233

dosage, 1, 15, 17, 56, 57, 98, 203, 208

drug abuse, 69, 75, 90, 93

drug addict, 76

drug addiction, 76

drug dependence, 67

drug side effects, 202

drug therapy, 57, 58, 62, 155, 203

drug toxicity, 203

drug treatment, 33, 70, 73, 74, 81, 90

drug use, 69, 73, 76, 83, 90, 191

drugs, 14, 35, 70, 71, 73, 74, 75, 76, 80, 81, 84, 88, 90, 91, 92, 150, 196, 197, 202, 239, 247

DSM, 5, 6, 8, 12, 13, 53, 61, 72, 92, 96, 131, 134, 140, 182, 219, 228

DSM-II, 92

DSM-III, 92

DSM-IV, 61, 72, 96, 131, 134, 140, 219, 228

duration, 42, 96

duties, 31

dyslexia, 186

E

ears, 13, 16, 201

eating, 29, 81, 134, 196, 218, 228, 237, 238, 240, 241, 244, 247

eating disorders, 218, 240, 244, 247

ecology, 159

economic disadvantage, 226

educational system, 71

EEG, 15, 29, 35, 62, 203, 223, 230, 237, 247

EEG activity, 29

ego, 215, 220, 222, 228, 233, 235, 236, 245, 247

egocentrism, 136

elaboration, 165

elementary school, 3, 53, 125, 138, 191, 219, 227, 241, 247

elementary students, 48

embryo, viii, 98, 101

embryogenesis, 3, 53, 66

emergence, 127, 174, 188, 191

emotion, 38, 43, 114, 116, 140, 141, 222, 229, 230, 234, 236, 245, 247

emotional distress, 201

emotional experience, 220, 234

emotional information, 230

emotional stability, 99

emotions, viii, 10, 20, 46, 116, 117, 200, 201, 213, 223, 229, 230, 231, 235, 244, 247

empathy, 136, 149, 239, 247

employment, 75, 84, 110, 121, 169, 217

encephalitis, 14

encephalopathy, 182, 188, 193, 194

encoding, 2, 166, 171, 219, 221

encouragement, 75, 84, 107, 174

endocrine, 14, 20, 203

endocrine disorders, 14

endocrinologist, 17, 209

energy, 18, 109, 209

England, 177

enlargement, 98

enrollment, 70, 87, 190

environment, 2, 4, 6, 7, 17, 19, 33, 39, 41, 45, 46, 49,
    52, 55, 59, 62, 69, 80, 81, 84, 88, 118, 127, 138,
    139, 140, 143, 144, 159, 170, 171, 172, 187, 189,
    192, 194, 200, 207, 209, 213, 221, 226, 228, 231,
    235, 236

environmental factors, 4, 25, 41, 65, 136

environmental influences, 182

environmental issues, 79

environmental stimuli, 6, 108

enzymes, 2, 3

epidemiology, 23, 26, 65, 157, 159, 211

epigenetics, 2, 23

epilepsy, 53, 229

equilibrium, 59, 120

ethanol, 3, 20, 23, 28, 35, 36, 37, 38, 62, 64, 98, 101,
    137, 156, 226, 243, 247

ethnic groups, 1

ethnicity, 17, 31, 75, 208, 219, 221, 227

etiology, 4, 12, 17, 20, 66, 182, 186, 188, 205, 209

etiquette, 79

Europe, vii, 96

evening, 46

event-related potential, 238, 247

evidence, 5, 6, 8, 15, 19, 25, 40, 41, 43, 51, 52, 65,
    104, 130, 131, 133, 141, 142, 165, 166, 181, 182,
    202, 212, 213, 216, 219, 223, 226, 229, 231, 236

evoked potential, 243, 247

evolution, 59, 237, 247

examinations, 52, 85

excitation, 202

excitotoxicity, 60

exclusion, 118

excuse, 111

executive functions, 164, 166, 167, 168, 169, 174,
    175, 177, 233

executive processes, 156

exercise, 106, 120

expectations, 14, 41, 46, 47, 75, 79, 80, 86, 105, 106,
    111, 112, 117, 119, 146, 162, 170, 180, 191, 205,
    217

expertise, 90, 148

experts, 79

explicit memory, 221, 241, 247

exposure, vii, viii, 1, 2, 4, 5, 6, 8, 9, 11, 13, 14, 15,
    16, 17, 18, 19, 20, 21, 22, 23, 25, 26, 27, 28, 29,
    30, 34, 35, 36, 37, 38, 40, 44, 47, 52, 54, 55, 57,
    58, 61, 62, 64, 65, 66, 67, 69, 80, 86, 87, 89, 92,
    95, 97, 98, 100, 101, 102, 104, 106, 108, 111,
    113, 115, 119, 123, 128, 131, 133, 134, 137, 139,
    144, 154, 160, 161, 162, 164, 168, 171, 172, 175,
    176, 177, 179, 181, 183, 185, 186, 188, 190, 192,
    193, 194, 195, 209, 210, 211, 212, 217, 219, 220,

221, 222, 224, 225, 228, 233, 235, 236, 237, 238,
    239, 240, 241, 242, 243, 247

expression, 35, 38, 52, 126, 127, 128, 129, 134, 136,
    137, 138, 139, 142, 143, 217, 219, 221, 222, 223,
    227, 230, 234

externalizing behavior, 223, 231, 234, 236

externalizing disorders, 228

extinction, 240, 247

F

facial expression, 80, 240, 247

failure, 28, 44, 79, 85, 109, 110, 111, 119, 129, 134,
    136, 221

failure to thrive, 28, 44

faith, 76, 167

false positive, 182

family, 11, 16, 20, 32, 57, 62, 66, 74, 76, 77, 78, 81,
    82, 83, 84, 85, 86, 88, 89, 90, 106, 108, 110, 112,
    115, 118, 139, 145, 151, 152, 155, 170, 174, 180,
    184, 185, 186, 187, 188, 189, 190, 191, 192, 193,
    194, 195, 197, 202, 204, 205, 206, 207, 210, 216,
    222, 225, 227, 228, 230

family functioning, 205

family history, 11, 20, 108, 186, 187, 190, 228

family life, 194

family members, 77, 84, 151, 189, 190, 197, 205

family physician, 202, 204

family planning, 76, 85, 86, 88, 90

family relationships, 225

family studies, 222

family support, 145, 195

family system, 16

family therapy, 32, 58, 66

FAS, vii, 2, 3, 4, 6, 8, 9, 10, 13, 15, 16, 17, 18, 23,
    26, 27, 31, 32, 33, 34, 37, 48, 51, 52, 56, 64, 66,
    69, 70, 73, 87, 91, 95, 96, 97, 98, 99, 100, 101,
    102, 130, 133, 139, 144, 157, 158, 159, 161, 175,
    176, 177, 181, 182, 188, 191, 194, 199, 200, 201,
    204, 205, 206, 207, 208, 209, 210, 211, 217, 218,
    220, 221, 222, 223, 226, 227, 228, 233, 234, 244,
    247

fast food, 152

fatigue, 120, 205, 232

FDA, 202

fear, 107, 108, 116, 204, 205

febrile seizure, 55

federal funds, 183

feedback, 44, 143, 165, 169

feelings, 10, 16, 17, 20, 86, 109, 116, 122, 129, 138,
    145, 201, 209, 213, 229, 231, 232, 234

females, 54, 126, 134, 135, 141, 144, 229, 234

fertilization, 3, 27

fetal alcohol syndrome, 21, 22, 23, 34, 35, 37, 38, 48, 62, 63, 64, 65, 66, 69, 91, 93, 101, 102, 124, 155, 157, 158, 159, 160, 175, 176, 177, 178, 196, 210, 211, 216, 217, 218, 227, 237, 238, 240, 241, 242, 243, 244, 245, 247
fetal growth, 27
fetus, 1, 4, 25, 30, 31, 95, 97, 98
fibromyalgia, 234
figure-ground, 223
financial stability, 90
financial support, 206
financing, 32, 207
Finland, 230, 232
fish, 114
flexibility, 110, 116, 219, 236
flight, 42, 113, 234
floating, 200
fluoxetine, 17, 57, 208
focusing, 168, 171, 183, 194, 228, 234
folate, 3, 31, 34
folic acid, 31
food, 27, 44, 103, 113, 119
forgetting, 108
forgiveness, 120
fragility, 120
France, 1, 3
freedom, 117
friends, 81, 106, 138, 139, 143, 151
friendship, 77, 139
frontal cortex, 4, 20, 28, 38
frontal lobe, 60, 106, 133, 220, 222
frustration, 85, 86, 136, 149, 200
fuel, 140
fulfillment, 106
functional approach, 163
funding, 16, 84, 183
furniture, 42

G

gait, 9, 18, 19, 29, 212
ganglion, 4, 11, 60
gangs, 83
gender, 3, 17, 31, 56, 84, 165, 204, 208, 217, 221, 232
gene, 2, 3, 23, 52, 62, 63
gene expression, 3
gene silencing, 3
general intelligence, 132
generalization, 150, 170, 174
generalized anxiety disorder, 55
generation, viii, 30, 33, 59, 110, 202, 222
genes, 2, 3, 21, 59, 62, 65, 210

genetic disorders, 13
genetic endowment, 2
genetic factors, 4
genetic traits, 4
genetics, 37
Georgia, 21, 210
Germany, 223
gestation, vii, 17, 61, 62, 87, 98, 189, 208, 237, 247
gestational age, 36
gestures, 140
girls, 4, 100, 144, 203, 241, 247
glial cells, 22, 60
glucose, 15, 67, 106, 203
glutamate, 60
goals, 7, 75, 77, 78, 79, 85, 121, 164, 165, 166, 168, 169, 170, 171
goal-setting, 86
gold, 181
government, viii
grades, 227
grants, 79
grief, 89, 205, 234
group processes, 149, 150
group therapy, 150, 173
groups, 4, 29, 85, 89, 99, 108, 115, 121, 122, 133, 140, 146, 149, 150, 165, 167, 169, 188, 205, 219
growth, 1, 8, 9, 15, 17, 19, 27, 28, 56, 57, 74, 87, 91, 92, 95, 97, 98, 100, 105, 122, 130, 137, 161, 181, 182, 187, 191, 194, 201, 208, 209, 212, 218, 220
growth hormone, 57
guidance, 206, 236
guidelines, 36, 65, 91, 151, 153, 170, 172, 173, 174, 175, 181, 217
guilt, 126, 226, 227
guilty, 145, 205

H

habituation, 29, 44, 52, 54, 134, 204
hallucinations, 9, 19, 203, 212
hands, 18, 78, 80, 89, 209
handwriting, 43, 119
happiness, 123
harm, 76, 81
harmful effects, 161
HE, 195
headache, 201, 232
headache,. 201, 232
healing, 119, 121, 122
health, viii, 15, 17, 26, 30, 32, 53, 63, 64, 72, 73, 76, 79, 81, 85, 90, 95, 96, 108, 110, 135, 148, 149, 180, 182, 183, 186, 188, 206, 209, 244, 245, 247
health care, 15, 17, 32, 73, 79, 81, 85, 209

health problems, 108, 135, 188
health services, 244, 247
heart rate, 36
heavy drinking, 98, 108
height, 9, 15, 17, 18, 32, 100, 187, 196, 208, 211, 212
helplessness, 129
hemiplegia, 53
hepatitis, 85
heroin, 89, 216
high school, 16, 17, 70, 141, 146, 147, 190, 208, 216, 227
higher education, 226
hip, 97
hippocampus, 5, 16, 52, 59
histone, 2, 3
HIV, 14
homelessness, 70, 110
homework, 104, 111, 150
honesty, 115
hopelessness, 232, 239, 247
hormone, 17, 62, 208
hospitals, 149
host, 1, 10, 70, 72
hostility, 219
housing, 71, 77, 78, 79, 80, 83, 84, 85, 89, 111, 121, 207
human brain, 60
human condition, 238, 247
human development, 137, 140
husband, 77, 189
hydrocephalus, 4, 98
hygiene, 105, 106, 107, 119, 122, 134
hyperactivity, 29, 40, 48, 53, 54, 61, 62, 63, 64, 65, 66, 67, 96, 99, 101, 112, 131, 133, 134, 136, 137, 139, 155, 158, 159, 160, 162, 176, 178, 179, 194, 195, 218, 219, 238, 242, 247
hypersensitivity, 55, 58, 108, 133
hyperventilation, 7
hypoglycemia, 97
hypoplasia, 4, 9, 12, 18, 19, 29, 97, 212
hypothesis, 29, 52, 108, 109, 120, 134
hypoxia, 14

I

ibuprofen, 36
ICD, 6
ideas, viii, 3, 47, 86, 167, 169, 170, 206, 221
identification, 31, 111, 119, 120, 127, 159, 161, 179, 182, 188
identity, 17, 31, 180, 205, 208, 226
illicit substances, 69

images, 43, 64, 187, 230
imagination, 103
imbalances, 106
immunoglobulin, 4
immunoreactivity, 22
imprinting, viii, 2, 22, 52
impulsive, viii, 7, 42, 52, 131, 162, 200, 207, 219, 235
impulsivity, 4, 5, 7, 11, 13, 16, 17, 29, 44, 57, 96, 117, 118, 126, 132, 133, 136, 139, 150, 159, 179, 191, 193, 208, 215, 220, 242, 247
inattention, 9, 15, 17, 18, 40, 52, 112, 131, 132, 133, 208, 209, 235
incarceration, 10, 106, 123, 132, 142, 228
incidence, 3, 31, 72, 73, 76, 85, 126, 127, 133, 134, 137, 182, 186, 191, 219, 222, 223, 226, 227, 242, 247
inclusion, 227
income, 71, 74, 80
independence, 77, 110, 122
indication, 76, 97, 103, 142
indicators, 44, 71, 95, 99
indices, 219, 223, 236
indirect effect, 238, 247
indirect measure, 229
individual character, 136
individual characteristics, 136
individual differences, 25, 43, 241, 247
industry, 85, 227
infancy, vii, viii, 6, 11, 14, 21, 25, 29, 32, 35, 38, 44, 51, 55, 62, 63, 96, 100, 101, 125, 137, 140, 157, 184, 186, 189, 204, 206, 210, 224
infants, vii, viii, 1, 2, 11, 26, 28, 29, 30, 31, 32, 33, 35, 38, 44, 45, 51, 53, 57, 62, 81, 97, 98, 133, 137, 160, 188, 218, 224, 238, 247
infection, 196
infectious disease, 14
inferences, 45, 166, 223
infinite, 112, 217
information processing, 221
informed consent, 58
ingestion, 36, 217
inheritance, 2, 22
inhibition, 54, 130, 131, 132, 134, 139, 150, 174, 218, 219, 220, 222, 229, 233, 234, 235, 239, 247
injury, vii, 57, 81, 89, 128, 131, 140, 179, 180, 181, 182, 186, 188, 189, 191, 196, 202, 231
innocence, 143
input, 39, 42, 43, 44, 45, 46, 99, 112, 117, 192, 193, 219
insecurity, 99
insight, 10, 20, 104, 213, 229, 234, 235
instability, 55, 58, 99, 201, 202

instinct, 107
institutions, 216
instruction, 99, 149
instruments, 5, 31, 223, 228, 231
insurance, 6, 17, 85, 209
integration, viii, 6, 15, 32, 39, 40, 41, 43, 44, 45, 46,
   47, 48, 58, 113, 116, 119, 151, 165, 187, 204,
   205, 206
integrity, 60, 105, 116, 220
intellect, 243
intellectual disabilities, 158
intelligence, 96, 100, 102, 115, 201, 219, 220, 243,
   244, 247
intensity, 33, 42, 44, 113, 116, 117, 230, 231
intent, 122, 128, 153, 231
intentionality, 220
intentions, 107, 130, 169
interaction, 10, 20, 33, 45, 51, 53, 134, 150, 166,
   175, 180, 187, 204, 213, 222, 225, 231
interactions, 44, 107, 153, 154, 162, 164, 165, 166,
   167, 168, 169, 171, 175, 177, 180, 184, 187, 192,
   215, 219, 221
interdependence, 77
interest, 2, 126, 139, 140, 141, 142, 144, 162, 188,
   190, 194
internal working models, 220
internalization, 132
internalizing, 223
International Classification of Diseases, 95
interpersonal relations, 74, 193, 194
interpersonal relationships, 74, 193, 194
interpersonal skills, 135, 143
interpretation, 106, 114, 186, 219
interval, 27
intervention, 22, 26, 30, 33, 34, 45, 46, 48, 49, 56,
   58, 65, 70, 72, 73, 74, 76, 77, 78, 79, 86, 87, 88,
   89, 91, 92, 104, 106, 108, 118, 119, 136, 137,
   139, 143, 144, 151, 153, 164, 168, 170, 174, 176,
   178, 185, 189, 193, 195, 211, 215, 234
intervention strategies, 45
interview, 61, 89, 185, 186, 187, 192, 216
intimacy, 139, 142, 143
intuition, 123
ipsilateral, 229
IQ scores, 29, 98, 178, 192
Ireland, vii
iron, 97
irritability, 26, 218
isolation, 27, 113, 123, 126, 169, 179, 180, 182, 218

J

job skills, 190

jobs, 105, 108, 111, 200, 216
joints, 97
Jordan, 92
judgment, 9, 10, 16, 20, 88, 90, 96, 108, 111, 114,
   116, 130, 180, 188, 190, 213
junior high school, 216, 227
justice, 111, 159
juveniles, 83, 128, 146

K

kidney, 12, 27, 95, 202, 204
kidneys, 12, 27
kindergarten, 219, 220
kindergarten children, 219
knowledge, vii, 58, 59, 76, 84, 85, 123, 126, 129,
   138, 153, 164, 166, 167, 168, 169, 180, 186, 206

L

labor, 112
labour, 14
lack of opportunities, 129
land, 120, 216
language, viii, 5, 8, 10, 15, 19, 20, 26, 32, 41, 52, 58,
   88, 96, 97, 100, 105, 109, 130, 160, 161, 162,
   163, 164, 165, 166, 167, 168, 169, 170, 171, 172,
   174, 175, 176, 177, 178, 180, 187, 188, 190, 192,
   199, 200, 201, 206, 207, 213, 221, 222, 229, 239,
   243, 247
language development, 5, 239, 247
language impairment, 175, 207
language processing, 100, 200
language proficiency, 52
language skills, 169, 171, 172, 190
latency, 29, 52, 224
later life, 215, 218, 224, 227, 231
laterality, 188
laughing, 134
law enforcement, 135, 186
lead, 4, 14, 15, 58, 119, 127, 134, 136, 150, 204,
   215, 219, 225, 226, 230, 231, 234, 236
learning, 2, 5, 10, 20, 26, 27, 36, 39, 40, 41, 43, 46,
   52, 53, 54, 55, 57, 80, 96, 99, 100, 101, 105, 108,
   125, 128, 130, 137, 138, 139, 143, 144, 150, 151,
   155, 158, 159, 162, 168, 170, 171, 172, 174, 177,
   178, 180, 185, 186, 188, 190, 193, 194, 195, 199,
   201, 213, 219, 220, 221, 240, 241, 243, 247
learning difficulties, 99, 130, 162, 243, 247
learning disabilities, 2, 40, 101, 108
learning environment, 99, 171
learning process, 143

learning task, 220
lesions, 14, 215, 221, 225, 233
life span, 135
lifespan, vii, 10, 11, 13, 26, 34, 44, 45, 52, 87, 90,
    92, 95, 96, 176, 207
lifestyle, 70, 85, 151, 159, 181, 190, 192, 219, 225
lifetime, viii, 73, 215
likelihood, 4, 69, 70, 82, 116, 144, 203
links, 164, 169, 225
listening, 108
liver, 3, 12, 14, 16, 56, 58, 203, 204
liver disease, 14
living arrangements, 149
living environment, 224, 236
local community, 84, 184, 186
localization, 238, 247
location, 43, 227
logistics, 185, 189
longitudinal study, 29, 157, 227, 237, 244, 247
long-term memory, 88
loyalty, 216
Luvox, 150
lying, 96, 104, 115, 116, 117

M

magazines, 152
magnesium, 31
magnetic resonance, 159
magnetic resonance imaging, 159
major depression, 72, 155, 228, 243, 247
major depressive disorder, 228, 232, 239, 247
males, 54, 134, 135, 139, 141, 154, 221, 229, 236,
    237, 247
malnutrition, 82
management, vii, viii, 9, 12, 15, 16, 27, 51, 57, 58,
    59, 60, 70, 72, 73, 83, 87, 111, 121, 127, 182,
    183, 184, 187, 189, 194, 199, 200, 202, 206, 207,
    215, 245, 247
manganese, 14
manipulation, 220
manners, 192
mapping, 3, 4
marijuana, 83, 126, 222, 242, 247
market, 113
marriage, viii, 33, 138, 217
Mars, 112
mathematics, 52, 201
maturation, 4, 106, 113, 163, 235, 236
meanings, 88
measurement, 187
measures, 56, 99, 100, 131, 156, 177, 219, 222, 223,
    229, 231, 232, 235, 241, 247

meat, viii
meconium, 28
media, 139, 144, 152
mediation, 159
medication, viii, 9, 12, 13, 15, 16, 17, 32, 51, 52, 55,
    56, 57, 58, 59, 60, 63, 64, 65, 76, 81, 83, 118,
    120, 150, 179, 188, 193, 194, 195, 202, 203, 204,
    207, 208, 209, 233
medulla, 98
medulla oblongata, 98
melatonin, 203
memory, 27, 52, 59, 88, 89, 90, 96, 105, 111, 113,
    114, 115, 116, 117, 119, 120, 121, 130, 148, 150,
    160, 170, 174, 177, 193, 200, 201, 220, 221, 229,
    241, 245, 247
memory retrieval, 221
men, 222, 229
meningitis, 14
mental development, 29
mental disorder, 25, 72, 153
mental health, viii, 6, 11, 15, 16, 21, 26, 62, 63, 72,
    76, 83, 96, 109, 111, 119, 126, 129, 134, 142,
    143, 147, 149, 151, 174, 180, 182, 183, 185, 186,
    188, 190, 195, 205, 206, 224, 225, 226, 231
mental health professionals, 126, 129, 143
mental illness, 22, 70, 83, 104, 105, 119, 122, 228
mental processes, 155
mental representation, 235
mental retardation, 9, 15, 21, 26, 52, 55, 56, 61, 63,
    69, 96, 98, 99, 100, 127, 143, 145, 155, 158, 159,
    199, 201, 202, 206, 210, 218
mental state, 166, 172
mental states, 166
mentoring, 90
mentorship, 16
mercury, 14
messages, 83, 113, 138
metabolic disorder, 14
metabolism, 3, 64, 67, 203
metacognition, 10, 20, 130, 213
methodology, 155
methylation, 2, 3
methylphenidate, 17, 18, 56, 57, 59, 61, 62, 63, 64,
    66, 67, 202, 208, 209
mice, 36, 38, 54
microcephaly, 4, 9, 18, 19, 29, 96, 97, 98, 100, 187,
    212
middle class, 82, 227
migration, 4, 27, 98, 181
military, 216
minors, 128
misunderstanding, 109, 126, 195, 203, 204
mitochondria, 60

mobility, 152
mode, 220, 231
model system, 66
modeling, 75, 80, 86, 92, 118, 129, 172, 178, 226
models, 35, 53, 62, 65, 75, 79, 152, 157, 172, 184, 188, 228
modern society, 233
money, 108, 111, 117, 121, 190
monitoring, 13, 43, 63, 152, 168, 169, 194, 207, 218, 227, 234
monograph, 217
mood, 8, 18, 22, 51, 53, 55, 57, 60, 76, 106, 112, 117, 119, 120, 133, 209, 211, 226, 228, 239, 247
mood disorder, 18, 22, 51, 53, 57, 60, 209, 211, 228, 239, 247
mood states, 76
moral reasoning, 132
morbidity, 11, 61, 203
morning, 108
morphogenesis, 98
morphological abnormalities, 223
morphology, 52, 155, 164, 195, 220
mortality, 4, 31, 35, 240, 247
Moscow, 23
mothers, 1, 21, 27, 28, 30, 34, 35, 37, 62, 70, 71, 72, 77, 80, 81, 84, 86, 87, 90, 91, 97, 98, 99, 101, 137, 138, 176, 190, 210, 218, 222, 223, 224, 225, 226, 227, 235, 237, 238, 239, 240, 241, 243, 244, 247
motion, 7, 79, 97, 217
motivation, 75, 84, 88, 106, 139, 140, 222, 236
motor actions, 43
motor activity, 7
motor control, 106, 113
motor skills, 26, 29, 43, 97, 113
movement, 28, 39, 42, 43, 44, 45, 46, 113
MRI, 4, 16, 17, 133, 187, 202, 208, 223
multidimensional, 63
multiple personality, 8
muscles, 98
music, 46, 80, 206
mutagen, 4

174, 176, 186, 197, 199, 201, 204, 205, 207, 209, 233
negative affectivity, 231
negative consequences, 174, 200, 233
negativity, 52
neglect, 7, 30, 32, 81, 82, 83, 144, 180, 187, 190, 191, 197, 221, 231, 235
negotiating, 79, 167, 169, 171
negotiation, 145, 147
neonates, 29, 35, 44, 52, 64, 133
nerve, 4, 12, 137
nervous system, 1, 40, 42, 44, 46, 47, 62, 65, 104, 109, 116, 119, 120, 122
network, 73, 77, 79, 83, 89, 90, 121
neurobiology, 41, 62, 243, 247
neurodegeneration, 4, 21, 60, 157, 210
neurogenesis, 27
neurologist, 15
neuromotor, 47, 119
neuronal cells, 98
neurons, 60
neurophysiology, 51, 55, 106
neuroprotective agents, 31
neuroscience, 53, 66
neurotransmission, 60
neurotransmitter, 1, 11, 26, 27, 51, 54, 55, 60, 106, 203
newspapers, 152
next generation, 33, 70, 207
nicotine, 14, 34, 66, 118, 160
nightmares, 197
noise, 80
non-clinical population, 222
norepinephrine, 54, 156
normal children, 132, 133, 155, 157
normal development, 117, 179, 194, 233
North America, 96
nucleus, 98, 106, 155, 157, 236
nursing, 75, 218, 231
nurturance, 180
nutrients, 31
nutrition, 9, 18, 34, 35, 37, 117, 120, 211

N

NAD, 3
NADH, 3
narratives, 165, 167, 169
National Institutes of Health, 38
Native Americans, 56
needs, 7, 15, 18, 33, 39, 44, 46, 49, 55, 78, 79, 80, 81, 84, 85, 86, 87, 88, 90, 109, 112, 122, 126, 142, 143, 147, 149, 150, 151, 153, 160, 166, 168,

O

observable behavior, 40, 167
observations, 29, 44, 45, 100, 166, 192, 219, 229, 232
occupational therapy, 48, 89
offenders, 111, 126, 127, 130, 132, 135, 149, 150, 151, 157, 158, 234
oil, 120
Oklahoma, 154

oocyte, 27
oppositional behaviour, 96
Oppositional Defiant Disorder, 200
organ, 12, 26, 27, 45, 100, 204
organization, 7, 27, 193, 200, 220, 229
otitis media, 12, 28, 221
outpatients, 232
output, 100, 180
overload, 105
oversight, 82
ovum, 27
oxidative stress, 3

P

pain, 42, 201, 204, 205
pancreatitis, 203
panic attack, 7, 55, 57, 203
panic disorder, 14
paradigm shift, 105
parameter, 181
parental care, 231
parental relationships, 231
parenthood, 58
parenting, 7, 16, 30, 31, 75, 78, 80, 81, 83, 84, 89,
    107, 108, 111, 115, 121, 122, 180, 186, 204, 226,
    231, 239, 247
parenting styles, 226
parents, 16, 17, 21, 22, 30, 32, 36, 38, 39, 46, 48, 58,
    65, 70, 83, 92, 93, 100, 110, 113, 126, 132, 133,
    138, 144, 151, 154, 167, 174, 186, 187, 189, 191,
    200, 201, 205, 206, 208, 211, 223, 226, 227, 231,
    242, 244, 247
parole, 147, 151
paroxetine, 233
partnership, 151
passive, 108, 192
pathology, 98, 182, 186, 231
pathophysiology, vii, 62
pathways, 3, 58, 59, 180, 217, 231
pediatrician, 17, 183, 202, 208, 217
peer conflict, 178
peer group, 162, 167, 171, 235
peer influence, 150
peers, 104, 138, 139, 141, 143, 145, 146, 162, 165,
    178, 191, 219, 223, 227, 245, 247
penalties, 147, 148
penis, 139
percentile, 9, 17, 18, 32, 192, 208, 209, 211, 212
perceptions, 45, 47, 48, 120, 172, 183, 189, 205
perceptual performance, 220
perinatal, 31, 35, 53, 64, 98
peripheral blood, 34

permit, 143, 166, 187
personal goals, 75, 169
personal history, 14
personal hygiene, 204
personality, 6, 11, 80, 159, 193, 200, 209, 216, 225,
    228, 232, 239, 247
personality disorder, 159, 200, 209
perspective, 40, 45, 46, 47, 64, 85, 96, 100, 102, 104,
    116, 155, 165, 166, 167, 168, 169, 172, 227, 233
PET, 240, 247
pharmacology, 59, 63, 210
pharmacotherapy, 61, 66
phenomenology, 222
phenotype, 98, 112, 224, 228, 236, 244, 247
philtrum, 9, 13, 18, 95, 192, 211
phonology, 164
phospholipids, 38
photographs, 152
physical abuse, 30, 32, 129, 136, 227, 234
physical aggression, 133
physical environment, 43
physical therapist, 41, 48, 188
physical well-being, 120
physiology, 29, 65, 138
pia mater, 98
pilot study, 64, 86, 89, 156
planning, 16, 18, 43, 74, 78, 79, 85, 86, 103, 108,
    111, 112, 113, 132, 166, 170, 174, 179, 182, 184,
    185, 200, 209, 220, 222
plasticity, 235
pleasure, 121, 137
PM, 35, 195, 234, 247
police, 82, 144, 145, 146, 147
polymorphism, 63
pools, 152
poor, 9, 10, 13, 16, 18, 19, 20, 29, 39, 41, 43, 44, 45,
    46, 49, 70, 78, 79, 88, 96, 97, 105, 107, 108, 110,
    115, 117, 118, 121, 130, 131, 132, 176, 188, 190,
    194, 204, 212, 213, 217, 226, 231, 234
population, viii, 2, 3, 6, 12, 13, 26, 31, 33, 40, 57, 58,
    69, 71, 72, 76, 80, 87, 127, 129, 132, 137, 143,
    149, 152, 153, 155, 159, 162, 166, 179, 183, 185,
    188, 194, 195, 200, 201, 202, 203, 204, 206, 224,
    226, 228, 232, 233, 239, 243, 247
positive relation, 227
positive relationship, 227
post traumatic stress disorder, 30, 235
posttraumatic stress, 237, 247
post-traumatic stress disorder, 233
posture, 43, 109, 166
potato, 32
poverty, 53, 75, 103, 107
power, 238, 247

precocious puberty, 203
prediction, 100, 232
predictors, 36, 53, 100
preference, 190
prefrontal cortex, 22, 233
pregnancy, vii, 1, 2, 15, 17, 18, 25, 27, 28, 29, 30,
    31, 34, 35, 36, 37, 53, 61, 63, 64, 69, 70, 72, 73,
    82, 83, 85, 86, 88, 89, 90, 91, 95, 96, 97, 99, 133,
    137, 161, 177, 184, 185, 186, 189, 190, 191, 196,
    207, 208, 209, 216, 218, 222, 224, 225, 226, 228,
    230, 239, 242, 244, 247
premature death, 4
prematurity, 35
preparation, 34, 59, 134
preschool, 33, 36, 44, 132, 133, 158, 242, 247
preschool children, 33, 36, 44, 133, 158
preschoolers, 45, 129, 133, 177, 218, 220, 240, 247
pressure, 81, 145, 146, 147
prevention, 23, 34, 63, 64, 85, 123, 149, 150, 151,
    156, 157, 159, 175, 183, 211
primate, 62
priming, 11
principle, 118, 202
prisoners, 132, 146
prisons, 131, 146
privacy, 136
private practice, 125
probability, 12, 144
probation officers, 151
probe, 148, 220, 230
problem drinkers, 37
problem solving, 171, 178, 186, 219
problem-solving, 116, 119, 156, 172, 206
processing deficits, 167
production, 3, 150, 165, 178, 191, 192, 221, 222,
    230, 231
profanity, 138
professions, 75, 112
prognosis, 58, 72
program, 30, 73, 74, 76, 77, 81, 82, 83, 84, 85, 91,
    92, 105, 111, 115, 125, 150, 151, 174, 175, 183,
    190, 197, 216, 236
programming, 35, 91, 180
prolactin, 233
prosocial behavior, 245, 247
protective factors, 70
protein synthesis, 60
proteins, 3, 4, 20, 22, 60
protocol, 181, 182, 184, 220
Prozac, 150
psychiatric diagnosis, 72, 223
psychiatric disorders, 2, 3, 4, 6, 7, 8, 11, 14, 30, 51,
    61, 92, 239, 247

psychiatric illness, 72
psychiatrist, 15, 32
psychodynamic perspective, 217, 236
psychoeducational program, 149
psychological development, 99
psychological distress, 72
psychological variables, 99
psychologist, 87, 110, 126, 148
psychology, 26, 41, 108, 185, 222, 228
psychopathology, 52, 53, 62, 65, 66, 102, 175, 210,
    223, 227, 228, 229, 239, 244, 247
psychopathy, 226
psychopharmacology, 64
psychosis, 14, 223, 241, 247
psychosomatic, 17, 200, 209, 232, 244, 247
psychostimulants, 17, 55, 56, 59, 66, 150, 202, 208
psychotherapy, 122, 200, 207, 234, 235, 241, 243,
    247
psychotropic drugs, 58
psychotropic medications, 17, 194, 209
ptosis, 98
PTSD, 8, 30, 180, 185, 186, 187, 188, 194, 233, 244,
    247
puberty, 138, 139, 142, 144
public health, viii, 53, 69
pulse, 55
punishment, 115, 241, 247
pyridoxine, 31

Q

quality of life, 90
quality of service, 87
questioning, 148, 230

R

race, 70, 75, 95
radar, 105
radiation, 216
rain, 247
range, vii, viii, 2, 11, 25, 39, 43, 44, 53, 73, 85, 86,
    96, 97, 99, 106, 113, 118, 128, 139, 148, 151,
    161, 162, 181, 190, 191, 215, 217, 219, 220, 222,
    223, 229, 230, 231, 233, 235, 236
rape, 126, 128, 140
rapists, 156, 159
rating scale, 56
ratings, 45, 101, 133, 157, 219, 241, 247
reaction time, 35, 66, 92, 160
reading, 52, 103, 159, 190, 191, 192, 193, 197, 221
reading comprehension, 192

reading disability, 159
reading disorder, 52
reading skills, 190
realism, 21, 209
reality, 75, 86, 112, 114, 116, 120, 121, 164, 182, 183, 200
reasoning, 79, 88, 96, 99, 100, 103, 105, 114, 116, 117, 118, 159, 222
rebelliousness, 108
recall, 141, 220, 221, 233
recalling, 169
reception, 41
receptors, 2, 5, 11, 22, 54, 57, 60, 67, 156
recidivism, 156
reciprocity, 235
recognition, viii, 30, 32, 33, 110, 116, 122, 180, 183, 186, 192, 221, 234
recollection, 116
reconstruction, 243, 247
recovery, 32, 73, 74, 75, 78, 79, 81, 82, 92, 108, 205
recurrence, 127, 146
reduction, 3, 22, 58, 76, 92, 102, 138, 140, 188, 233
refining, 161
reflection, 217, 232
reflexes, 29, 45, 218
refugees, 244, 247
regression, 234
regulation, 29, 37, 46, 52, 60, 62, 64, 113, 133, 218, 219, 229, 231, 235, 243, 247
rehabilitation, 111, 112, 180, 235
reinforcement, 236
rejection, 109, 143, 204, 219, 234
relational theory, 74
relationship, 6, 7, 48, 73, 74, 77, 79, 83, 88, 99, 107, 108, 114, 121, 139, 142, 149, 150, 158, 196, 206, 216, 225, 227
relationships, 7, 77, 84, 105, 107, 111, 112, 114, 116, 117, 119, 121, 126, 129, 138, 143, 145, 157, 159, 180, 187, 194, 200, 217, 223, 226, 230, 232, 233, 236
relatives, 139, 151
relaxation, 46
relevance, vii, 3, 100
reliability, 176
REM, 29
remembering, 115, 116, 147, 174
remission, 154
repetitions, 171
replacement, 216
replication, 73
resentment, 7
resilience, 116, 145, 235
resistance, 86, 98, 193

resolution, 81, 185
resources, 71, 111, 149, 180, 182, 183, 185, 188, 192, 228, 236
respiratory, 97
responsibility, 81, 105, 106, 117, 146, 151, 153, 236
responsiveness, 13
retardation, 1, 9, 18, 19, 95, 98, 100, 128, 159, 211, 212, 220
retention, 89, 150
retribution, 107
retrieval, 27, 110, 222
returns, 190
rewards, 104, 122
rice, 32
rights, 31, 89, 105, 146, 147, 190
risk, 4, 7, 16, 17, 21, 23, 31, 34, 35, 40, 53, 55, 58, 61, 66, 69, 70, 71, 72, 73, 75, 76, 80, 81, 82, 87, 90, 91, 92, 97, 111, 127, 132, 136, 144, 147, 148, 150, 152, 158, 168, 179, 187, 188, 190, 193, 194, 203, 204, 207, 208, 210, 211, 224, 226, 231, 235, 238, 239, 240, 242, 247
risk assessment, 127, 148
risk factors, 40, 70, 127, 144, 231, 238, 240, 247
risk-taking, 188
risperidone, 203
RNA, 2, 3
role playing, 204
role-playing, 172, 174
routines, 45, 46, 49, 121, 171, 173, 205, 216
routing, 118

S

safety, 7, 44, 57, 58, 123, 151
sample, 34, 86, 99, 100, 130, 134, 223, 225, 226, 228, 238, 242, 245, 247
sanctions, 128, 143, 146, 236
satisfaction, 234, 239, 247
Scandinavia, 64
scarce resources, 71, 179
scatter, 80
scheduling, 134, 151
schizophrenia, 3, 22, 72
school, 10, 17, 20, 32, 33, 42, 44, 45, 46, 47, 52, 62, 63, 71, 75, 83, 87, 100, 103, 104, 108, 110, 113, 125, 126, 132, 134, 138, 141, 152, 154, 156, 161, 162, 163, 164, 165, 166, 168, 169, 173, 175, 176, 177, 178, 179, 180, 185, 189, 190, 191, 193, 195, 197, 198, 200, 201, 204, 209, 213, 219, 220, 221, 224, 228, 235
school activities, 44, 162
school failure, 103
school performance, 10, 20, 132, 213

schooling, 58

scientific knowledge, 53

scientific method, 131

scores, 56, 62, 72, 90, 99, 100, 110, 192, 220, 222, 226, 230, 231, 232, 233

search, 120, 166, 169, 232, 233

security, 7, 147

seed, 107

segregation, 147

seizure, 5, 9, 14, 15, 18, 19, 20, 26, 55, 59, 203, 209, 212, 242, 247

selecting, 78, 162, 165, 166, 168, 169, 171

selective memory, 104

self, 20, 31, 34, 35, 37, 39, 45, 55, 74, 75, 78, 82, 92, 99, 105, 107, 108, 109, 110, 111, 112, 113, 115, 118, 119, 120, 122, 123, 129, 130, 132, 133, 134, 136, 138, 139, 140, 148, 149, 150, 154, 155, 169, 177, 199, 204, 205, 209, 215, 216, 218, 220, 221, 224, 226, 227, 228, 231, 233, 234, 235, 236, 240, 242, 243, 247

self-awareness, 149, 204

self-concept, 233

self-confidence, 99

self-control, 109, 130, 136, 149, 150, 154, 235

self-efficacy, 75, 78, 82

self-esteem, 132, 204, 216

self-monitoring, 155

self-mutilation, 231

self-regulation, 105, 112, 113, 132, 136, 139, 177, 240, 247

self-report data, 148

self-worth, 227

semantics, 164, 176

sensation, 9, 19, 39, 40, 41, 42, 44, 45, 46, 49, 212

sensations, 9, 19, 32, 39, 42, 46, 140, 212, 231

sensitivity, 41, 44, 58, 60, 113, 120, 200, 206, 225, 236, 241, 247

sensitization, 11, 14

sensory experience, 42, 141

sensory systems, 39

sentencing, 83

separation, 7, 117, 129, 224, 238, 247

septic shock, 216

sequencing, 43, 88, 119, 132, 150, 220

series, 8, 23, 27, 47, 56, 141, 186, 187, 221, 222, 231, 232, 239, 247

serotonin, 60

serum, 15, 233

service provider, 79, 80, 81, 87, 90

services, 12, 16, 31, 33, 70, 73, 74, 77, 79, 82, 84, 88, 89, 90, 92, 110, 119, 122, 127, 144, 146, 149, 151, 160, 162, 183, 185, 186, 198

severity, 8, 53, 98, 100, 112, 185, 223, 227, 228, 231, 232, 234

sex, 85, 126, 127, 128, 129, 130, 135, 136, 139, 140, 142, 144, 145, 146, 147, 148, 149, 150, 151, 152, 153, 155, 156, 157, 158, 160

sex offenders, 127, 128, 129, 130, 135, 136, 145, 146, 148, 149, 150, 151, 153, 155, 156, 157, 160

sexual abuse, 4, 8, 16, 30, 70, 71, 129, 139, 145, 204, 207, 227, 231

sexual assaults, 128

sexual behavior, 10, 126, 127, 128, 129, 132, 133, 134, 135, 136, 137, 138, 139, 140, 141, 143, 144, 148, 150, 152, 154, 160, 224, 234

sexual behaviour, 96

sexual contact, 140

sexual development, 126, 127, 204

sexual deviancy, 127, 128, 129, 143, 144, 148, 153, 158

sexual experiences, 138, 156

sexual health, 151

sexual motivation, 146

sexual offending, 128, 135, 143, 145, 146, 150, 151, 154, 237, 247

sexual pathology, 126

sexual recidivism, 156

sexual violence, 147

sexuality, 126, 127, 128, 129, 138, 139, 142, 143, 150, 152, 153, 156

sexually transmitted diseases, 69, 85, 138, 204

shame, 82, 107, 123

shape, 4, 118, 154, 170, 237, 247

sharing, 207

short-term memory, 88, 221, 237, 247

sibling, 192

siblings, 139, 187, 189, 190, 192, 194

side effects, 56, 61, 85, 202, 204

sign, 19, 111, 119, 212

signals, 60, 107, 114, 137

similarity, 97, 131, 143

sites, 70, 73, 91, 156, 183, 184

skeleton, 130

skills, 5, 10, 16, 20, 27, 30, 31, 43, 45, 46, 77, 79, 80, 83, 84, 87, 88, 129, 130, 131, 134, 137, 139, 140, 142, 144, 145, 146, 147, 149, 150, 151, 164, 167, 168, 169, 170, 172, 174, 175, 191, 192, 193, 201, 213, 223, 235

skills training, 149

skin, 44

sleep disturbance, 29

smokers, 226

smoking, 82, 92, 103, 118, 133, 226, 228, 237, 239, 244, 247

snoring, 197

sobriety, 190
social activities, 142, 143, 144, 151
social adjustment, 75, 176
social behavior, 58, 137, 141, 164, 167, 168, 171,
    172, 223, 240, 247
social class, 219
social cognition, 5, 16, 52, 132, 137, 138, 164, 166,
    167, 168, 201
social competence, 164, 172, 174, 175, 219
social context, 130, 162
social environment, 45, 138
social exchange, 168
social ills, 71
social information processing, 164
social learning, 143, 176
social life, 166
social perception, 10, 20, 130, 213
social problems, 96, 125, 162, 170, 171, 172, 174,
    223
social relations, 166, 177, 206
social relationships, 166, 177, 206
social services, 32, 76, 84, 90, 206
social situations, 7, 165, 166, 168, 170, 172, 174,
    201
social skills, 5, 104, 129, 142, 144, 146, 150, 167,
    193
social skills training, 142, 144
social status, 219
social support, 239, 247
social withdrawal, 134
socialization, 5, 16, 127, 128, 129, 135, 138, 139,
    142, 143, 145, 149, 150, 153, 201, 218, 224
socioeconomic status, 223, 227
soil, 235
somatization, 231, 235, 238, 241, 247
somatization disorder, 235
South Africa, 3
special education, 16, 100, 125, 141, 190, 191, 193,
    201, 207
species, 229, 240, 247
specificity, 31, 62, 136
spectrum, 20, 21, 22, 23, 34, 36, 38, 40, 55, 61, 65,
    66, 70, 91, 93, 98, 101, 104, 108, 112, 113, 124,
    158, 161, 162, 175, 176, 178, 186, 195, 201, 209,
    210, 211, 226, 229, 234, 242, 244, 247
speculation, 234
speech, 17, 32, 41, 99, 112, 132, 154, 155, 162, 169,
    192, 201, 208, 221, 222, 223, 228, 230
speed, 103, 110, 221
spelling, 221
spinal cord, 98
spine, 63
sports, 119

stability, 36, 193, 194, 195, 225, 238, 247
staffing, 85, 87
stages, 75, 79, 205, 225
standard deviation, 192
standards, 107
state control, 29
statistics, 128, 134
stereotypes, 143
stigma, 186
stimulant, 57, 58, 63, 64, 159, 193, 194
stimulus, 78, 105, 130, 219
stock, 140
storage, 88, 221, 222
strabismus, 27
strategies, viii, 21, 35, 47, 70, 75, 76, 80, 82, 85, 86,
    87, 88, 132, 157, 165, 166, 168, 169, 170, 171,
    174, 176, 182, 199, 205, 210, 220, 236
street drugs, 186, 194
strength, 119, 120, 174, 229
stress, 43, 52, 57, 58, 63, 109, 113, 115, 117, 140,
    180, 193, 210, 215, 224, 226, 231, 234
stressors, 7, 8, 11, 30, 53, 85, 180
striatum, 133
structural changes, 56
structural defects, 222
structure formation, 245, 247
structuring, 148, 151
students, 3, 173, 175, 176, 227, 231
substance abuse, 30, 35, 58, 69, 70, 71, 72, 75, 77,
    79, 80, 83, 84, 89, 92, 110, 123, 141, 151, 182,
    186, 189, 190, 195, 197, 226, 228, 236
substance use, 61, 72, 104, 109, 224, 242, 247
substrates, 217
sugar, 120
suicidal ideation, 83, 232
suicide, 226
suicide attempts, 226
Sun, 93
superego, 220
supervision, 143, 146, 149, 151, 152, 153, 192, 224
supervisor, 75, 89, 111
supervisors, 76, 82, 87
supply, 107, 118, 225
support services, 186
suprachiasmatic nucleus, 11
surprise, 82, 100, 117
survival, 224
susceptibility, 3, 4, 25
suspects, 81
Sweden, 99
symbols, 221
symptom, 72, 96, 131, 132, 179, 181, 202, 227, 232,
    234, 245, 247

symptoms, 4, 6, 13, 26, 29, 40, 41, 44, 53, 54, 56, 57, 58, 67, 83, 96, 98, 100, 113, 126, 131, 132, 133, 134, 139, 143, 150, 179, 182, 188, 201, 202, 225, 228, 230, 231, 233, 234, 238, 240, 243, 247
synapse, 59
synaptic plasticity, 4, 23
synaptic vesicles, 60
synchronization, 230, 237, 247
syndrome, 12, 23, 34, 37, 48, 61, 62, 63, 64, 66, 95, 96, 97, 100, 101, 102, 157, 158, 159, 160, 175, 177, 178, 182, 202, 211, 217, 227, 237, 240, 242, 243, 247
synergistic effect, 25
synthesis, 60
systems, 26, 27, 41, 42, 46, 54, 84, 88, 90, 110, 111, 112, 122, 134, 182, 203, 204

T

tactics, 145
talent, 206
tardive dyskinesia, 188
targets, 23, 171
teachers, 46, 104, 105, 126, 139, 143, 167, 189, 191, 193, 195, 201
teaching, 80, 103, 107, 128, 129, 149, 170, 171, 172, 173, 178, 204
team members, 183
technology, 183, 187
teenagers, 143, 152
teeth, 115
telephone, 79, 152
television, 138, 139, 152
temperament, 51, 232
temporal lobe, 5, 200, 203, 223
temporal lobe epilepsy, 200
tension, 138
teratogen, 25, 69, 95, 162, 225
teratology, 37, 102, 237, 247
testosterone, 150
thallium, 14
theory, 41, 47, 48, 76, 90, 104, 120, 129, 166, 169, 178, 224, 225, 244, 245, 247
therapeutic interventions, 10
therapeutic process, 76, 152
therapists, 39, 41, 45, 46, 151, 234
therapy, viii, 32, 35, 48, 58, 108, 126, 139, 141, 150, 160, 180, 182, 185, 187, 188, 189, 193, 199, 200, 202, 204, 205, 206, 207, 229, 234
thiamin, 31
thinking, 46, 86, 110, 113, 116, 136, 144, 150, 161, 165, 167, 169, 172, 175, 215, 229
Third Reich, 245, 247

threat, 180, 234
threshold, viii, 5, 20, 26, 29, 35, 40, 191, 203, 209, 220, 221, 236
thresholds, 46
thyroid, 14, 55, 188, 203
time, 3, 9, 11, 18, 27, 30, 32, 40, 42, 56, 57, 72, 75, 76, 77, 78, 79, 81, 83, 84, 85, 89, 98, 99, 100, 104, 106, 108, 109, 110, 111, 113, 114, 116, 117, 120, 123, 125, 126, 142, 143, 144, 145, 146, 147, 148, 153, 164, 170, 185, 186, 187, 192, 193, 194, 197, 198, 200, 202, 205, 206, 211, 216, 219, 224, 226, 227, 228, 233, 235, 236
time constraints, 79
timing, 1, 96, 98, 169, 179, 185
tissue, 31, 98
tobacco, 61, 103, 196
toddlers, 26, 28, 30, 32, 33, 38, 45, 160, 218, 225
toxic effect, 4, 31, 203
toxicity, 203, 204
toxin, 179, 224
toys, 43, 44, 46, 137
trade, 181
traffic, 112, 114
training, 41, 76, 80, 87, 111, 122, 123, 129, 143, 146, 148, 149, 150, 153, 155, 175, 176, 178, 210
traits, 61, 99, 105, 135, 217, 219, 229, 232, 233, 235
trajectory, 215
transcription, viii, 3, 25
transection, 229
transference, 234
transferrin, 28
transition, 76, 88
transition period, 88
transmission, 3, 11, 57, 225, 245, 247
transportation, 79, 83, 88
trauma, 53, 57, 121, 122, 156, 180, 185, 186, 200, 210, 225, 231, 233, 240, 243, 247
traumatic brain injury, 104, 176, 177
treatment methods, 149
tremor, 9, 19, 192, 212
trend, 219, 223, 226, 230, 232
trial, 145, 147, 148, 193, 195
triggers, 85, 121, 150, 203, 234
trust, 77, 81, 83, 226
trustworthiness, 107
tryptophan, 18, 203, 209
TSH, 15
tubal ligation, 89

U

UK, viii, 36, 53, 65, 66, 178
ultrasound, 28

unemployment, 103
unhappiness, 233
United States, 25, 34, 70, 90, 91
universality, 206
university students, 231
unmasking, 55, 58
urban centers, 182
urine, 54, 60, 82, 197

V

validity, 145, 157, 159, 242, 243, 247
values, 115, 121
variable, 40, 45, 164, 183
variables, 96, 98, 99, 100, 166, 189, 195, 219, 221,
    227, 228, 238, 239, 247
variation, 23, 29, 131, 151, 154
ventricular septal defect, 27
vessels, 12
victimization, 130, 139, 144, 145, 146, 193, 206
victims, 71, 106, 127, 141, 152, 158, 234
village, 191
violence, 71, 75, 136, 144, 147, 234
vision, 39, 49, 114
visual attention, 201
visual stimuli, 32, 99, 230
vitamin A, 31
vitamin D, 31
vocabulary, 201, 227
vocational training, 125
voice, 79, 82, 125
volunteer work, 121
vulnerability, 54, 65, 129, 144, 146, 217, 227, 229,
    236

W

waking, 197

walking, 17, 32, 84, 111, 139, 208
water, 7, 32, 120, 200, 216
weakness, 120
wealth, 205, 217
wear, 42, 44, 79, 141
wearing apparel, 140
weight gain, 63, 97
welfare, 17, 71, 75, 82, 84, 89, 209
well-being, 74, 76
white matter, 98
wind, 46, 115, 123
windows, 80, 119
winter, 200
withdrawal, 7, 29, 35, 37, 42, 216
women, vii, 4, 12, 28, 30, 31, 33, 34, 35, 36, 60, 63,
    64, 69, 70, 71, 72, 73, 74, 80, 81, 83, 84, 86, 87,
    88, 89, 91, 92, 101, 111, 123, 130, 142, 186, 206,
    218, 226, 229, 234, 240, 242, 247
workers, 82, 111, 121, 190
working memory, 4, 5, 9, 10, 14, 16, 19, 26, 27, 52,
    130, 132, 166, 168, 169, 200, 213, 220, 235
writing, 43, 153, 192, 206

Y

yield, 110, 164
young adults, 11, 36, 58, 132, 149, 155, 206, 207,
    220
young men, vii
young women, vii, 71, 72, 87, 90, 91, 126

Z

zinc, 3, 31, 35
Zoloft, 150
zygote, 27